An illustrated guide to
Skin Lymphoma

To our colleagues, students, teachers and especially our patients

An illustrated guide to
Skin Lymphoma

Lorenzo Cerroni MD
Department of Dermatology
University of Graz, Medical School
Graz
Austria

Kevin Gatter BM, DPhil, MRCPath
Nuffield Department of Clinical Laboratory Sciences
John Radcliffe Hospital
Oxford
UK

Helmut Kerl MD
Department of Dermatology
University of Graz, Medical School
Graz
Austria

Second edition

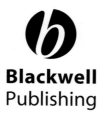

Blackwell
Publishing

© 1998, 2004 by Blackwell Publishing Ltd
Blackwell Publishing Inc., 350 Main Street, Malden, Massachusetts 02148-5020, USA
Blackwell Publishing Ltd, 9600 Garsington Road, Oxford OX4 2DQ, UK
Blackwell Publishing Asia Pty Ltd, 550 Swanston Street, Carlton, Victoria 3053, Australia

The right of the Authors to be identified as the Authors of this Work has been asserted in accordance with the Copyright, Designs and Patents Act 1988.

First published 1998
Second edition 2004
4   2007

Library of Congress Cataloging-in-Publication Data
Cerroni, Lorenzo.
    An illustrated guide to skin lymphoma / Lorenzo Cerroni, Kevin Gatter, Helmut Kerl.—2nd ed.
      p. ; cm.
    Includes bibliographical references and index.
    ISBN 978-1-4051-1376-2 (alk. paper)
    1. Skin—Cancer. 2. Lymphomas.
    [DNLM: 1. Skin Neoplasms—diagnosis. 2. Skin Neoplasms—therapy. 3. Lymphoma—pathology.
WR 500 C417i 2004] I. Gatter, Kevin. II. Kerl, Helmut. III. Title.

    RC280.S5C47 2004
    616.99'477—dc22

                                                                    2004000860

ISBN 978-1-4051-1376-2

A catalogue record for this title is available from the British Library

Set in 10/12pt Minion by Graphicraft Limited, Hong Kong
Printed and bound in India by Replika Press Pvt. Ltd

Commissioning Editor: Stuart Taylor
Editorial Assistant: Katrina Chandler
Production Editor: Fiona Pattison
Production Controller: Kate Charman

For further information on Blackwell Publishing, visit our website:
www.blackwellpublishing.com

The publisher's policy is to use permanent paper from mills that operate a sustainable forestry policy, and which has been manufactured from pulp processed using acid-free and elementary chlorine-free practices. Furthermore, the publisher ensures that the text paper and cover board used have met acceptable environmental accreditation standards.

Contents

Preface

The positive response to the first edition of this book was most gratifying. However, even as we were completing it, we knew already that advances in the fields of haematopathology in general and of cutaneous lymphomas in particular meant we should need to review many concepts and beliefs in the light of new discoveries and novel interpretations in the future. This of course mirrors exactly what is happening daily in all other fields of medicine. In fact, in the last few years many entities have been further characterized and some have been newly described. In addition, the field of cutaneous lymphomas has been revolutionized by advances in the use of immunohistological, molecular genetics and *in situ* hybridization techniques. In this context, for the second edition of our book we have completely re-written most of the chapters rather than just edited them.

Besides updating concepts and interpretation of single disease entities, we have added completely new chapters such as those on cutaneous manifestations in myelogenous leukaemia and on cutaneous lymphoproliferative disorders in immunocompromised patients. Some chapters have been deleted and replaced by new ones that are completely changed (especially those on cutaneous T-cell lymphomas other than mycosis fungoides). In addition, several entities that were not included in the first edition have been added in some of the chapters. Finally, we have greatly expanded the chapter on mycosis fungoides, the single disease entity that represents by itself more than 50% of all cases of cutaneous lymphoma. In short, this is more a new book than a second edition of the old one.

One of the criticisms of the first edition was the absence of in-text citations. We have now added this feature, and in addition expanded greatly the number of references. The sections on clinical features, therapy and prognosis have also been greatly expanded in every chapter in order to provide guidelines for the management of patients with cutaneous lymphomas.

The great strength of the first edition of this book was the high quality and large number of illustrations. In this second edition we have increased the number of illustrations by 50%; in addition, many of the figures printed in the first edition have been replaced by better ones. This was possible due to the fine efforts of those working at Blackwell Publishing: we are greatly indebted to Stuart Taylor, Katrina Chandler and Fiona Pattison for the help and support provided in the preparation of this second edition.

Of course, the decision as to whether or not our efforts have produced a valid work—one that can be of help in the diagnosis and management of patients with cutaneous lymphomas—rests with the readers. We hope that you will find it helpful and that your patients will profit from it as, in the end, this is the only consideration that counts in medicine.

Graz and Oxford, January 2004
Lorenzo Cerroni
Helmut Kerl
Kevin Gatter

Acknowledgements

We would like to thank once again the many clinicians and patients who provided the essential material and information necessary to prepare the book.

We would like to express special thanks to Uli Schmidbauer, who prepared superb histopathological and immunohistochemical sections, and to Werner Stieber, who was responsible for the excellent quality of the clinical pictures.

Chapter 1 Introduction

It is becoming increasingly evident that primary cutaneous lymphomas represent distinct clinical and histopathological subtypes of extranodal lymphomas [1–7]. They can be defined as neoplasms of the immune system, characterized by a proliferation of either T or B lymphocytes which show a particular tropism for the skin. Extracutaneous spread with lymph node involvement can be observed during the course of the disease.

Primary cutaneous lymphomas should be separated from secondary skin manifestations of extracutaneous (usually nodal) lymphomas, which represent metastatic disease and are characterized by a different prognosis and treatment. Because the histopathology of primary and secondary cutaneous lymphomas may be similar or identical [8], complete staging investigations are needed to establish this distinction.

The standard definition of primary cutaneous lymphomas is disease confined solely to the skin for at least 6 months after complete staging procedures have been performed [4]. Recently, two of the authors (LC, HK) proposed changing the definition to 'no extracutaneous manifestations of the disease at presentation' [7]. The main reason for adopting this definition is the need to classify the disease accurately, and treat patients accordingly, at presentation, without waiting for 6 months.

Classification of cutaneous lymphomas

Clinical and biological differences between nodal and cutaneous lymphomas have prompted the development of specialized classification schemes. In 1997, a European Organization for Research and Treatment of Cancer (EORTC) Cutaneous Lymphoma Study Group panel proposed a new classification of cutaneous lymphomas based on recognized clinicopathological entities (Table 1.1) [4]. Although this classification is easily assimilated into the widely accepted general lymphoma classification (the World Health Organization—WHO system; Table 1.2), as both are based on clinicopathological entities, some conceptual differences exist [9]. The skin classification is obviously expanded in certain areas to allow a detailed description of individual types of cutaneous lymphoma. At the time of writing, a combined EORTC/WHO classification of skin lymphomas is being prepared.

In the following chapters we describe the clinicopathological characteristics of lymphomas arising in the skin, with special emphasis on primary cutaneous lymphomas. A guideline for treatment is also included. In addition, a short discussion of the inflammatory diseases that simulate lymphomas (cutaneous pseudolymphomas) is provided.

Examination of patients

Primary cutaneous lymphomas represent an heterogeneous group of diseases with different clinicopathological presentations and prognostic features. In order to classify patients correctly, it is crucial that a complete clinical history is obtained and integrated with histopathological, immunophenotypical and molecular data. To take but one example, lesions of type B lymphomatoid papulosis show histopathological features that may be indistinguishable from those observed in mycosis fungoides, and differentiation in these cases can only be achieved by correlation with the clinical picture.

As a general rule, complete staging investigations at presentation include physical examination, laboratory investigations, chest X-ray, ultrasound of lymph nodes and visceral organs, computerized tomography (CT) scans and bone marrow biopsy. Positron emission tomography is also being increasingly used for staging of patients with cutaneous lymphoma. Patients with patch-stage mycosis fungoides or lymphomatoid papulosis do not require extensive investigations. The necessity of bone marrow biopsy in patients with cutaneous marginal zone lymphoma is questionable.

Surgical techniques

Surgical specimens should be carefully removed, paying particular attention not to crush the tissue. Shave biopsies must

Table 1.1 Classification of cutaneous lymphomas (EORTC Cutaneous Lymphoma Study Group).

T-cell lymphomas	B-cell lymphomas
Indolent behaviour	*Indolent behaviour*
Mycosis fungoides	Follicle centre lymphoma
Mycosis fungoides with follicular mucinosis	Immunocytoma
Pagetoid reticulosis	(marginal zone B-cell lymphoma)
Large cell cutaneous T-cell lymphoma, CD30$^+$	
anaplastic	
immunoblastic	
pleomorphic	
Lymphomatoid papulosis	
Aggressive behaviour	*Intermediate behaviour*
Sézary syndrome	Large B-cell lymphoma of the leg
Large cell T-cell lymphoma, CD30$^-$	
immunoblastic	
pleomorphic	
Provisional entities*	*Provisional entities**
Granulomatous slack skin	Intravascular large B-cell lymphoma
CTCL, pleomorphic, small/medium-sized	Plasmacytoma
Subcutaneous panniculitis-like T-cell lymphoma	

CTCL, cutaneous T-cell lymphoma.
*This group includes cutaneous lymphomas with insufficient data to delineate clear-cut clinicopathological entities.

be avoided. Punch biopsies, although sometimes insufficient for a definitive diagnosis, may be performed in special instances (early lesions of mycosis fungoides).

Histopathology, immunophenotype and molecular genetics

Histopathology

Sections should be cut with a maximum thickness of 4 μm and subsequently stained with haematoxylin and eosin (H&E), periodic acid–Schiff (PAS) and, if possible, Giemsa. High-quality sections are necessary for a correct diagnosis.

Immunophenotype

Modern immunohistochemical techniques allow the study of phenotypical patterns on routinely fixed, paraffin-embedded tissue sections [10–12]. The use of proteolytic enzymes (trypsin) has been widely replaced by other antigen demasking methods such as microwave heating of sections. In short, tissue sections are placed in a microwave heater and heated up to 100°C for 10–15 min, and then slowly cooled off before application of the first antibody. Microwave heating can be substituted by pressure cooking or by overnight incubation

of sections at 80°C. A list of antibodies reactive with lymphocyte subsets and accessory cells (macrophages, dendritic reticulum cells and interdigitating cells) in routinely fixed, paraffin-embedded tissue sections is reported in Table 1.3.

Molecular genetics

Analysis of the T-cell receptor (TCR) and immunoglobulin heavy-chain (J_H) genes has provided a new and important technique for the study of cutaneous lymphomas. Early in their differentiation, T and B lymphocytes rearrange their TCR and J_H genes, respectively [13,14]. Analysis of the gene rearrangement by Southern blot or polymerase chain reaction (PCR) techniques provides clues to the clonality of a given infiltrate. The PCR technique presents two main advantages: (i) DNA can be extracted from routinely fixed tissues; and (ii) the sensitivity is higher (5–10% of clonal cells within a mixed cell population can be detected by Southern blot analysis, compared to 1% by PCR). Benign (reactive) lymphoid proliferations are characterized by a polyclonal pattern of TCR and/or J_H gene rearrangement. In contrast, malignant lymphomas reveal a monoclonal population of lymphocytes, identified as an additional band with the Southern blot method and as a single band with the PCR technique. Although these methods are effective and reliable, they have some limitations: benign inflammatory dermatoses

Table 1.2 The WHO classification of tumours of haematopoietic and lymphoid tissues.

B-cell neoplasms
Precursor B-cell neoplasms
Precursor B-lymphoblastic leukaemia–lymphoma

Mature B-cell neoplasms
Chronic lymphocytic leukaemia/small lymphocytic lymphoma
B-cell prolymphocytic leukaemia
Lymphoplasmacytic lymphoma
Splenic marginal zone lymphoma
Hairy cell leukaemia
Plasma cell myeloma
Solitary plasmacytoma of bone
Extraosseous plasmacytoma
Extranodal marginal zone B-cell lymphoma of mucosa-associated lymphoid tissue (MALT lymphoma)
Nodal marginal zone B-cell lymphoma
Follicular lymphoma
Mantle cell lymphoma
Diffuse large B-cell lymphoma
Mediastinal (thymic) large B-cell lymphoma
Intravascular large B-cell lymphoma
Primary effusion lymphoma
Burkitt lymphoma/leukaemia

B-cell proliferations of uncertain malignant potential
Lymphomatoid granulomatosis
Post-transplant lymphoproliferative disorder, polymorphic

T- and NK-cell neoplasms
Precursor T-cell neoplasms
Precursor T-lymphoblastic leukaemia/lymphoma
Blastic NK-cell lymphoma (neoplasm of uncertain lineage and stage of differentiation)

Mature T- and NK-cell neoplasms
T-cell prolymphocytic leukaemia
T-cell large granular lymphocytic leukaemia
Aggressive NK-cell leukaemia
Adult T-cell leukaemia/lymphoma
Extranodal NK/T-cell lymphoma, nasal type
Enteropathy-type T-cell lymphoma
Hepatosplenic T-cell lymphoma
Subcutaneous panniculitis-like T-cell lymphoma
Mycosis fungoides
Sézary syndrome
Anaplastic large cell lymphoma, primary cutaneous
Peripheral T-cell lymphoma, unspecified
Angioimmunoblastic T-cell lymphoma
Anaplastic large cell lymphoma

T-cell proliferation of uncertain malignant potential
Lymphomatoid papulosis

Hodgkin lymphoma
Nodular lymphocyte-predominant Hodgkin lymphoma
Nodular sclerosis classical Hodgkin lymphoma
Lymphocyte-rich classical Hodgkin lymphoma
Mixed cellularity classical Hodgkin lymphoma
Lymphocyte-depleted classical Hodgkin lymphoma

may rarely present a monoclonal pattern, and a 'germline' or polyclonal pattern may be observed in clear-cut lymphomas. In addition, lack of sensitivity may give rise to negative results in many cases of early cutaneous T- or B-cell lymphoma.

A common pitfall in molecular analysis of cutaneous lymphoproliferative disorders is the presence of 'pseudomonoclonal' rearrangement of the J_H gene in cutaneous lymphoid infiltrates characterized by the presence of only a few B lymphocytes. In fact, it is not uncommon to observe this phenomenon in lesions of cutaneous T-cell lymphoma with reactive B lymphocytes. A good rule is to perform at least two (better three) separate extractions of DNA from different sections of the biopsy tissue, and to run one independent PCR assay for every extraction. In this way, different 'pseudomonoclonal' bands will be observed, thus showing overall a polyclonal pattern.

Molecular analyses are also widely used in haematology to identify particular genetic aberrations characteristic of a specific clinicopathological entity, such as the interchromosomal 14;18 translocation typical of nodal follicular lymphoma or the t(2;5) of nodal anaplastic large cell lymphoma. Unfortunately, as yet only a few specific genetic alterations have been identified in primary cutaneous lymphomas.

Other methods in the study of cutaneous lymphoid infiltrates

Fluorescence *in situ* hybridization technique

Chromosomal abnormalities are becoming increasingly important in the study and classification of haematopoietic neoplasms. In recent years, new methods have been developed for evaluation of tissue specimens fixed in formalin and embedded in paraffin, allowing the investigation of routine biopsy samples and archive material. The fluorescence *in situ* hybridization (FISH) technique is based on the same principle as the Southern blot method, relying on the annealing of single-stranded DNA to complementary DNA.

Depending on the probes selected, the FISH method can be used to detect different types of chromosomal abnormalities, including monosomy, trisomy and other aneuploidies, as well as translocations and deletions. The use of FISH applied to routinely processed tissue specimens identified a hitherto unknown t(14;18)(q32;q21) involving the J_H and MALT1 genes in a subset of cases of primary cutaneous marginal zone B-cell lymphomas [15].

Microarrays

The recent development of techniques of comparative genomic hybridization, and the identification of over 19 000 human genes by the Human Genome Project, allows one to

Table 1.3 Panel of antibodies for immunohistological analysis of cutaneous lymphomas on routinely fixed, paraffin-embedded tissue sections.

Antigen	Immunostaining	Suggested clone	Pre-treatment
CD1a	Langerhans cells, precursor T cells	010*	C/D
CD2	T cells	271†	C/D
CD3	T cells	PS1†	B/C/D
CD3ε	T cells (epsilon chain of CD3)	PC3/188 A‡	C/D
CD4	T-helper cells	IF6†	C/D
CD5	T cells; B-CLL	4C7†	C/D
CD7	T cells	272†	C/D
CD8	T-cytotoxic cells	C8/144B‡	C/D
CD10	CALLA; germinal centre cells	270†	C/D
CD15	Hodgkin cells	C3D-1‡	A/B
CD20	B cells	L26‡	A/C/D
CD21	Follicular dendritic cells	IF8‡	C/D
CD30	Activated T and B cells, Hodgkin cells	Ber-H2‡	B/C/D
CD31	Endothelial cells	JC70A‡	B/C/D
CD34	Precursor cells	QBend 10‡	C/D
CD43	T cells	DF-T1‡	C/D
CD45	Leucocyte common antigen	2B11‡	A/B
CD45RA	Naive T cells	4KB5‡	C/D
CD45RO	Memory T cells	UCHL1‡	C/D
CD56	NK cells, NCAM	1B6‡	C/D
CD57	NK cells	TB01§	C/D
CD68	Histiocytes, macrophages	KP1‡ or PGM1‡	B/C/D
CD79a	B cells	JCB117‡	C/D
CD99	Precursor cells	mic-2‡	C/D
CD138	Plasma cells	Mi15‡	C/D
Ig heavy-chains	B cells (IgA, IgD, IgG, IgM)	Polyclonal‡	C/D
Ig light-chains	B cells (kappa, lambda)	Polyclonal‡	B/C/D
Ki-67	Proliferating cells	MIB-1‡	C/D
Cytokeratin	Epithelial cells	MNF116‡	B/C/D
EMA	Epithelial membrane antigen	E29‡	A
S100 protein	Langerhans cells, interdigitating reticulum cells	Polyclonal‡	B/C/D
TdT	Precursor cells	8-1 E4¶	C/D
TCR-β	α/β T cells	b-F1‖	C/D
TIA	Cytotoxic T cells	TIA-1**	C/D
Granzyme-B	Cytotoxic T cells	Gr-B7††	C/D
Perforin	Cytotoxic T cells	358-020‡‡	C/D
Bcl-2	T and B cells	124‡	C/D
Bcl-6	B cells, germinal centre	PG-B6p‡	C/D
ALK protein	Anaplastic large cell lymphoma	ALK-1‡	C/D
Myeloperoxidase	Myeloid cells	MPO-7‡	B
Anti-HLA-DR	HLA-DR	CR3/43‡	C/D
Cyclin-D1	B cells, mantle cell lymphoma	DCS-6§§	C/D

A, nil; B, enzyme; C, microwave; D, pressure cooking.
*Immunotech.
†Novocastra.
‡Dako.
§Serotec.
¶Sigma.
‖Endogen.
**Coulter.
††Monosan.
‡‡Ancell.
§§NeoMarkers.

check copy numbers and expression profiles of thousands of genes in a single experiment (microarray technology), thus providing important new information on the genetic profiles of human cancers [16]. Microarrays can be used to detect copy numbers of given genes (DNA microarrays), gene expression (RNA microarrays), RNA-inhibitor expression (RNAi microarray) and proteins (proteomics).

Using these methods, different subgroups of patients with nodal diffuse large B-cell lymphoma have been recently identified, as well as prognostic categories of patients with diffuse large B-cell lymphoma after treatment [17,18]. In the skin, microarray studies have been used to characterize infiltrates of B-cell lymphomas and to elucidate their relationship to nodal counterparts, and to evaluate genetic features of mycosis fungoides [19–21]. As this area of study is rapidly expanding, many more data will be gathered in the near future on different diagnostic and prognostic features of cutaneous lymphomas.

Laser-based microdissection

Microdissection of tissue specimens using a laser beam to isolate single cells or structures has been increasingly used in recent years in the study and characterization of cutaneous lymphoid infiltrates by PCR [22–27]. The main advantage over conventional microdissection techniques lies in the selective destruction of tissue by laser-beam energy. This obtains a contamination-free sample, with DNA from cells other than the target population totally destroyed. Most routine histological or immunohistological stains can be used. As the laser is suitable for analysis of routinely fixed specimens, there is no need for fresh-frozen tissue. Archival material stored in paraffin blocks can therefore be easily evaluated.

References

1 Kerl H, Kresbach H. Lymphoretikuläre Hyperplasien und Neoplasien der Haut. In: Schnyder UW, ed. *Spezielle Pathologische Anatomie*. Berlin: Springer Verlag, 1979: 351–480.

2 Burg G, Braun-Falco O. *Cutaneous Lymphomas, Pseudolymphomas and Related Disorders*. Berlin: Springer Verlag, 1983.

3 Kerl H, Cerroni L, Burg G. The morphologic spectrum of T-cell lymphomas in the skin: a proposal for a new classification. *Semin Diagn Pathol* 1991; **8**: 55–61.

4 Willemze R, Kerl H, Sterry W *et al.* EORTC classification for primary cutaneous lymphomas: a proposal from the Cutaneous Lymphoma Study Group of the European Organization for Research and Treatment of Cancer. *Blood* 1997; **90**: 354–71.

5 Edelson RL. Cutaneous T-cell lymphoma. *J Dermatol Surg Oncol* 1980; **6**: 358–68.

6 Isaacson PG, Norton AJ. Cutaneous lymphoma. In: Isaacson PG, Norton AJ, eds. *Extracutaneous Lymphomas*. Edinburgh: Churchill Livingstone, 1994: 131–91.

7 Fink-Puches R, Zenahlik P, Bäck B *et al.* Primary cutaneous lymphomas: applicability of current classification schemes (European Organization for Research and Treatment of Cancer, World Health Organization) based on clinicopathologic features observed in a large group of patients. *Blood* 2002; **99**: 800–5.

8 Lennert K, Feller AC. *Histopathology of Non-Hodgkin's Lymphomas*, 2nd edn. Berlin: Springer Verlag, 1992.

9 Jaffe ES, Harris NL, Stein H, Vardiman JW, eds. *World Health Organization Classification of Tumours: Tumours of Haematopoietic and Lymphoid Tissues*. Lyon: IARC Press, 2001.

10 Cerroni L, Smolle J, Soyer HP, Martinez Aparicio A, Kerl H. Immunophenotyping of cutaneous lymphoid infiltrates in frozen and paraffin-embedded tissue sections: a comparative study. *J Am Acad Dermatol* 1990; **22**: 405–13.

11 Cerroni L, Kerl H. Diagnostic immunohistology: cutaneous lymphomas and pseudolymphomas. *Semin Cutan Med Surg* 1999; **18**: 64–70.

12 Gatter KC. Diagnostic immunocytochemistry: achievements and challenges. *J Pathol* 1989; **159**: 183–90.

13 Van Dongen JJM, Wolvers-Tettero ILM. Analysis of immunoglobulin and T cell receptor genes. I. Basic and technical aspects. *Clin Chim Acta* 1991; **198**: 1–91.

14 Van Dongen JJM, Wolvers-Tettero ILM. Analysis of immunoglobulin and T cell receptor genes. II. Possibilities and limitations in the diagnosis and management of lymphoproliferative diseases and related disorders. *Clin Chim Acta* 1991; **198**: 93–174.

15 Streubel B, Lamprecht A, Dierlamm J *et al.* t(14;18)(q32;q21) involving *IGH* and *MALT1* is a frequent chromosomal aberration in MALT lymphoma. *Blood* 2003; **101**: 2335–9.

16 Pollack JR, Perou CM, Alizadeh AA *et al.* Genome-wide analysis of DNA copy-number changes using cDNA microarrays. *Nat Genet* 1999; **23**: 41–6.

17 Alizadeh AA, Eisen MB, Davis RE *et al.* Distinct types of diffuse large B-cell lymphoma identified by gene expression profiling. *Nature* 2000; **403**: 503–11.

18 Rosenwald A, Wright G, Chan WC *et al.* The use of molecular profiling to predict survival after chemotherapy for diffuse large-B-cell lymphoma. *N Engl J Med* 2002; **346**: 1937–47.

19 Storz MN, van de Rijn M, Kim YH *et al.* Gene expression profiles of cutaneous B cell lymphoma. *J Invest Dermatol* 2003; **120**: 865–70.

20 Tracey L, Villuendas R, Dotor AM *et al.* Mycosis fungoides shows concurrent deregulation of multiple genes involved in the TNF signaling pathway: an expression profile study. *Blood* 2003; **102**: 1042–50.

21 Tracey L, Villuendas R, Ortiz P *et al.* Identification of genes involved in resistance to interferon-α in cutaneous T-cell lymphoma. *Am J Pathol* 2002; **161**: 1825–37.

22 Cerroni L, Minkus G, Pütz B, Höfler H, Kerl H. Laser beam microdissection in the diagnosis of cutaneous B-cell lymphoma. *Br J Dermatol* 1997; **136**: 743–6.

23 Cerroni L, Arzberger E, Pütz B *et al.* Primary cutaneous follicle center cell lymphoma with follicular growth pattern. *Blood* 2000; **95**: 3922–8.

24 Cerroni L, Arzberger E, Ardigó M, Pütz B, Kerl H. Monoclonality of intraepidermal T lymphocytes in early mycosis fungoides detected

by molecular analysis after laser-beam-based microdissection. *J Invest Dermatol* 2000; **114**: 1154–7.

25 Gellrich S, Wilks A, Lukowsky A *et al*. T cell receptor-γ gene analysis of CD30[+] large atypical individual cells in CD30[+] large primary cutaneous T-cell lymphomas. *J Invest Dermatol* 2003; **120**: 670–5.

26 Steinhoff M, Hummel M, Anagnostopoulos I *et al*. Single-cell ana-lysis of CD30[+] cells in lymphomatoid papulosis demonstrates a common clonal T-cell origin. *Blood* 2002; **100**: 578–84.

27 Gellrich S, Rutz S, Golembowski S *et al*. Primary cutaneous follicle center cell lymphomas and large B-cell lymphomas of the leg descend from germinal center cells: a single cell polymerase chain reaction analysis. *J Invest Dermatol* 2001; **117**: 1512–20.

Part 1 Cutaneous T-cell lymphomas

In contrast to the situation in the lymph nodes, where B-cell lymphomas represent the majority of non-Hodgkin lymphomas, in the skin, T-cell lymphomas are the most frequent group of malignant lymphomas, and mycosis fungoides is by far the most frequent single entity, alone representing approximately 50–60% of all primary cutaneous lymphomas. The peculiar clinicopathological and prognostic aspects of cutaneous T-cell lymphomas are well recognized, and prompted the inclusion in the World Health Organization (WHO) classification of haematopoietic neoplasms of many of the entities listed in the European Organization for Research and Treatment of Cancer (EORTC) classification for primary cutaneous lymphomas [1,2]. Although the utility of the EORTC scheme has been validated in one large study, some uncommon entities of the cytotoxic NK/T-cell lymphomas are not listed there [3].

In recent years, progress in immunohistochemistry and molecular genetics has allowed the reclassification of many of the cases diagnosed in the past as unusual variants of mycosis fungoides: disseminated pagetoid reticulosis, mycosis fungoides 'a tumeur d'emblee', and other cases of mycosis fungoides showing an aggressive course and short survival. It has been demonstrated that many of these cases belong to the recently described group of cytotoxic lymphomas, including mainly nasal-type NK/T-cell lymphoma, cutaneous γ/δ T-cell lymphoma, and epidermotropic aggressive CD8+ T-cell lymphoma. To this group of disorders belong also cases classified in the past as 'malignant histiocytosis'. Many of the cytotoxic lymphomas are today well characterized, and cutaneous lesions can be studied on routinely fixed sections of tissue.

It should be noted that, with some exceptions, cytomorphological features of neoplastic cells are of less importance in the classification of cutaneous T-cell lymphomas, and that a precise diagnosis can be achieved only by integration of clinical features with histopathological, immunophenotypical and molecular ones. In fact, most cutaneous T-cell lymphomas (including mycosis fungoides) are characterized by a proliferation of small-, medium- or large-sized pleomorphic T lymphocytes. Thus, the distinction of rare entities of cutaneous T-cell lymphoma from mycosis fungoides can be achieved only by careful taking of the clinical history and clinical examination of the patients. In addition, although in mycosis fungoides the size of the neoplastic cells has a prognostic value and the onset of large cell transformation bears a worse prognosis (see Chapter 2), in many other entities of cutaneous T-cell lymphoma the size of the neoplastic cells is not a prognostic indicator, as the biological behaviour is independent of the cytomorphological features. Thus, for example, a nasal-type NK/T-cell lymphoma with predominance of small pleomorphic lymphocytes has a very aggressive behaviour and bears a poor prognosis; in contrast, lymphomatoid papulosis and CD30+ anaplastic large cell lymphoma have an indolent behaviour and an excellent prognosis in spite of the marked atypia and the large size of the neoplastic cells.

Many controversies still exist in the field of cutaneous T-cell lymphomas. The definition of Sézary syndrome, for example, varies in different centres, and is still a matter of discussion. Criteria for the early diagnosis of mycosis fungoides, as well as the exact nosological classification of variants of it such as so-called small-plaque parapsoriasis, are also a matter of discussion. Exact definitions and diagnostic criteria for some subtypes of cytotoxic lymphomas are still lacking, and many overlaps exist among different entities. The entity of small–medium pleomorphic T-cell lymphoma is not widely accepted, and needs to be verified by studying larger numbers of patients [4]. Molecular data gathered from microarray studies may give us some of the answers to these questions in the near future.

References

1 Willemze R, Kerl H, Sterry W *et al*. EORTC classification for primary cutaneous lymphomas: a proposal from the Cutaneous Lymphoma Study Group of the European Organization for Research and Treatment of Cancer. *Blood* 1997; **90**: 354–71.

2 Jaffe ES, Harris NL, Stein H, Vardiman JW, eds. *World Health Organization Classification of Tumours: Tumours of Haematopoietic and Lymphoid Tissues.* Lyon: IARC Press, 2001.

3 Fink-Puches R, Zenahlik P, Bäck B *et al.* Primary cutaneous lymphomas: applicability of current classification schemes (European Organization for Research and Treatment of Cancer, World Health Organization) based on clinicopathologic features observed in a large group of patients. *Blood* 2002; **99**: 800–5.

4 Kerl H, Cerroni L. Controversies in cutaneous lymphomas. *Semin Cutan Med Surg* 2000; **19**: 157–600.

Chapter 2 Mycosis fungoides

Mycosis fungoides represents the most common type of cutaneous T-cell lymphoma [1,2]. It is also a long-standing entity, having been described almost two centuries ago, in 1806, by the French dermatologist Alibert. Traditionally, it is divided into three clinical phases: patch, plaque and tumour stages. The clinical course can be protracted over years or decades. The term 'mycosis fungoides' should be restricted to the classic so-called 'Alibert–Bazin' type of the disease, characterized by the typical slow evolution and protracted course. More aggressive entities (e.g. mycosis fungoides 'a tumeur d'emblee'), characterized by an onset with plaques and tumours, an aggressive course and a bad prognosis, are better classified among the recently described group of cutaneous cytotoxic T- (NK/T-) cell lymphomas (see Chapter 6).

In the past, mycosis fungoides has been considered as an 'incurable', albeit slowly progressive disease, that inevitably ended with the death of the patient. Recently, an early form of mycosis fungoides has been recognized, consisting of subtle patches of the disease [3–5]. These patients have relatively mild stable disease, which questions the traditional concept of the inevitability of disease progression until death.

The aetiology of mycosis fungoides remains unknown. A genetic predisposition may have a role in some cases, and a familial occurrence of the disease has been reported in a few instances [6,7]. Association with long-term exposure to various allergens has also been advocated, as well as exposure to environmental agents and association with chronic skin disorders and viral infections [8–12]. Recently, seropositivity for cytomegalovirus (CMV) has been observed at unusually high frequencies in patients with mycosis fungoides, suggesting a role for this virus in the pathogenesis of the disease [13]. In some countries, mycosis fungoides-like disorders are clearly associated with viral infections (human T-cell lymphotrophic virus I [HTLV-I]-associated adult T-cell lymphoma–leukaemia), but the search for viral particles in patients with mycosis fungoides has so far been unsuccessful [14]. Genetic alterations have been identified mainly in late stages of the disease, and their importance for disease initiation is unclear [15–20].

Mycosis fungoides has been described in patients with other haematological disorders, especially lymphomatoid papulosis and Hodgkin lymphoma. In occasional patients, the same clone has been detected in mycosis fungoides and associated lymphomas, raising questions about a common origin of the diseases [21–24]. In addition, patients with mycosis fungoides are at higher risk of developing a second (non-haematological) malignancy [25].

A staging classification system for mycosis fungoides was proposed in 1979 by the Mycosis Fungoides Cooperative Group (TNMB staging) (Table 2.1) [26]. This system takes into account the percentage of body area covered by lesions, and the presence of lymph node or visceral involvement. Although the presence of malignant circulating cells in the blood should be recorded for each patient, these data are not used for staging. More recently, a new staging classification for mycosis fungoides has been proposed in the World Health Organization (WHO) classification of haematopoietic neoplasms (Table 2.2) [27].

Some centres specializing in the study and management of skin lymphomas do not utilize the TNM or WHO staging schemes, but classify mycosis fungoides according to the type of skin lesions (patches, plaques and tumours) and the presence or absence of large cell transformation and/or extracutaneous involvement. Table 2.3 summarizes a clinical staging system for patients with mycosis fungoides.

In this scheme, stage I disease is confined to the skin and characterized morphologically by patches only. Survival is extremely long in these patients (usually decades), and non-aggressive treatments should be applied. Most patients in this stage die of unrelated causes. Patients with stage II in this scheme also have disease limited to the skin, but characterized morphologically by the presence of plaques, tumours or erythroderma, or by large cell transformation histopathologically. The disease in these patients is inevitably progressive, and treatment should be more aggressive. Stage III patients have extracutaneous disease and should be managed with aggressive treatment options.

Staging investigations are not necessary in early stage mycosis fungoides (patch stage). Patients with plaques, tumours or erythroderma should be screened for extracutaneous

Table 2.1 TNMB staging of mycosis fungoides [26].

Skin

T_1	Patches, papules or plaques covering < 10% of the skin surface
T_2	Patches, papules or plaques covering > 10% of the skin surface
T_3	Tumours
T_4	Generalized erythroderma

Lymph nodes

N_0	No clinically abnormal lymph nodes; histology negative
N_1	Clinically abnormal peripheral lymph nodes
N_{1o}	histology not performed
N_{1n}	histology negative
N_{1r}	histology reactive
N_{1d}	dermopathic lymphadenitis
N_2	No clinically abnormal peripheral lymph nodes; histology positive
N_3	Clinically abnormal peripheral lymph nodes; histology positive

Visceral organs

M_0	No visceral involvement
M_1	Visceral involvement

Blood

B_0	< 5% of atypical circulating cells
B_1	> 5% of atypical circulating cells

Stage

Ia	$T_1 N_0 M_0$
Ib	$T_2 N_0 M_0$
IIa	$T_{1-2} N_1 M_0$
IIb	$T_3 N_{0-1} M_0$
III	$T_4 N_{0-1} M_0$
IVa	$T_{1-4} N_{2-3} M_0$
IVb	$T_{1-4} N_{0-3} M_1$

Table 2.2 Clinical staging of mycosis fungoides according to the WHO [27].

Stage	
I	Disease confined to the skin
Ia	Limited patches/plaques
Ib	Disseminated patches/plaques
Ic	Tumours
II	Enlarged lymph nodes (histology negative)
III	Lymph node involvement (histology positive)
IV	Visceral involvement

Table 2.3 Clinical staging for patients with mycosis fungoides (Department of Dermatology, University of Graz).

Stage	
Ia	Patches < 10% of body area
Ib	Patches > 10% of body area
IIa	Plaques
IIb	Tumours
IIc	Erythroderma
IId	Large cell morphology
III	Lymph node involvement and/or visceral dissemination

Clinical features

Lesions of mycosis fungoides can be divided morphologically into patches, plaques and tumours. Itching is often a prominent symptom. Erythroderma may develop in the course of the disease, rendering distinction from Sézary syndrome difficult without a proper clinical history (see also Erythrodermic mycosis fungoides, page 25; and Chapter 3).

Patch stage

Patches of mycosis fungoides are characterized by variably large, erythematous, finely scaling lesions with a predilection for the buttocks and other sun-protected areas (Figs 2.1 & 2.2). Loss of elastic fibres and atrophy of the epidermis may confer on the lesions a typical wrinkled appearance, and terms such as 'parchment-like' or 'cigarette paper-like' have been used to describe them (Fig. 2.3). Sometimes, these single patches have a yellowish hue, conferring a 'xanthomatous'-like aspect to the lesions (xanthoerythroderma perstans) (Fig. 2.4). In early phases, a 'digitate' pattern can be observed (alone or in combination with larger patches; see also Small-plaque parapsoriasis, page 22) (Fig. 2.5).

involvement (laboratory investigations, sonography of lymph nodes, computerized tomography (CT) scan of thorax and abdomen, bone marrow biopsy, examination of the peripheral blood). Although the presence of a monoclonal population of T lymphocytes within the peripheral blood has been observed by polymerase chain reaction (PCR) technique in some patients with early mycosis fungoides, in many of these cases the clone was different from that detected in the skin lesions [28–31]. In addition, the prognostic value of the detection of monoclonality in the peripheral blood is unclear. It has been suggested that flow cytometry analysis is highly effective in demonstrating and quantifying small numbers of circulating tumour cells in patients with mycosis fungoides [32].

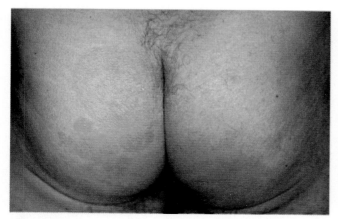

Fig. 2.1 Mycosis fungoides, patch stage. Early patches on the buttocks.

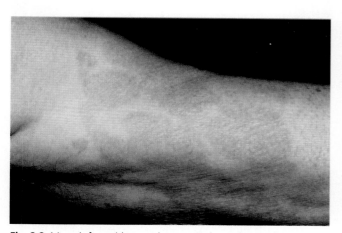

Fig. 2.2 Mycosis fungoides, patch stage. Early patches on the arm.

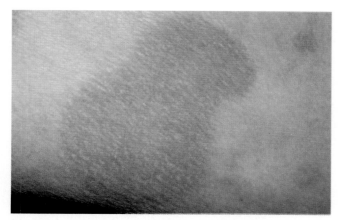

Fig. 2.3 Mycosis fungoides, patch stage. Detail of a patch. Note finely wrinkled surface.

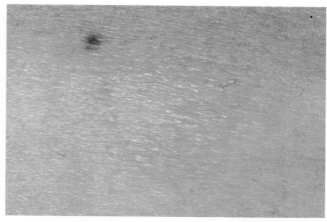

Fig. 2.4 Mycosis fungoides, patch stage. Detail of a yellowish patch with clinical features of 'xanthoerythroderma perstans'.

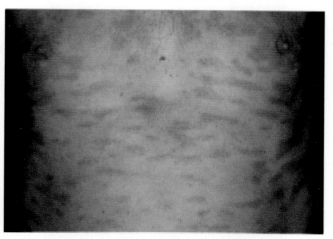

Fig. 2.5 Mycosis fungoides, patch stage. So-called 'digitate dermatosis'. Histological examination of two patches revealed in both a band-like infiltrate diagnostic of mycosis fungoides.

Plaque stage

Plaques of mycosis fungoides are characterized by infiltrated, scaling, reddish brown lesions (Figs 2.6 & 2.7). Typical patches are usually observed contiguous to plaques or at other sites on the body (Fig. 2.8). Plaques of mycosis fungoides should be distinguished from flat tumours of the disease (Figs 2.9 & 2.10). Flat infiltrated lesions should be biopsied in order to allow histopathological examination and a precise classification of the lesions.

Tumour stage

In tumour-stage mycosis fungoides a combination of patches, plaques and tumours is usually found, but tumours may also be observed in the absence of other lesions (Figs 2.11 & 2.12).

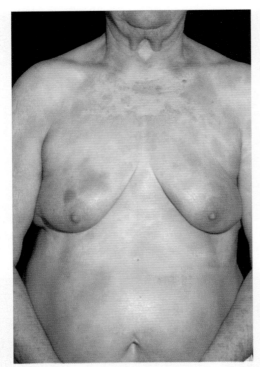

Fig. 2.6 Mycosis fungoides, plaque stage. Patches and plaques on the trunk.

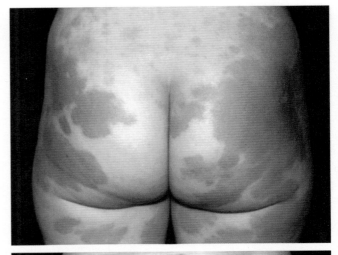

(a)

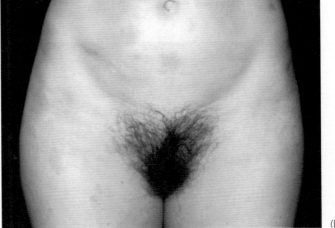

(b)

Fig. 2.8 Mycosis fungoides, plaque stage. (a) Patches and early plaques on the buttocks. (b) Note concomitant small patches ('parapsoriasis en plaques') on the abdomen and upper legs.

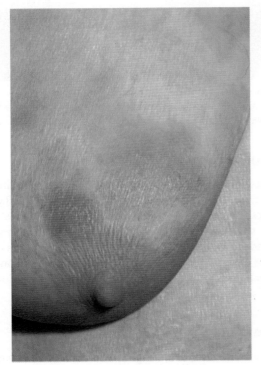

Fig. 2.7 Mycosis fungoides, plaque stage. Small plaque near the nipple surrounded by infiltrated scaly patches (detail of Fig. 2.6).

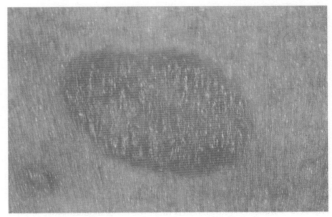

Fig. 2.9 Mycosis fungoides, plaque stage. Detail of a plaque.

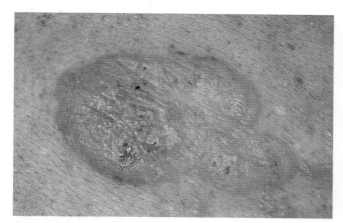

Fig. 2.10 Mycosis fungoides, tumour stage. Detail of a flat tumour with small crusts and scales.

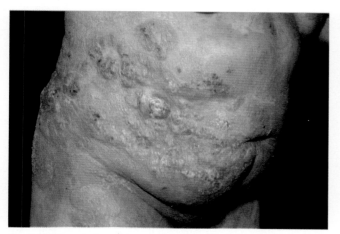

Fig. 2.11 Mycosis fungoides, tumour stage. Patches, plaques and tumours.

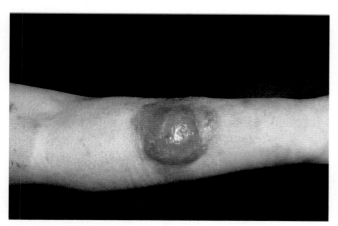

Fig. 2.12 Mycosis fungoides, tumour stage. Large ulcerated tumour on the right arm. Note patches and plaques in the vicinity of the tumour.

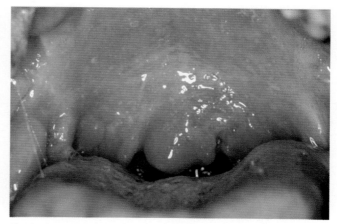

Fig. 2.13 Mycosis fungoides, tumour stage. Involvement of the buccal mucosa.

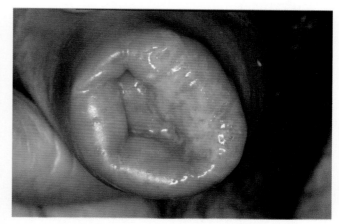

Fig. 2.14 Mycosis fungoides, tumour stage. Involvement of the genital mucosa.

Tumours may be solitary or, more often, localized or generalized. Ulceration is common.

In tumour-stage mycosis fungoides unusual sites of involvement may be observed, such as the mucosal regions (Figs 2.13 & 2.14). As oral and genital mucosae are frequently involved in cytotoxic T/NK-cell lymphomas, care should be taken to classify these cases correctly. Careful clinical history taking, re-evaluation of previous biopsies, and complete phenotypical and genotypical investigations are mandatory to make the diagnosis of mucosal involvement in mycosis fungoides.

Extracutaneous involvement

Lymph nodes, lung, spleen and liver are the most frequent sites of extracutaneous involvement in mycosis fungoides, but specific lesions can arise in all organs [33,34]. The bone marrow is usually spared. Lymph node involvement may be difficult to differentiate histopathologically from dermatopathic lymphadenopathy, and it has been suggested that, irrespective of the histopathological features, enlarged lymph nodes represent a bad prognostic sign. Because of the presence of ulcerated tumours and of immunodeficiency (caused both by the lymphoma and the many treatments typically administered to these patients during the course of the disease), septicaemia and/or pneumonia are the major causes of death.

Association with other diseases

Mycosis fungoides can be observed in association with other haematological disorders such as lymphomatoid papulosis, CD30+ anaplastic large cell lymphoma and Hodgkin lymphoma. The onset of these disorders may precede, be concomitant with, or occur later than the diagnosis of mycosis fungoides. In a few patients, molecular analyses revealed that the same neoplastic clone of T lymphocytes was present in mycosis fungoides and associated lymphomas [21–24]. It may be extremely difficult (if not impossible) to differentiate tumour-stage mycosis fungoides from lesions of lymphomatoid papulosis and CD30+ anaplastic large cell lymphoma (see Chapter 4). It may well be that at least some of the cases reported as lymphomatoid papulosis or cutaneous CD30+ anaplastic large cell lymphoma arising after the onset of mycosis fungoides in fact represent lesions of tumour-stage mycosis fungoides with expression of CD30. In this context, it should be noted that spontaneous regression (usually partial regression) of single tumours of mycosis fungoides can be observed.

As well as these haematological disorders, specific infiltrates of mycosis fungoides can be observed in benign and malignant skin tumours such as melanocytic naevi, malignant melanoma and seborrhoeic keratoses among others (Fig. 2.15) [35]. In these cases, the association of the two diseases represents an example of 'collision tumours'.

Histopathology, immunophenotype and molecular genetics

Mycosis fungoides is a cutaneous T-cell lymphoma characterized cytomorphologically by the proliferation of small- to medium-sized pleomorphic ('cerebriform') lymphocytes (Fig. 2.16). Intraepidermal collections of lymphocytes ('Pautrier's microabscesses'), considered for decades to be the hallmark of the disease, are present only in a minority of early patches of mycosis fungoides and can be absent from more advanced lesions too. Parenthetically, the first descrip-

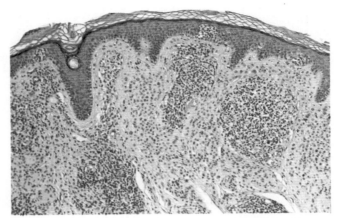

Fig. 2.15 Mycosis fungoides. Specific infiltrate of the disease within a pre-existent melanocytic naevus. Note nests of intraepidermal lymphocytes.

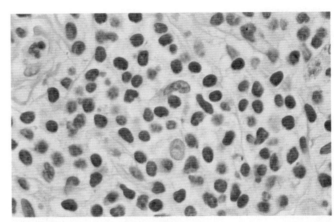

Fig. 2.16 Cytomorphology of mycosis fungoides reveals predominance of small- and medium-sized pleomorphic ('cerebriform') lymphocytes.

tion of the 'microabscesses' is not by Pautrier but by Jean Ferdinand Darier several decades before [36]. Pautrier was puzzled by the attribution of this observation to himself and acknowledged that the intraepidermal collections of lymphocytes should have been termed 'Darier's nests' instead (a term that was used in the 1920s) [36].

It should be emphasized that, although precise histopathological criteria for the diagnosis of early mycosis fungoides have been identified (Table 2.4), a definitive diagnosis can only be made, in many cases, after careful correlation with the clinical features of the disease. Further problems can arise when biopsies are taken after different types of local treatment that alter the histopathological features of the lesions. In unclear cases, a useful approach is to take biopsies from morphologically different lesions, to repeat biopsies after a 2-week period without local treatment, and to perform repeat biopsies on recurrent lesions. Repeat biopsies on recurrent

Table 2.4 Histopathological criteria for the diagnosis of early mycosis fungoides.

Epidermis

Intraepidermal collections of lymphocytes ('Pautrier's microabscesses'/'Darier's nests')

Lymphocytes aligned along the dermo-epidermal junction

Intraepidermal lymphocytes larger than lymphocytes in the dermis

'Disproportionate' epidermotropism (epidermotropic lymphocytes with only scant spongiosis)

Intraepidermal lymphocytes with 'haloed' nuclei

Dermis

Expanded papillary dermis with slight fibrosis and coarse bundles of collagen

Band-like or patchy lichenoid infiltrate of lymphocytes

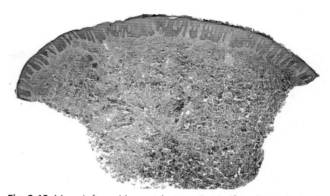

Fig. 2.18 Mycosis fungoides, patch stage. Psoriasiform hyperplasia of the epidermis.

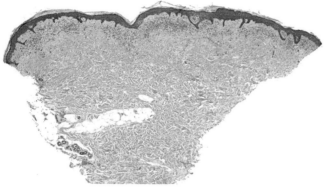

Fig. 2.17 Mycosis fungoides, patch stage. Band-like infiltrate of lymphocytes within an expanded papillary dermis.

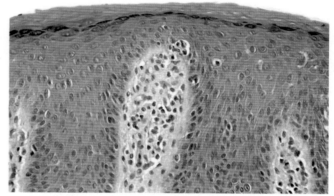

Fig. 2.19 Mycosis fungoides, patch stage. Note a small intraepidermal collection of lymphocytes (detail of Fig. 2.18).

lesions should also be performed to check whether the features are stable or changing (occurrence of large cell transformation). Recently, a scoring system for the diagnosis of mycosis fungoides has been proposed, combining the clinical aspect with the immunophenotypical and molecular features of the infiltrate [37]. However, in our view the diagnosis of mycosis fungoides can be achieved in most cases by accurate clinicopathological correlation.

Histopathology

Early lesions of mycosis fungoides reveal a patchy lichenoid or band-like infiltrate in an expanded papillary dermis (Fig. 2.17). A psoriasiform hyperplasia of the epidermis may be seen (Figs 2.18 & 2.19), but in most cases the epidermis is normal. Small lymphocytes predominate, and atypical cells can be observed only in a minority of cases. Epidermotropism of solitary lymphocytes is usually found, but Darier's nests (Pautrier's microabscesses) are rare (Fig. 2.20). Useful

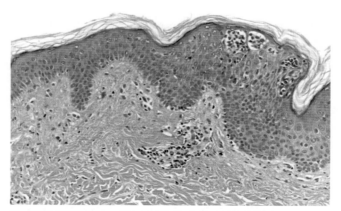

Fig. 2.20 Mycosis fungoides, patch stage. Scant superficial perivascular infiltrate of lymphocytes and intraepidermal collections of lymphocytes ('Darier's nests', 'Pautrier's microabscesses'). Note perivascular distribution of the infiltrate within the papillary dermis.

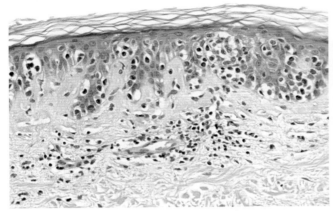

Fig. 2.21 Mycosis fungoides, patch stage. Epidermotropic lymphocytes with nuclei larger than those of the lymphocytes within the superficial dermis. Note also lymphocytes with clear halo around the nuclei ('haloed lymphocytes').

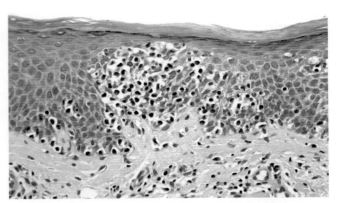

Fig. 2.23 Mycosis fungoides, patch stage. 'Disproportionate' epidermotropism (presence of many intraepidermal lymphocytes on the background of only scant spongiosis of the epidermis).

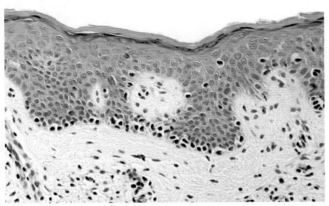

Fig. 2.22 Mycosis fungoides, patch stage. Epidermotropism of solitary lymphocytes aligned along the basal layer of the epidermis.

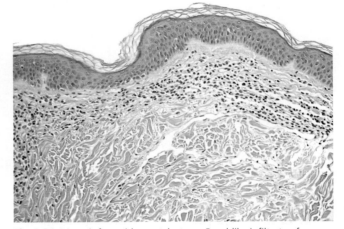

Fig. 2.24 Mycosis fungoides, patch stage. Band-like infiltrate of lymphocytes within a thickened fibrotic papillary dermis. Note complete absence of epidermotropism.

diagnostic clues are the presence of epidermotropic lymphocytes with nuclei slightly larger than those of lymphocytes within the upper dermis and/or the presence of lymphocytes aligned along the basal layer of the epidermis (Figs 2.21 & 2.22) [3–5,38–42]. Also useful is the presence of many intraepidermal lymphocytes in areas with scant spongiosis (Fig. 2.23). In this context, it should be emphasized that in a few cases (approximately 5% of the total) epidermotropism may be missing (Fig. 2.24). The papillary dermis shows a moderate to marked fibrosis with coarse bundles of collagen and a band-like or patchy lichenoid infiltrate of lymphocytes. Dermal oedema is usually not found.

Unusual histopathological patterns of mycosis fungoides in early phases include the presence of a perivascular (as opposed to band-like) superficial infiltrate (Fig. 2.20), prominent spongiosis simulating the picture of acute contact

dermatitis (Fig. 2.25), an interface dermatitis, sometimes with several necrotic keratinocytes (Fig. 2.26), marked pigment incontinence with melanophages in the papillary dermis (Fig. 2.27), prominent epidermal hyperplasia simulating the picture of lichen simplex chronicus (Fig. 2.28) and prominent extravasation of erythrocytes (Fig. 2.29). A pattern characterized by a markedly flattened epidermis, a lichenoid infiltrate in the dermis and increased dilated vessels in the papillary dermis is the histopathological counterpart of poikilodermatous mycosis fungoides (Fig. 2.30) (see page 26).

Plaques of mycosis fungoides are characterized by a dense band-like infiltrate within the upper dermis (Fig. 2.31). Intraepidermal lymphocytes arranged in Darier's nests (Pautrier's microabscesses) are a common finding at this

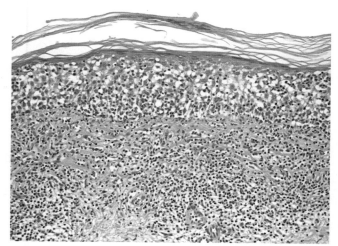

Fig. 2.25 Mycosis fungoides, patch stage. Prominent spongiosis of the epidermis associated with several epidermotropic lymphocytes. Note also the presence of a band-like infiltrate of lymphocytes within an expanded fibrotic papillary dermis.

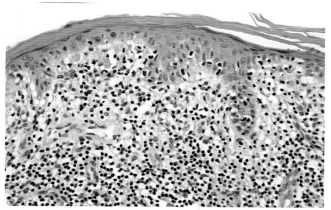

Fig. 2.26 Mycosis fungoides, patch stage. Vacuolization of basal keratinocytes ('interface dermatitis') with several necrotic keratinocytes.

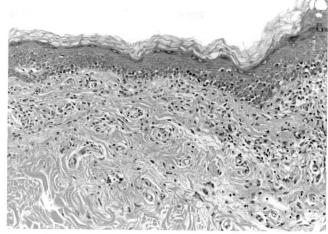

Fig. 2.27 Mycosis fungoides, patch stage. Note epidermotropic lymphocytes and several melanophages within the papillary dermis.

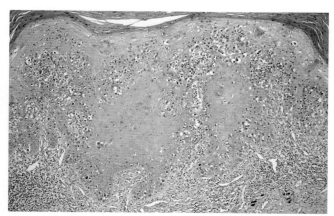

Fig. 2.28 Mycosis fungoides, patch stage. The epidermis shows a prominent pseudocarcinomatous hyperplasia. Note epidermotropic lymphocytes with atypical nuclei.

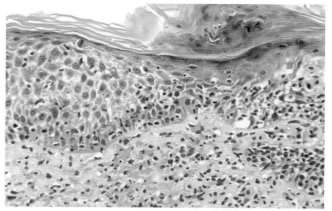

Fig. 2.29 Mycosis fungoides, patch stage. Prominent extravasation of erythrocytes in 'purpuric' mycosis fungoides. Note also spongiosis and epidermotropic lymphocytes.

stage (Fig. 2.32). Cytomorphologically, small pleomorphic (cerebriform) cells predominate (Fig. 2.16). In some cases, plaques or flat tumours of mycosis fungoides may present with a predominantly interstitial infiltrate (Fig. 2.33). This peculiar presentation can give rise to diagnostic problems, and has been designated 'interstitial mycosis fungoides' [43]. Immunohistology confirms that interstitial cells are T lymphocytes, thus being a helpful clue for the differential diagnosis with the interstitial variant of granuloma annulare (Fig. 2.34). Intersitial mycosis fungoides is usually a manifestation of either the plaque or tumour stage of the disease.

In tumours of mycosis fungoides, a dense nodular or diffuse infiltrate is found within the entire dermis, usually involving the subcutaneous fat (Fig. 2.35). Epidermotropism

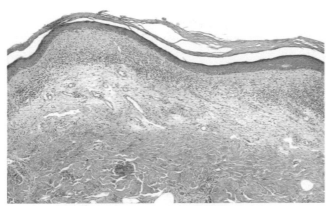

Fig. 2.30 Mycosis fungoides, patch stage. Prominent atrophy of the epidermis with loss of rete ridges and epidermotropic lymphocytes within the lower layers (poikilodermatous mycosis fungoides). Note band-like infiltrate of lymphocytes within a fibrotic papillary dermis and increased number of telangiectatic vessels.

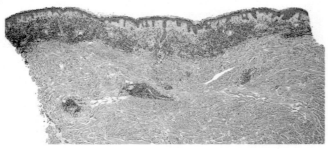

Fig. 2.31 Mycosis fungoides, plaque stage. Dense band-like infiltrate of lymphocytes within the superficial dermis. Note small perivascular aggregates of lymphocytes in the mid-dermis.

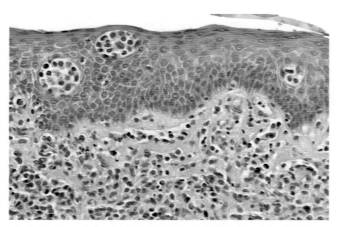

Fig. 2.32 Mycosis fungoides, plaque stage. Intraepidermal collections of lymphocytes ('Darier's nests' or 'Pautrier's microabscesses').

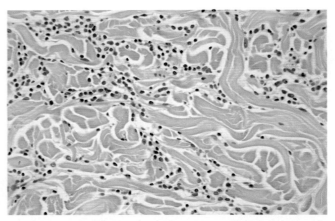

Fig. 2.33 Interstitial mycosis fungoides. Note neoplastic cells arranged in intertwining cords within the collagen, simulating the histopathological picture of the interstitial variant of granuloma annulare.

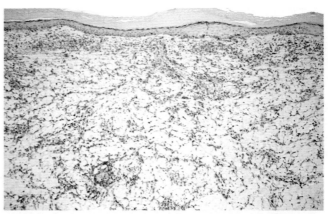

Fig. 2.34 Interstitial mycosis fungoides. Staining for CD3 reveals that all interstitial cells are T lymphocytes.

may be lost. Flat tumours are characterized histopathologically by dense infiltrates confined to the superficial and mid parts of the dermis (Fig. 2.36). Angiocentricity and/or angiodestruction can be observed in some cases [44].

A peculiar histopathological presentation of mycosis fungoides characterized by marked involvement of hyperplastic sweat glands has been termed 'syringotropic' mycosis fungoides (Fig. 2.37). In some of these cases, syringometaplasia can be observed. Involvement of the epidermis may be missing in syringotropic mycosis fungoides, thus creating problems in the histopathological diagnosis of this variant of the disease.

Large cell transformation

In later stages, patients with mycosis fungoides usually develop lesions with many large cells (immunoblasts, large

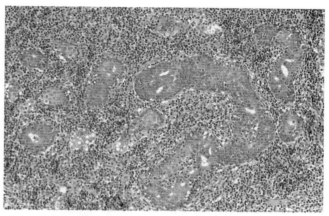

Fig. 2.37 Syringotropic mycosis fungoides. Neoplastic lymphocytes arranged predominantly around and within sweat glands. Note syringometaplasia.

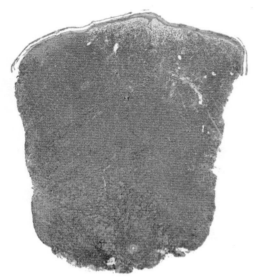

Fig. 2.35 Mycosis fungoides, tumour stage. Dense nodular infiltrates of lymphocytes within the entire dermis involving the subcutaneous fat.

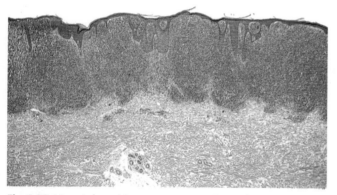

Fig. 2.36 Mycosis fungoides, tumour stage. Histopathology of a flat tumour showing a dense diffuse infiltrate of lymphocytes within the superficial dermis involving the mid-dermis.

pleomorphic cells or large anaplastic cells) (Fig. 2.38) [45–47]. Large cell transformation in mycosis fungoides is defined as the presence of large cells exceeding 25% of the infiltrate, or of large cells forming microscopic nodules, and has been detected in more than 50% of patients with tumour-stage mycosis fungoides [45]. Clusters of large cells may be observed sometimes in plaques of mycosis fungoides (usually in patients having tumours on other sites of the body), and rarely even in thin patches of the disease (these patients too usually also have plaques and tumours of mycosis fungoides at other sites of the body) (Fig. 2.39).

Tumours with a large cell morphology may or may not express CD30. Expression of the antigen does not have any prognostic significance in these patients. Large cell transformation of mycosis fungoides bears a poor prognosis, and usually heralds the terminal stage of the disease.

Immunophenotype

Mycosis fungoides is characterized by an infiltrate of α/β T-helper memory lymphocytes (βF1+, CD3+, CD4+, CD5+, CD8-, CD45RO+) (Fig. 2.40) [48,49]. Only a minority of cases exhibit a T-cytotoxic (βF1+, CD3+, CD4-, CD5+, CD8+) or γ/δ (βF1-, CD3+, CD4-, CD5+, CD8+) lineage that show no clinical and/or prognostic differences (Fig. 2.41) [50]. In these cases, correlation with the clinical features is crucial, in order to rule out skin involvement by aggressive cytotoxic lymphomas such as CD8+ epidermotropic T-cell lymphoma or γ/δ T-cell lymphoma (see Chapter 6). In late stages there may be a (partial) loss of pan-T-cell antigen expression. In plaque and tumour lesions, neoplastic T cells may express the CD30 antigen.

Recently, it has been suggested that a low CD8 : CD3 ratio in skin infiltrates supports the histopathological diagnosis of mycosis fungoides, but this finding should be confirmed by larger studies [51].

Cytotoxic-associated markers such as TIA-1 and granzyme B are negative in mycosis fungoides, although occasionally in late stages of the disease some positivity may be observed [52]. These cases should not be classified as cytotoxic lymphomas (see Chapter 6), but as tumour-stage mycosis fungoides with cytotoxic phenotypes. A similar phenotype may also be seen in early lesions of the rare γ/δ+ mycosis fungoides, which besides cytotoxic proteins also express CD56 (Fig. 2.42).

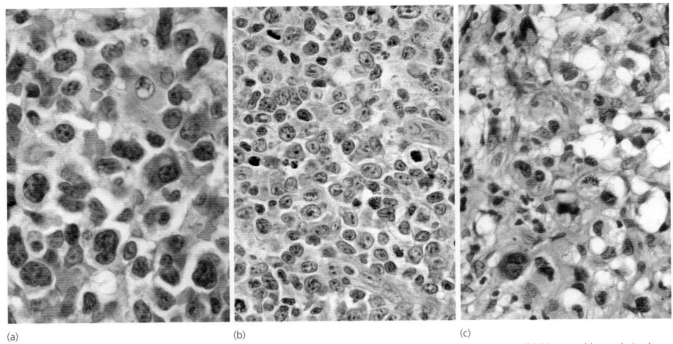

(a)   (b)   (c)

Fig. 2.38 Mycosis fungoides with large cell transformation. (a) Medium- and large-sized pleomorphic lymphocytes. (b) T immunoblasts admixed with pleomorphic lymphocytes. (c) Large anaplastic cells predominate.

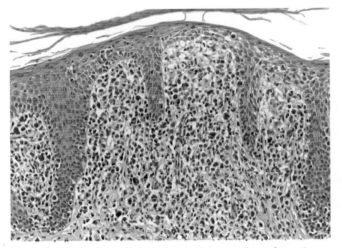

Fig. 2.39 Plaque of mycosis fungoides with large cell transformation.

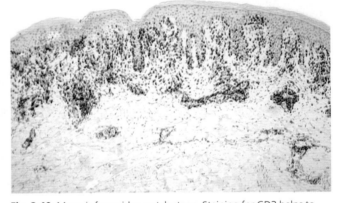

Fig. 2.40 Mycosis fungoides, patch stage. Staining for CD3 helps to highlight intraepidermal T lymphocytes.

Molecular genetics

There are no specific abnormalities commonly associated with mycosis fungoides. Using cDNA microarray analysis, a signature of 27 genes, including oncogenes and other genes involved in the control of apoptosis, has been recently identified in cases of early- and late-stage mycosis fungoides [53]. Oncogenes such as *p16* and *p53* do not show alterations in early lesions, but are often mutated in late (tumour) phases of the disease. Amplification and overexpression of *JUNB* has been found in one study [54].

Rearrangement of the T-cell receptor (TCR) gene is commonly found in plaques and tumours, but is present in only approximately 50% of early (patch) lesions [55,56]. Development of 'patient-specific' DNA probes can identify the neoplastic clone in lesions that are not specific histopathologically [57–59].

The presence of a monoclonal population of T lymphocytes has been detected in the peripheral blood in patients

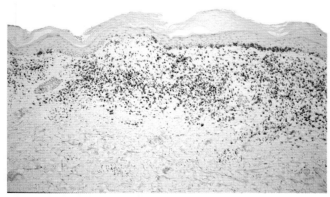

Fig. 2.41 Mycosis fungoides, patch stage. Positive staining for CD8 in the CD8+ variant of mycosis fungoides.

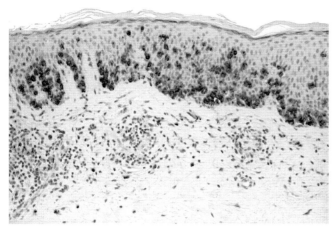

Fig. 2.42 Mycosis fungoides, patch stage. Positive staining for CD56 in the γ/δ+ variant of mycosis fungoides.

with early-stage mycosis fungoides [28–30]. In many of these patients, the clone was different from that detected within the skin, but in some cases the same clone was present both in the peripheral blood and in the cutaneous lesions of mycosis fungoides, even after successful treatment and complete clinical remission [28,30,31]. The exact diagnostic and prognostic value of molecular genetic analysis of the TCR gene rearrangement within the peripheral blood in patients with early mycosis fungoides is still unclear [60].

Histopathological differential diagnosis

The histopathological diagnosis of early mycosis fungoides may be extremely difficult. In some instances, differentiation from inflammatory skin conditions (e.g. psoriasis, chronic contact dermatitis) may be impossible on histopathological grounds alone. In these cases, clinical correlation is crucial to make a definitive diagnosis. Immunohistological features are not distinctive, and are similar to those observed in many inflammatory skin conditions [48,49]. Staining for CD3 or CD4 may help by highlighting epidermotropic T lymphocytes (Fig. 2.40).

It has been suggested that in early stages of mycosis fungoides, in contrast to benign (inflammatory) cutaneous infiltrates of T lymphocytes, there is a loss of expression of the T-cell-associated antigen CD7 [61,62]. This finding has not been confirmed by other studies showing normal CD7+ populations in early mycosis fungoides [48,55]. In addition, T lymphocytes in some cases of benign inflammatory dermatosis can also show partial loss of CD7 [63,64]. At present, the value of CD7 staining in the differential diagnosis of cutaneous T-cell infiltrates is unclear [65]. Immunohistochemical analysis of the TCRs has also been advocated for differentiation of early mycosis fungoides from chronic benign inflammatory conditions. The TCR consists of a constant and a variable region. Two types of TCR may be distinguished with respect to the constant regions: α/β and γ/δ heterodimers. Analysis of these receptors shows, in most cases of early mycosis fungoides, an α/β phenotype (βF1+/TCRδ1−), similar to that seen in benign cutaneous T-cell infiltrates [66]. More interesting results have been obtained from the analysis of the variable regions of TCR. In benign T-cell infiltrates these differ from one cell to another, whereas malignant proliferations usually exhibit a monoclonal expression of these determinants. Jack *et al.* [67] showed a monoclonal population in 10 out of 16 cases of plaque- or tumour-stage mycosis fungoides using antibodies specific for the Vβ8 and the Vβ5 determinants. However, monoclonality could not be demonstrated in patch-stage mycosis fungoides. It has been suggested that the frequent expression of the same variable region in different cases of mycosis fungoides may reflect similarities in the aetiology and/or pathogenesis (a distinct population of virus-infected cells) of this condition [67].

Molecular analysis of TCR gene rearrangement is a further criterion helpful in the differentiation of mycosis fungoides from benign skin conditions [55,56]. It must be underlined that early lesions of mycosis fungoides reveal a monoclonal rearrangement only in approximately 50% of cases, and that several benign dermatoses have been shown to harbour a monoclonal population of T lymphocytes (e.g. lichen planus and lichen sclerosus among others) [68–70]. The reason for the low sensitivity of gene rearrangement analysis in mycosis fungoides may reside in the very low number of neoplastic lymphocytes in early phases of the disease, and it has been shown that the sensitivity can be increased upon microdissection of the specimen [71]. Attempts to increase the sensitivity of PCR techniques by refining the detection methods have been described [72], but they are often too complex for routine examination of biopsy specimens. Moreover, increasing sensitivity has an adverse effect on the specificity of PCR techniques. At present, therefore, the presence or absence of a monoclonal pattern of TCR gene rearrangement cannot be considered as a crucial criterion in the early diagnosis of mycosis fungoides.

Clinical and histopathological variants

Several clinical and/or histopathological variants of mycosis fungoides have been described (Table 2.5) [73,74]. Patients with these variants often also show features of 'classic' mycosis fungoides at other sites of the body.

Many of the clinicopathological variants listed in Table 2.5 are quite rare. In the past some of them were separated from mycosis fungoides and considered as distinct entities (e.g. small-

Table 2.5 Clinicopathological variants of mycosis fungoides.

Acanthosis nigricans-like mycosis fungoides
Angiocentric/angiodestructive mycosis fungoides
Bullous (vesiculobullous) mycosis fungoides
Dyshidrotic mycosis fungoides
Erythrodermic mycosis fungoides
Follicular (pilotropic) mycosis fungoides
Granulomatous mycosis fungoides
Granulomatous slack skin
Hyperpigmented mycosis fungoides
Hypopigmented mycosis fungoides
Ichthyosis-like mycosis fungoides
Interstitial mycosis fungoides
'Invisible' mycosis fungoides
Mucinous mycosis fungoides
Mycosis fungoides palmaris et plantaris
Mycosis fungoides with eruptive infundibular cysts
Mycosis fungoides with follicular mucinosis
Mycosis fungoides with large cell transformation
Pagetoid reticulosis (Woringer–Kolopp type)
Papular mycosis fungoides
Papuloerythroderma Ofuji
Perioral dermatitis-like mycosis fungoides
Pigmented purpura-like mycosis fungoides
Poikilodermatous mycosis fungoides (poikiloderma vasculare
    atrophicans)
Pustular mycosis fungoides
Small-plaque parapsoriasis
Syringotropic mycosis fungoides
Unilesional (solitary) mycosis fungoides
Verrucous/hyperkeratotic mycosis fungoides
Zosteriform mycosis fungoides

Table 2.6 Historical terms used for mycosis fungoides.*

Erythrodermie pityriasique en plaques disseminées
Parakeratosis variegata
Parapsoriasis en plaques
Parapsoriasis lichenoides
Parapsoriasis variegata
Poikiloderma vasculare atrophicans
Premycotic erythema
Prereticulotic poikiloderma
Retiform type of parapsoriasis
Xanthoerythroderma perstans

*Some of these terms are still used today in some centres.

plaque parapsoriasis, pagetoid reticulosis, granulomatous slack skin, papuloerythroderma Ofuji), but they are now known to be variants of mycosis fungoides. In the following text the main characteristics of some of these forms are summarized.

In addition to these variants, a plethora of terms has been used in the past for mycosis fungoides (Table 2.6), and some of them are still in use today. The use of these terms has brought much confusion to this field, and should be strongly discouraged.

Small-plaque parapsoriasis

The presence of small patches of disease is common in patients with otherwise 'classic' mycosis fungoides. Some patients present only with small, sometimes 'digitated' patches, typically located on the trunk and upper extremities (Fig. 2.5). In the past, cases characterized by small lesions alone were variously diagnosed as 'digitate' dermatosis, chronic superficial scaly dermatitis or small-plaque parapsoriasis (the term is a misnomer, for these patients never present with plaques). Molecular genetic techniques revealed that in some of these lesions a monoclonal population of T lymphocytes could be found.

At present there is a lack of agreement concerning the exact relationship of small-plaque parapsoriasis and mycosis fungoides: some think that they represent one and the same disease, whereas others maintain that they are completely unrelated [75,76]. In Graz, we have encountered patients with small patches of 'parapsoriasis en plaques' who decades later developed the plaques and tumours of mycosis fungoides, leading us to conclude that small-plaque parapsoriasis represents an early manifestation of the disease. It is important to underline that these patients should not be treated aggressively, as progression of the disease is rare and, when it happens, takes place only after a very long period of time.

It should be clearly stated that these authors (in line with most others) do not believe that 'large plaque parapsoriasis' is a peculiar variant of mycosis fungiodes, but rather represents one of the most typical presentations of the disease. In this sense we have not listed 'large plaque parapsoriasis' among the clinicopathological variants of mycosis fungiodes.

Mycosis fungoides with follicular mucinosis/follicular (pilotropic) mycosis fungoides

Some patients with mycosis fungoides present with follicular papules and plaques characterized histopathologically by abundant deposits of mucin within hair follicles that are surrounded by a more or less dense infiltrate of T lymphocytes (Figs 2.43 & 2.44) [77]. The hair follicles are infiltrated by the lymphocytes (pilotropism). The epidermis between affected follicles may be spared or involved by the disease ('epidermal mucinosis') (Fig. 2.45). Alopecia resulting from destruction of the follicles is common (alopecia mucinosa), either generalized or localized (Fig. 2.46). Itching is severe and represents a major problem in this variant of mycosis fungoides, and may be non-responsive to standard treatments.

A variant of mycosis fungoides with marked involvement of the hair follicles but without deposition of mucin has also been described (pilotropic mycosis fungoides) (Fig. 2.47); its relationship with follicular mucinosis-associated mycosis fungoides is unclear, but it seems that pilotropic mycosis fungoides represents a distinct clinicopathological variant of the disease [78].

In patients with marked involvement of the hair follicles, with or without deposition of mucin, a localized eruption of small infundibular cysts and comedones infiltrated by neoplastic T lymphocytes can be observed (mycosis fungoides with eruptive cysts and comedones) (Figs 2.48 & 2.49). The clinical picture is similar to that observed in 'milia en plaques'.

We believe that 'idiopathic generalized follicular mucinosis' represents a variant of mycosis fungoides with marked

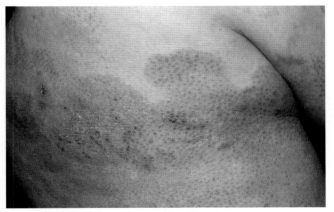

Fig. 2.43 Mycosis fungoides with follicular mucinosis. Follicular erythematous papules and plaques on the thigh.

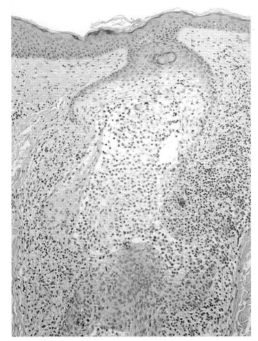

Fig. 2.44 Mycosis fungoides with follicular mucinosis. Mucin deposits within a hair follicle with destruction of the follicle. Note lymphocytes infiltrating the hair follicle ('pilotropism').

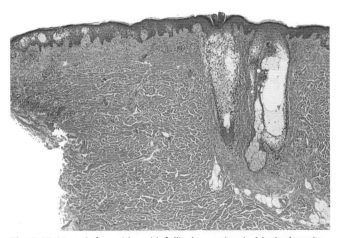

Fig. 2.45 Mycosis fungoides with follicular mucinosis. Mucin deposits within two hair follicles as well as within the interfollicular epidermis ('epidermal mucinosis'). Note also patchy lichenoid infiltrate of lymphocytes with epidermotropism.

deposition of mucin within hair follicles, and cases of progression to late-stage mycosis fungoides and death have been well documented [77]. We have also observed patients with clear-cut mycosis fungoides-associated follicular mucinosis who went into clinical remission after conventional

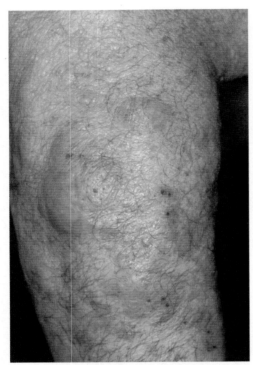

Fig. 2.46 Mycosis fungoides with follicular mucinosis. Note partial loss of hairs within the affected skin ('alopecia mucinosa') and superficial erosions representing scratch artefacts resulting from intense itching.

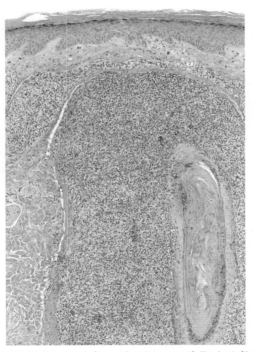

Fig. 2.47 Pilotropic mycosis fungoides. Dense perifollicular infiltrate of lymphocytes without deposits of mucin within the hair follicle.

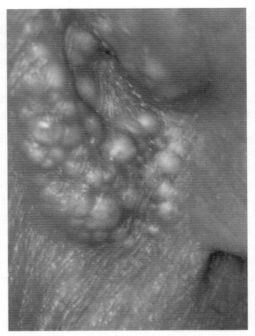

Fig. 2.48 Mycosis fungoides with eruptive cysts and comedones. Retroauricular eruption of small epidermal cysts (milia).

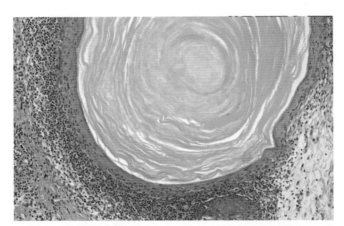

Fig. 2.49 Mycosis fungoides with eruptive cysts and comedones. Dense infiltrate of lymphocytes involving the wall of the cysts.

treatments, and who subsequently relapsed with skin lesions showing clinical and histopathological features of 'idiopathic' follicular mucinosis, again suggesting that this condition represents a variant of mycosis fungoides. Even 'benign' localized follicular mucinosis may represent a variant of mycosis fungoides, conceptually and biologically similar to localized pagetoid reticulosis and 'unilesional' mycosis fungoides [77].

Some authors report a worse prognosis in mycosis fungoides associated with follicular mucinosis in comparison to patients with 'common' mycosis fungoides [79].

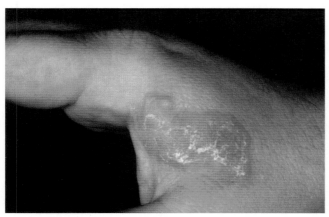

Fig. 2.50 Localized pagetoid reticulosis. Erythematous plaque on the right hand. (Courtesy of Professor W. Sterry, Berlin.)

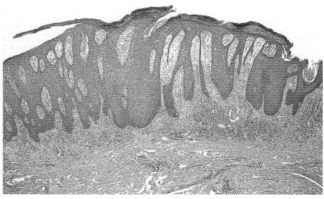

Fig. 2.52 Localized pagetoid reticulosis. Hyperplastic epidermis with prominent epidermotropism of lymphocytes.

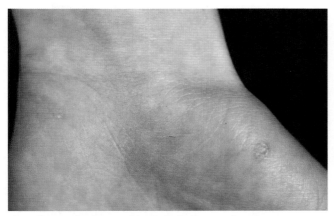

Fig. 2.51 Localized pagetoid reticulosis. Two small erythematous papules on the left hand simulating clinically the picture of a wart.

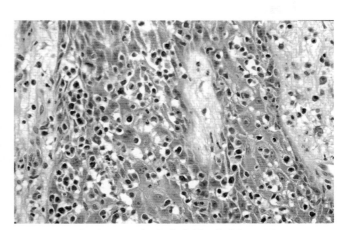

Fig. 2.53 Localized pagetoid reticulosis (detail of Fig. 2.52).

Localized pagetoid reticulosis (Woringer–Kolopp type)/unilesional (solitary) mycosis fungoides

Localized pagetoid reticulosis is a variant of mycosis fungoides presenting with solitary psoriasiform scaly erythematous patches or plaques, usually located on the extremities (Fig. 2.50). The clinical picture can be deceptive, simulating that of benign conditions such as warts or eczematous dermatitis (Fig. 2.51) [80]. The histological picture shows a markedly hyperplastic epidermis with striking epidermotropism of T lymphocytes (Figs 2.52 & 2.53). Intraepidermal lymphocytes are characterized usually by medium-sized pleomorphic nuclei. Both T-helper and T-cytotoxic phenotypes have been described.

The term pagetoid reticulosis should be restricted to solitary lesions only (Woringer–Kolopp type) [1,2]. Patients presenting with the 'generalized' form of pagetoid reticulosis

(Ketron–Goodman type) probably have either classic mycosis fungoides or, more frequently, one of the recently described primary cutaneous cytotoxic NK/T-cell lymphomas (aggressive epidermotropic CD8+ T-cell lymphoma, γ/δ cutaneous T-cell lymphoma, NK/T-cell lymphoma—nasal type) (see Chapter 6).

The prognosis of patients with solitary pagetoid reticulosis is excellent, and involvement of internal organs has never been observed. In a few patients, development of 'classic' mycosis fungoides has been documented. The treatment of choice is surgical excision or local radiotherapy.

Besides localized pagetoid reticulosis, a solitary variant of mycosis fungoides with clinicopathological features similar to 'common' mycosis fungoides has been described (Fig. 2.54) [81–83]. It is as yet unclear whether the prognosis for these patients is better, but in some instances development of generalized lesions of mycosis fungoides has been observed over time.

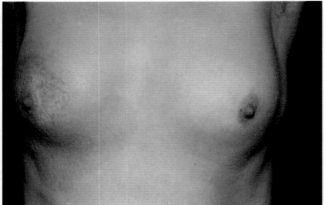

Fig. 2.54 Solitary lesion of mycosis fungoides located on the breast.

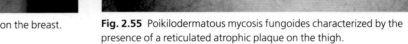

Fig. 2.55 Poikilodermatous mycosis fungoides characterized by the presence of a reticulated atrophic plaque on the thigh.

Erythrodermic mycosis fungoides

Patients with mycosis fungoides may develop erythroderma during the course of their disease. Rarely, swelling of the lymph nodes and the presence of circulating neoplastic cells (Sézary cells) are observed as well, thus showing complete overlap of clinical features with Sézary syndrome (see Chapter 3). The histopathological and phenotypical features are identical to those of conventional mycosis fungoides. After successful treatment, patients may relapse with conventional patches, plaques or tumours of mycosis fungoides or with new flares of erythroderma.

These cases probably should not be classified as Sézary syndrome but as erythrodermic mycosis fungoides, and the diagnosis of Sézary syndrome should be reserved for those patients presenting with the typical features of this disease from the onset.

Poikilodermatous mycosis fungoides (poikiloderma vasculare atrophicans)

Poikilodermatous mycosis fungoides is characterized clinically by atrophic red–brown macules and patches with prominent telangiectasias (Fig. 2.55). Sites of predilection are the breast and buttocks. Histology reveals an atrophic epidermis with the loss of rete ridges, an interface dermatitis with a superficial band-like infiltrate of lymphocytes and a thickened papillary dermis (Fig. 2.30). Necrotic keratinocytes may be a prominent finding. Widely dilated capillaries are present within the superficial dermis. This variant of the disease has been referred to as the 'lichenoid' type of mycosis fungoides.

Hypopigmented mycosis fungoides/ hyperpigmented mycosis fungoides

Patients with mycosis fungoides may develop hypopig-

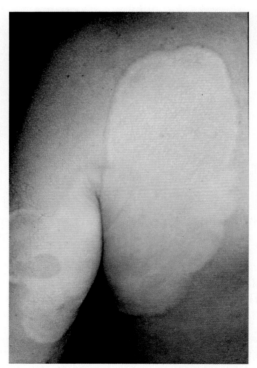

Fig. 2.56 Hypopigmented patch of mycosis fungoides on the right shoulder. Note elevated, slightly erythematous margin.

mented patches and plaques (Fig. 2.56). These lesions may be misinterpreted clinically as those of pityriasis versicolor, pityriasis alba or vitiligo. Histology reveals features typical of mycosis fungoides. Hypopigmented mycosis fungoides is observed more frequently in dark-skinned individuals, and is one of the most frequent variants seen in children [84,85]. Repigmentation usually takes place after successful treatment of the lesions.

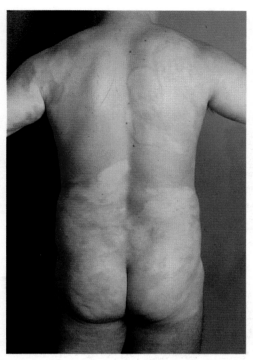

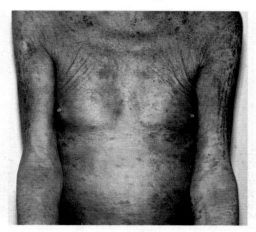

Fig. 2.58 Hyperpigmented mycosis fungoides ('melanoerythroderma'). Note diffuse reddish brown colour with multiple areas of marked hyperpigmentation.

Fig. 2.57 Hypopigmented mycosis fungoides covering large parts of the body. Note erythematous areas as well.

Although hypopigmented lesions may present as the sole manifestation of mycosis fungoides, in many cases, especially in white people, careful examination of the patients will detect the presence of erythematous lesions as well (Fig. 2.57). Interestingly, patients with hypopigmented mycosis fungoides tend to develop more hypopigmented lesions during the course of the disease, suggesting that this is indeed an unusual variant of mycosis fungoides.

A predominant CD8+ phenotype has been described in patients with hypopigmented mycosis fungoides, possibly underlying some pathogenetic similarities to vitiligo [84]. However, a CD4+ phenotype can also be observed.

Rarely, the clinical picture of mycosis fungoides may be characterized by markedly hyperpigmented lesions, corresponding histopathologically to the presence of pigment incontinence and abundant melanophages in the papillary dermis (Figs 2.27 & 2.58). Generalized hyperpigmented lesions have been described as 'melanoerythroderma' and are seen more frequently in patients with Sézary syndrome.

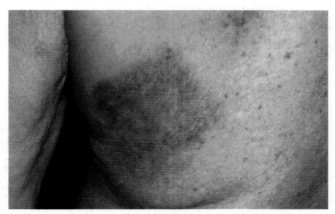

Fig. 2.59 Purpuric mycosis fungoides. Same patient as Fig. 2.29. The patient also had 'conventional' patches of mycosis fungoides elsewhere on the trunk.

Pigmented purpura-like mycosis fungoides

In some patients, lesions of mycosis fungoides are characterized clinically by a purpuric hue, and histopathologically by the presence of many extravasated erythrocytes (Figs 2.29 & 2.59). Differential diagnosis of these cases from lichenoid purpura and lichen aureus can be difficult on histopathological grounds, and correlation with the clinical features is crucial (see Chapter 20). The distinction of purpuric mycosis fungoides from purpuric dermatoses has been rendered more difficult in recent years by the introduction of the term 'atypical pigmented purpura', and of the concept of a possible relationship between some purpuric dermatoses and mycosis fungoides [86–89]. Patients with 'pigmented purpura' progressing into mycosis fungoides probably had purpuric mycosis fungoides from the outset [89,90]. In this context, it should be emphasized that lichen aureus and lichenoid purpura are wholly benign disorders which should be clearly differentiated from mycosis fungoides.

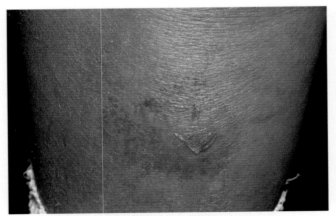

Fig. 2.60 Bullous mycosis fungoides. Note ruptured bulla with superficial erosion.

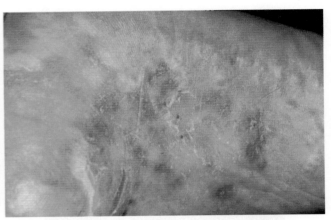

Fig. 2.62 Dyshidrotic mycosis fungoides. Dyshidrotic vesicles and small erosions on the soles.

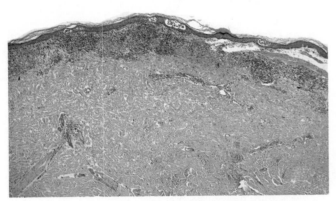

Fig. 2.61 Bullous mycosis fungoides. Subepidermal bulla with dense band-like infiltrate of lymphocytes in the papillary dermis and epidermotropism.

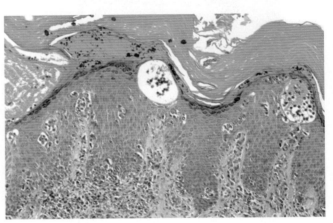

Fig. 2.63 Dyshidrotic mycosis fungoides. Histology reveals epidermotropic lymphocytes, some within intraepidermal vesicles.

Bullous (vesiculobullous) mycosis fungoides/dyshidrotic mycosis fungoides

Some patients with mycosis fungoides present with vesicular or bullous lesions, these last usually associated with large superficial erosions (Fig. 2.60) [91]. Bullous lesions may be brought about by cleavage at the dermo-epidermal junction, or by the confluence of intraepidermal vesicles (Fig. 2.61). A 'dyshidrotic' variant of the disease located at the palms and soles has also been described (Figs 2.62 & 2.63) [92,93]. Typical lesions of mycosis fungoides are commonly present near to the vesicular and bullous ones.

The reason(s) for the formation of vesicular and bullous lesions is unclear. Some patients may present with pre-existent dyshidrotic or vesicular dermatitis and subsequent colonization by neoplastic cells. In other patients, a direct cytotoxic effect may be responsible for the detachment of the epidermis from the dermis, or pronounced spongiosis may lead to vesiculation, and eventually larger blisters may develop resulting from the confluence of vesicles. In some patients, the onset of bullous lesions has been related to the use of interferon-α [94].

Granulomatous mycosis fungoides/ granulomatous slack skin

Granulomatous mycosis fungoides is an unusual histological variant of mycosis fungoides described first by Ackerman and Flaxman in 1970, who reported a patient with tumour-stage mycosis fungoides with huge giant cells scattered within the dermal infiltrate [95]. A granulomatous pattern can be observed in different lesions of mycosis fungoides, including patches, plaques and tumours, and in some cases even within affected lymph nodes (Figs 2.64 & 2.65) [96]. Granuloma-

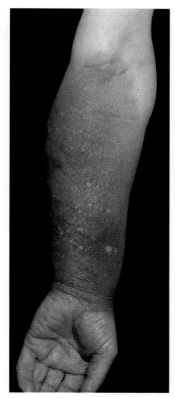

Fig. 2.64 Granulomatous mycosis fungoides. Note reddish brown plaque with several papules and small nodules on the arm.

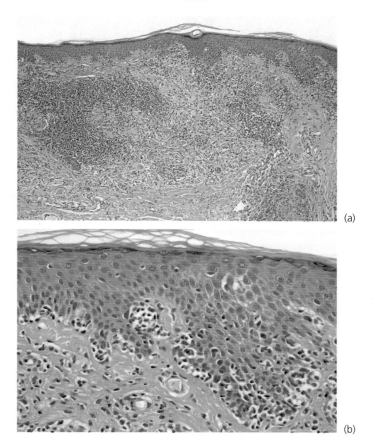

(a)

(b)

Fig. 2.65 Granulomatous mycosis fungoides. (a) Dense lymphoid infiltrate admixed with large epithelioid granulomas in the dermis. (b) Note focal epidermotropism of lymphocytes.

tous lesions may either precede, be concomitant with or follow 'classic' mycosis fungoides. Especially if the first manifestation of the disease shows prominent granulomatous features, the diagnosis of mycosis fungoides may be missed, and the histopathological picture may be misinterpreted as that of a 'granulomatous dermatitis'. Histopathologically, granulomatous mycosis fungoides may also be difficult or even impossible to distinguish from other cutaneous T-cell lymphomas with granulomatous features (Sézary syndrome, small/medium pleomorphic T-cell lymphoma) [73,96], and clinicopathological correlation is crucial for the diagnosis.

A rare variant of granulomatous mycosis fungoides is represented by 'granulomatous slack skin', which is characterized clinically by the occurrence of bulky pendulous skin folds, usually located in flexural areas (Fig. 2.66) [73,98–102]. Granulomatous slack skin is considered to be a specific manifestation of mycosis fungoides in most cases [96]. The granulomatous infiltrate in granulomatous slack skin is usually diffuse and involves the deep subcutaneous tissues, in contrast to the patchy, more superficial granulomas observed in 'conventional' granulomatous mycosis fungoides. Giant cells with many nuclei are a common finding (Fig. 2.67). Elastophagocytosis is also typically present.

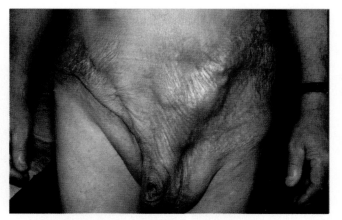

Fig. 2.66 Granulomatous slack skin. Prominent atrophy of the skin with bulky pendulous skin folds in the lower abdomen and inguinal region. (Courtesy of Professor Giovanni Borroni, Pavia, Italy.)

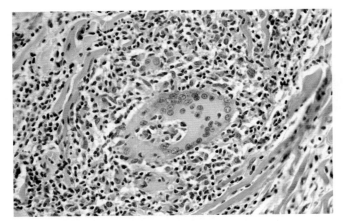

Fig. 2.67 Granulomatous slack skin. Histiocytic giant cell with several intracellular leucocytes, surrounded by a dense infiltrate of lymphocytes.

Although it has been suggested that a granulomatous reaction is associated with a good prognosis in patients with mycosis fungoides [103], patients doing badly have also been reported [73,104]. In addition, the amount of the granulomatous reaction is often variable in different biopsies from a single patient, suggesting that the term 'granulomatous mycosis fungoides' should be used as a description of histopathological specimens, and not as a classification of disease in a given patient [105].

Papular mycosis fungoides

In some patients with mycosis fungoides, small papules represent the predominant morphological expression of the disease, and small and/or large patches are absent (Figs 2.68 & 2.69). The absence of typical manifestations of the disease renders the clinical diagnosis very difficult. Moreover, differentiation from type B lymphomatoid papulosis can only be

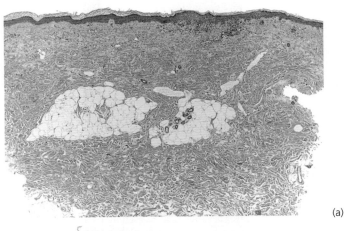

(a)

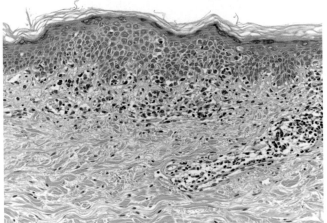

(b)

Fig. 2.69 Papular mycosis fungoides. (a) Histology reveals an infiltrate confined to a small portion of the specimen. (b) Detail shows typical changes of mycosis fungoides.

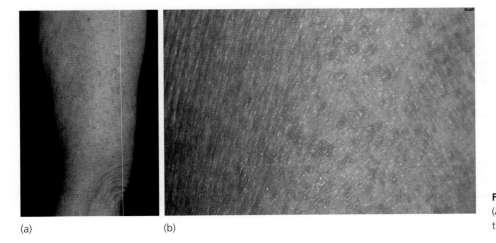

(a)   (b)

Fig. 2.68 Papular mycosis fungoides. (a) Note small erythematous papules on the arm. (b) Detail of the papules.

achieved by short-term follow-up of the patient, as the histopathological features may be indistinguishable (see Chapter 4). In fact, papular lesions of mycosis fungoides do not show the spontaneous regression typical of type B lymphomatoid papulosis.

'Invisible' mycosis fungoides

Normal-looking skin in patients with mycosis fungoides may show histopathological, electron microscopical, immuno- phenotypical and/or molecular genetic evidence of neoplas- tic lymphocytes [106–108]. These cases have been termed 'invisible' mycosis fungoides in the literature, because the lesions are clinically inapparent. The presence of such histo- logical features in normal-looking skin has been documented at the first diagnosis of mycosis fungoides, in patients with mycosis fungoides at sites distant from erythematous lesions and in patients in complete clinical remission after treatment [106–108].

The finding of specific infiltrates of mycosis fungoides in skin that looks clinically normal poses two main questions: the first relates to the extent of the area treated by skin- targeted therapies, and the second concerns the proper monitoring of patients after treatment.

Mycosis fungoides in children

Mycosis fungoides is the most common form of cutaneous lymphoma in childhood and adolescence (Fig. 2.70) [109]. In general, mycosis fungoides is rare in patients younger than 20 years of age, but the true incidence may be higher than generally assumed, because there is often a reluctance to per- form biopsies in children, and the diagnosis can be delayed for several years [110,111]. The hypopigmented variant of mycosis fungoides appears with unusually high frequency in this age group, especially in children with dark skin [84,110,112]. In addition, a distinct percentage of young patients with mycosis fungoides have localized pagetoid reticulosis (Woringer–Kolopp type), suggesting that this variant of mycosis fungoides may occur more frequently in childhood. The clinical presentation in these cases can be deceiving, and often lesions will be biopsied only after pro- longed local treatment [80]. Other variants observed in children include follicular mucinosis-associated mycosis fungoides, CD8+ mycosis fungoides, and a variant simulat- ing clinically pityriasis lichenoides et varioliformis acuta [77,113–117].

The overall outlook for children or adolescents with myco- sis fungoides is difficult to predict and it has been maintained that mycosis fungoides is more aggressive in childhood, with a higher frequency of extracutaneous involvement [110,113]. Other reports have suggested that the natural history of the disease is comparable with that seen in adults [114,117–120]. Indeed, it may be that at least some of the cases reported in the past as 'atypical' or 'aggressive' mycosis fungoides in chil- dren represent examples of cytotoxic T/NK-cell lymphomas, which usually show a more aggressive course with a poor prognosis. Overall, it seems likely that the onset of lesions of mycosis fungoides in childhood will increase the probability of disease progression during the lifetime of the patient.

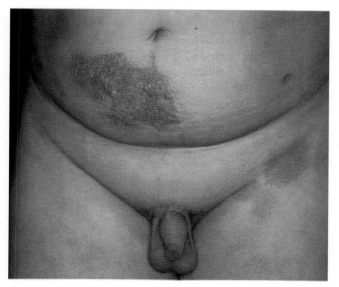

Fig. 2.70 Mycosis fungoides in a 14-year-old boy. The patient also had lesions of hypopigmented mycosis fungoides on the back.

Treatment

The standard treatment of early lesions of mycosis fungoides includes psoralen in association with UVA irradiation (PUVA), interferon-α2a, retinoids, or a combination of these three modalities [121,122]. Several other treatments have been used in the past (and are still in use at present), includ- ing UVB irradiation (or narrow-band UVB—311 nm) and topical application of chemotherapeutic agents [123–126]. In many cases, patients with localized patches of the disease can be treated with local steroid ointments [127]. Localized variants of the disease have also been treated by laser vapor- ization [128]. The administration of total body irradiation [129,130], proposed by some authors as a first-line treat- ment, should probably be restricted to patients with mycosis fungoides in the later stages. It should be noted that the administration of placebo as a topical vehicle devoid of active principle was found to produce an objective response in 24% of patients with early mycosis fungoides in a double-blind randomized study [131].

Although interferon-α is well tolerated and shows good results in most patients with early mycosis fungoides, resistance to this drug has been observed, hindering its use in many patients. Analysis of these patients showed that multiple genes involved in signal transduction, apoptosis, transcription regulation and cell growth are implicated in the mechanism of resistance [132]. Interferon treatment may be improved by the use of pegylated compounds but large studies are still lacking.

Recently, many new protocols have been introduced for the treatment of early mycosis fungoides, including photodynamic therapy with 5-aminolaevulinic acid, new retinoids such as bexarotene (Targretin®, administered orally or topically) and tazarotene (administered topically), new chemotherapeutic drugs for topical use, and immune response modifiers such as imiquimod [133–140]. At present there are insufficient data to evaluate the efficacy of these new modalities in terms of remission and recurrence rates. Combinations of different protocols have not yet shown clear-cut advantages in terms of overall survival [141].

The notion that a proportion of patients with patch-stage mycosis fungoides shows complete clinical response upon local application of placebo suggests that in early phases the disease may be controlled with a watchful waiting strategy.

In the late stages, in addition to PUVA, retinoids and interferon-α2a, conventional systemic chemotherapy (CHOP), extracorporeal photopheresis and radiotherapy have been applied [129,142]. Autologous bone marrow transplantation showed good results with complete clinical responses, but recurrence within short periods of time is the rule [143]. Allogeneic stem cell transplantation has been performed in a few patients and seems to be a promising treatment modality, perhaps with potential for cure resulting from a graft-vs.-tumour response [144,145]. However, toxicity is still very high, and it is unclear whether allogeneic stem cell transplantation should be considered as a treatment option for early tumour-stage mycosis fungoides. New chemotherapeutic or immunological agents, including gemcitabine, fludarabine, temozolomide, pegylated liposomal doxorubicin (Caelyx), pentostatin, anti-CD52 antibody (alemtuzumab, Campath-IH), interleukin 12 (IL-12), DAB_{389}–IL-2 fusion protein (Ontak, denileukin diftitox) and trimetrexate, have also been used in a few patients [146–152]. Recently, some patients have also been treated with different types of tumour vaccines [153,154]. In the future, cancer-related genes may be the target for immunotherapeutic strategies in mycosis fungoides [155]. Treatment of advanced (tumour-stage) mycosis fungoides remains unsatisfactory, and the disease usually progresses in spite of aggressive therapy.

An issue that has never been properly addressed in controlled studies, but that should be carefully evaluated, concerns the quality of life in patients with late-stage mycosis fungoides. Patients may have tumour-stage disease for several years, underlying the need for proper palliation and alleviation of symptoms.

Prognosis

Mycosis fungoides is a lymphoma of low-grade malignancy with prolonged survival, and progression from the clinical stage of patches to those characterized by plaques, tumours and extracutaneous spread usually takes place over many years to decades [1,2]. Development of plaques and/or tumours, or of large cell transformation, heralds the terminal stages of the disease (patients may survive several years with tumour-stage mycosis fungoides). As the disease arises more commonly in the elderly, most patients never progress to plaque or tumour stage, and die of unrelated causes [156,157]. It has been estimated that only 15–20% of patients die of their disease [158]. However, a small subset of patients experience a more rapidly aggressive course with extracutaneous spread and death resulting from complications of the disease (usually sepsis or other severe infections). Moreover, a substantial subset of patients are middle-aged or young adults, and a few are children, thus having a higher risk of progression during their lifetime.

The most important prognostic parameters are stage at diagnosis, absence of complete remission after first treatment, age and race (black patients have a worse prognosis, but this may be related to difficulties in gaining access to therapy) [156–159]. There are no significant differences in survival between stages Ia and Ib (TNM classification), or between patients with tumours and erythroderma [159,160]. Once extracutaneous spread takes place, prognostic parameters have no influence on survival, and the prognosis is bad [34]. The detection of a malignant clone in the blood is an independent prognostic criterion, whereas the exact implications of the detection of a clone in the skin alone in the early phases of the disease remain unclear [160–164]. The finding of an identical clone in the blood and skin seems to be an independent prognostic criterion [160,161,165]. Similarly, the finding of a monoclonal population of T lymphocytes in the lymph nodes of patients with mycosis fungoides has been linked to a worse prognosis compared to patients presenting with 'dermopathic lymphadenopathy' and no evidence of monoclonal rearrangement [166]. Although the influence of the presence of follicular mucinosis on survival is debated [77,79], it certainly complicates the treatment of these patients. Analysis of the histopathological features of biopsy specimens of early mycosis fungoides has so far failed to detect parameters that might predict the course of the disease [167].

Although most treatments are efficacious in the early phases, and long-term remissions can be achieved, it is unlikely that cures will be obtained, with the possible exception of the solitary variants of the disease (although life-long follow-up is still needed in these patients). The use of the PCR technique has been advocated for the detection of minimal residual disease after treatment, but the value of this method as a routine investigation needs to be confirmed by larger studies [168].

RÉSUMÉ

Clinical	Adults. Patches, plaques and tumours can be found. Preferential location: buttocks, other sun-protected areas (early phases). Rarely observed in children (but the most common cutaneous lymphoma in this age group!).
Morphology	Small pleomorphic (cerebriform) cells. During the course of the disease large cell transformation may occur indicating a worse prognosis (immunoblasts, large cell anaplastic, large cell pleomorphic).
Immunology	CD2, 3, 4, 5, 45RO + CD8, 45RA – CD30 may be positive in tumours with large cell morphology; cytotoxic markers (TIA-1) may be positive in late stages and rarely in early lesions.
Genetics	No specific abnormalities in early phases. Frequent abnormalities of *p53* and *p16* in advanced disease. Monoclonal rearrangement of the TCR is absent in about 50% of patients in early phases.
Treatment guidelines	*Early phases*: PUVA, interferon-α2a, retinoids (alone or in combination); topical chemotherapy; topical steroids; narrow-band UVB (311 nm); photodynamic therapy. *Advanced disease:* chemotherapy (single agent or multiagent); extracorporeal photopheresis; radiotherapy (including total body electron beam irradiation). *Experimental:* new retinoids (bexarotene); imiquimod; new chemotherapeutic drugs (gemcitabine, fludarabine, pegylated doxorubicin); pentostatin; allogeneic stem cell transplantation.

References

1 Willemze R, Kerl H, Sterry W *et al.* EORTC classification for primary cutaneous lymphomas: a proposal from the Cutaneous Lymphoma Study Group of the European Organization for Research and Treatment of Cancer. *Blood* 1997; **90**: 354–71.

2 Fink-Puches R, Zenahlik P, Bäck B *et al.* Primary cutaneous lymphomas: applicability of current classification schemes (European Organization for Research and Treatment of Cancer, World Health Organization) based on clinicopathologic features observed in a large group of patients. *Blood* 2002; **99**: 800–5.

3 Sanchez JL, Ackerman AB. The patch stage of mycosis fungoides: criteria for histologic diagnosis. *Am J Dermatopathol* 1979; **1**: 5–26.

4 Shapiro PE, Pinto FJ. The histologic spectrum of mycosis fungoides/Sezary syndrome (cutaneous T-cell lymphoma): a review of 222 biopsies, including newly described patterns and the earliest pathologic changes. *Am J Surg Pathol* 1994; **18**: 645–67.

5 Santucci M, Biggeri A, Feller AC, Massi D, Burg G. Efficacy of histologic criteria for diagnosing early mycosis fungoides: an EORTC Cutaneous Lymphoma Study Group investigation. *Am J Surg Pathol* 2000; **24**: 40–50.

6 Baykal C, Büyülbabani N, Kaymaz R. Familial mycosis fungoides. *Br J Dermatol* 2002; **146**: 1108–10.

7 Naji AA, Waiz MM, Sharquie KE. Mycosis fungoides in identical twins. *J Am Acad Dermatol* 2001; **44**: 532–3.

8 Morales MM, Olsen J, Johansen P *et al.* Viral infection, atopy and mycosis fungoides: a European multicentre case–control study. *Eur J Cancer* 2003; **39**: 511–6.

9 Whittemore AS, Holly EA, Lee IM *et al.* Mycosis fungoides in relation to environmental exposures and immune response: a case–control study. *J Natl Cancer Inst* 1989; **81**: 1560–7.

10 Fransway AF, Winkelmann RK. Chronic dermatitis evolving to mycosis fungoides: report of four cases and review of the literature. *Cutis* 1988; **41**: 330–5.

11 Tuyp E, Burgoyne A, Aitchison T, MacKie R. A case–control study of possible causative factors in mycosis fungoides. *Arch Dermatol* 1987; **123**: 196–200.

12 Tan RSH, Butterworth CM, McLaughlin H, Malka S, Samman PD. Mycosis fungoides: a disease of antigen persistence. *Br J Dermatol* 1974; **91**: 607–16.

13 Herne KL, Talpur R, Breuer-McHam J, Champlin R, Duvic M. Cytomegalovirus seropositivity is significantly associated with mycosis fungoides and Sezary syndrome. *Blood* 2003; **101**: 2132–5.

14 Bazarbachi A, Soriano V, Pawson R *et al.* Mycosis fungoides and Sezary syndrome are not associated with HTLV-I infection: an international study. *Br J Haematol* 1997; **98**: 927–33.

15 Karenko L, Sarna S, Kähkönen M, Ranki A. Chromosomal abnormalities in relation to clinical disease in patients with cutaneous T-cell lymphoma: a 5-year follow-up study. *Br J Dermatol* 2003; **148**: 55–64.

16 Dereure O, Levi E, Vonderheid EC, Kadin ME. Infrequent Fas mutations but no bax or p53 mutations in early mycosis fungoides: a possible mechanism for the accumulation of malignant T lymphocytes in the skin. *J Invest Dermatol* 2002; **118**: 949–56.

17 Mao X, Lillington D, Scarisbrick JJ *et al.* Molecular cytogenetic analysis of cutaneous T-cell lymphomas: identification of common genetic alterations in Sézary syndrome and mycosis fungoides. *Br J Dermatol* 2002; **147**: 464–75.

18 Scarisbrick JJ, Woolford AJ, Calonje E *et al.* Frequent abnormalities of the p15 and p16 genes in mycosis fungoides and Sezary syndrome. *J Invest Dermatol* 2002; **118**: 493–9.

19 Scarisbrick JJ, Woolford AJ, Russell-Jones R, Whittaker SJ. Allelotyping in mycosis fungoides and Sézary syndrome: common regions of allelic loss identified on 9p, 10q, and 17p. *J Invest Dermatol* 2001; **117**: 663–70.

20 Navas IC, Ortiz-Romero PL, Villuendas R *et al.* p16INK4a gene alterations are frequent in lesions of mycosis fungoides. *Am J Pathol* 2000; **156**: 1565–72.

21 Davis TH, Morton CC, Miller-Cassman R, Balk SP, Kadin ME. Hodgkin's disease, lymphomatoid papulosis, and cutaneous T-cell lymphoma derived from a common T-cell clone. *N Engl J Med* 1992; **326**: 1115–22.

22 Wood GS, Crooks CF, Uluer AZ. Lymphomatoid papulosis and associated cutaneous lymphoproliferative disorders exhibit a common clonal origin. *J Invest Dermatol* 1995; **105**: 51–5.

23 Joly P, Lenormand B, Bagot M *et al.* Sequential analysis of T-cell receptor gene rearrangement in skin biopsy specimens from 6 patients with Hodgkin disease, lymphomatoid papulosis, mycosis fungoides and CD30+ large cell lymphoma. *J Invest Dermatol* 1997; **109**: 485.

24 Zackheim HS, Jones C, LeBoit PE *et al.* Lymphomatoid papulosis associated with mycosis fungoides: a study of 21 patients including analyses for clonality. *J Am Acad Dermatol* 2003; **49**: 620–3.

25 Väkevä L, Pukkala E, Ranki A. Increased risk of secondary cancers in patients with primary cutaneous T cell lymphoma. *J Invest Dermatol* 2000; **115**: 62–5.

26 Bunn P, Lamberg S. Report of the committee on staging and classification of cutaneous T-cell lymphoma. *Cancer Treat Rep* 1979; **63**: 725–8.

27 Ralfkiaer E, Jaffe ES. Mycosis fungoides and Sézary syndrome. In: Jaffe ES, Harris NL, Stein H, Vardiman JW, eds. *World Health Organization Classification of Tumours: Tumours of Haematopoietic and Lymphoid Tissues.* Lyon: IARC Press, 2001: 216–20.

28 Dereure O, Balavoine M, Salles MT *et al.* Correlations between clinical, histologic, blood, and skin polymerase chain reaction outcome in patients treated for mycosis fungoides. *J Invest Dermatol* 2003; **121**: 614–7.

29 Muche JM, Lukowsky A, Asadullah K, Gellrich S, Sterry W. Demonstration of frequent occurrence of clonal T cells in the peripheral blood of patients with primary cutaneous T-cell lymphoma. *Blood* 1997; **90**: 1636–42.

30 Muche JM, Lukowsky A, Heim J *et al.* Demonstration of frequent occurrence of clonal T cells in the peripheral blood but not in the skin of patients with small plaque parapsoriasis. *Blood* 1999; **94**: 1409–17.

31 Delfau-Larue MH, Laroche L, Wechsler J *et al.* Diagnostic value of dominant T-cell clones in peripheral blood in 363 patients presenting consecutively with a suspicion of cutaneous lymphoma. *Blood* 2000; **96**: 2987–92.

32 Washington LT, Huh YO, Powers LC, Duvic M, Jones D. A stable aberrant immunophenotype characterizes nearly all cases of cutaneous T-cell lymphoma in blood and can be used to monitor response to therapy. *BMC Clin Pathol* 2002; **2**: 5.

33 Rappaport H, Thomas LB. Mycosis fungoides: the pathology of extracutaneous involvement. *Cancer* 1974; **34**: 1198–229.

34 de Coninck EC, Kim YH, Varghese A, Hoppe RT. Clinical characteristics and outcome of patients with extracutaneous mycosis fungoides. *J Clin Oncol* 2001; **19**: 779–84.

35 Kerl H, Cerroni L. Compare your diagnosis: seborrheic keratosis associated with mycosis fungoides. *Am J Dermatopathol* 1999; **21**: 94–5.

36 Cribier BJ. The myth of Pautrier's microabscesses. *J Am Acad Dermatol* 2003; **48**: 796–7.

37 Stevens SR, Ke MS, Birol A *et al.* A simple clinical scoring system to improve the sensitivity and standardization of the diagnosis of mycosis fungoides type cutaneous T-cell lymphoma: logistic regression of clinical and laboratory data. *Br J Dermatol* 2003; **149**: 513–22.

38 Smoller BR, Bishop K, Glusac E, Kim YH, Hendrickson M. Reassessment of histologic parameters in the diagnosis of mycosis fungoides. *Am J Surg Pathol* 1995; **19**: 1423–30.

39 Guitart J, Kennedy J, Ronan S *et al.* Histologic criteria for the diagnosis of mycosis fungoides: proposal for a grading system to standardize pathology reporting. *J Cutan Pathol* 2001; **28**: 174–83.

40 Yeh YA, Hudson AR, Prieto VG, Shea CR, Smoller BR. Reassessment of lymphocytic atypia in the diagnosis of mycosis fungoides. *Mod Pathol* 2001; **14**: 285–8.

41 Ming M, LeBoit PE. Can dermatopathologists reliably make the diagnosis of mycosis fungoides? If not, who can? *Arch Dermatol* 2000; **136**: 543–6.

42 Kamarashev J, Burg G, Kempf W, Hess Schmid M, Dummer R. Comparative analysis of histological and immunohistological features in mycosis fungoides and Sézary syndrome. *J Cutan Pathol* 1998; **25**: 407–12.

43 Su LD, Kim YH, LeBoit PE, Swetter SM, Kohler S. Interstitial mycosis fungoides, a variant of mycosis fungoides resembling granuloma annulare and inflammatory morphoea. *J Cutan Pathol* 2002; **29**: 135–41.

44 Fujiwara Y, Abe Y, Kuyama M *et al.* CD8+ cutaneous T-cell lymphoma with pagetoid epidermotropism and angiocentric and angiodestructive infiltration. *Arch Dermatol* 1990; **126**: 801–4.

45 Cerroni L, Rieger E, Hödl S, Kerl H. Clinicopathologic and immunologic features associated with transformation of mycosis fungoides to large-cell lymphoma. *Am J Surg Pathol* 1992; **16**: 543–52.

46 Vergier B, De Muret A, Beylot-Barry M *et al.* Transformation of mycosis fungoides: clinicopathologic and prognostic features of 45 cases. *Blood* 2000; **95**: 2212–8.

47 Diamandidou E, Colome-Grimmer MI, Fayad L, Duvic M, Kurzrock R. Transformation of mycosis fungoides/Sézary syndrome: clinical characteristics and prognosis. *Blood* 1998; **92**: 1150–9.

48 Willemze R, de Graaff-Reitsma CB, Cnossen J, van Vloten WA, Meijer CJLM. Characterization of T-cell subpopulations in skin and peripheral blood of patients with cutaneous T-cell lymphomas and benign inflammatory dermatoses. *J Invest Dermatol* 1983; **80**: 60–6.

49 Ralfkiaer E, Lange Wantzin G, Mason DY *et al.* Phenotypic characterization of lymphocyte subsets in mycosis fungoides: comparison

with large plaque parapsoriasis and benign chronic dermatoses. *Am J Clin Pathol* 1985; **84**: 610–9.

50 Tosca AD, Varelzidis AG, Economidou J, Stratigos JD. Mycosis fungoides: evaluation of immunohistochemical criteria for the early diagnosis of the disease and differentiation between stages. *J Am Acad Dermatol* 1986; **15**: 237–45.

51 Ortonne N, Buyukbabani N, Delfau-Larue MH, Bagot M, Wechsler J. Value of the CD8–CD3 ratio for the diagnosis of mycosis fungoides. *Mod Pathol* 2003; **16**: 857–62.

52 Vermeer MH, Geelen FAMJ, Kummer JA, Meijer CJLM, Willemze R. Expression of cytotoxic proteins by neoplastic T cells in mycosis fungoides increases with progression from plaque stage to tumor stage disease. *Am J Pathol* 1999; **154**: 1203–10.

53 Tracey L, Villuendas R, Dotor AM *et al.* Mycosis fungoides shows concurrent deregulation of multiple genes involved in the TNF signaling pathway: an expression profile study. *Blood* 2003; **102**: 1042–50.

54 Mao X, Orchard G, Lillington DM *et al.* Amplification and overexpression of JUNB is associated with primary cutaneous T-cell lymphomas. *Blood* 2003; **101**: 1513–9.

55 Böhncke WH, Krettek S, Parwaresch RM, Sterry W. Demonstration of clonal disease in early mycosis fungoides. *Am J Dermatopathol* 1992; **14**: 95–9.

56 Wood GS, Tung RM, Haeffner AC *et al.* Detection of clonal T-cell receptor gamma gene rearrangements in early mycosis fungoides/Sezary syndrome by polymerase chain reaction and denaturing gradient gel electrophoresis (PCR/DGGE). *J Invest Dermatol* 1994; **103**: 34–41.

57 Volkenandt M, Koch O, Wienecke R *et al.* Detection of monoclonal lymphoid subpopulations in clinical specimens by PCR and conformational polymorphism of cRNA molecules. *J Invest Dermatol* 1992; **98**: 508.

58 Volkenandt M, Soyer HP, Cerroni L, Bertino JR, Kerl H. Molecular detection of clone-specific DNA in histopathologically unclassified lesions of a patient with mycosis fungoides. *Arch Dermatol Res* 1992; **284**: 22–3.

59 Volkenandt M, Soyer HP, Cerroni L *et al.* Molecular detection of clone-specific DNA in hypopigmented lesions of a patient with early evolving mycosis fungoides. *Br J Dermatol* 1993; **128**: 423–8.

60 Jones D, Duvic M. The current state and future of clonality studies in mycosis fungoides. *J Invest Dermatol* 2003; **121**: ix–xi.

61 Wood GS, Abel EA, Hoppe RT, Warnke RA. Leu-8 and Leu-9 antigen phenotypes: immunological criteria for the distinction of mycosis fungoides from cutaneous inflammation. *J Am Acad Dermatol* 1986; **14**: 1006–13.

62 Ormsby A, Bergfeld WF, Tubbs RR, Hsi ED. Evaluation of a new paraffin-reactive CD7 T-cell deletion marker and a polymerase chain reaction-based T-cell receptor gene rearrangement assay: implications for diagnosis of mycosis fungoides in community clinical practice. *J Am Acad Dermatol* 2001; **45**: 405–13.

63 Payne CM, Spier CM, Grogan TM *et al.* Nuclear contour irregularities correlate with Leu-9-, Leu-8-cells in benign lymphoid infiltrates of the skin. *Am J Dermatopathol* 1988; **10**: 377–98.

64 Wood GS, Volterra AS, Abel EA, Nickoloff BJ, Adams RM. Allergic contact dermatitis: novel immunohistologic features. *J Invest Dermatol* 1986; **87**: 688–93.

65 Cerroni L, Kerl H. Diagnostic immunohistology: cutaneous lymphomas and pseudolymphomas. *Semin Cutan Med Surg* 1999; **18**: 64–70.

66 Michie SA, Abel EA, Hoppe RT, Warnke RA, Wood GS. Expression of T-cell receptor antigens in mycosis fungoides and inflammatory skin lesions. *J Invest Dermatol* 1989; **93**: 116–20.

67 Jack AS, Boylston AW, Carrel S, Grigor I. Cutaneous T-cell lymphoma cells employ a restricted range of T-cell antigen receptor variable region genes. *Am J Pathol* 1990; **136**: 17–21.

68 Lukowsky A, Muche JM, Sterry W, Audring H. Detection of expanded T cell clones in skin biopsy samples of patients with lichen sclerosus et atrophicus by T cell receptor-γ polymerase chain reaction assays. *J Invest Dermatol* 2000; **115**: 254–9.

69 Schiller PI, Flaig MJ, Puchta U, Kind P, Sander CA. Detection of clonal T cells in lichen planus. *Arch Dermatol Res* 2000; **292**: 568–9.

70 Citarella L, Massone C, Kerl H, Cerroni L. Lichen sclerosus with histopathologic features simulating early mycosis fungoides. *Am J Dermatopathol*, 2003; **25**: 463–5.

71 Cerroni L, Arzberger E, Ardigó M, Pütz B, Kerl H. Monoclonality of intraepidermal T lymphocytes in early mycosis fungoides detected by molecular analysis after laser-beam-based microdissection. *J Invest Dermatol* 2000; **114**: 1154–7.

72 Scheller U, Muche JM, Sterry W, Lukowsky A. Detection of clonal T cells in cutaneous T cell lymphoma by polymerase chain reaction: comparison of mutation detection enhancement polyacrylamide gel electrophoresis, temperature gradient gel electrophoresis and fragment analysis of sequencing gels. *Electrophoresis* 1998; **19**: 653–8.

73 LeBoit PE. Variants of mycosis fungoides and related cutaneous T-cell lymphomas. *Semin Diagn Pathol* 1991; **8**: 73–81.

74 Zackheim HS, McCalmont TH. Mycosis fungoides: the great imitator. *J Am Acad Dermatol* 2002; **47**: 914–8.

75 Ackerman AB, Schiff TA. If small plaque (digitate) parapsoriasis is a cutaneous T-cell lymphoma, even an 'abortive' one, it must be mycosis fungoides! *Arch Dermatol* 1996; **132**: 562–6.

76 Burg G, Dummer R, Nestle FO, Doebbeling U, Haeffner A. Cutaneous lymphomas consist of a spectrum of nosologically different entities including mycosis fungoides and small plaque parapsoriasis. *Arch Dermatol* 1996; **132**: 567–72.

77 Cerroni L, Fink-Puches R, Bäck B, Kerl H. Follicular mucinosis: a critical reappraisal of clinicopathologic features and association with mycosis fungoides and Sézary syndrome. *Arch Dermatol* 2002; **138**: 182–9.

78 Flaig MJ, Cerroni L, Schuhmann K *et al.* Follicular mycosis fungoides: a histopathologic analysis of nine cases. *J Cutan Pathol* 2001; **28**: 525–30.

79 van Doorn R, Scheffer E, Willemze R. Follicular mycosis fungoides, a distinct disease entity with or without associated follicular mucinosis. *Arch Dermatol* 2002; **138**: 191–8.

80 Scarabello A, Fantini F, Giannetti A, Cerroni L. Localized pagetoid reticulosis (Woringer–Kolopp disease). *Br J Dermatol* 2002; **147**: 806.

81 Cerroni L, Fink-Puches R, El-Shabrawi-Caelen L *et al.* Solitary skin lesions with histopathologic features of early mycosis fungoides. *Am J Dermatopathol* 1999; **21**: 518–24.

82 Oliver GF, Winkelmann RK. Unilesional mycosis fungoides: a distinct entity. *J Am Acad Dermatol* 1989; **20**: 63–70.

83 Heald PW, Glusac EJ. Unilesional cutaneous T-cell lymphoma: clinical features, therapy, and follow-up of 10 patients with a treatment-responsive mycosis fungoides variant. *J Am Acad Dermatol* 2000; **42**: 283–5.

84 El Shabrawi-Caelen L, Cerroni L, Medeiros LJ, McCalmont TH. Hypopigmented mycosis fungoides: frequent expression of a CD8+ T-cell phenotype. *Am J Surg Pathol* 2002; **26**: 450–7.

85 Ardigó M, Borroni G, Muscardin L, Kerl H, Cerroni L. Hypopigmented mycosis fungoides in Caucasian patients: a clinicopathologic study of 7 cases. *J Am Acad Dermatol* 2003; **49**: 264–70.

86 Toro JR, Sander CA, LeBoit PE. Persistent pigmented purpuric dermatitis and mycosis fungoides: simulant, precursor, or both? A study by light microscopy and molecular methods. *Am J Dermatopathol* 1997; **19**: 108–18.

87 Crowson AN, Magro CM, Zahorchak R. Atypical pigmentary purpura: a clinical, histopathologic, and genotypic study. *Hum Pathol* 1999; **30**: 1004–12.

88 Boyd AS, Vnencak-Jones CL. T-cell clonality in lichenoid purpura: a clinical and molecular evaluation of seven patients. *Histopathology* 2003; **43**: 302–3.

89 Barnhill RL, Braverman IM. Progression of pigmented purpura-like eruptions to mycosis fungoides: report of three cases. *J Am Acad Dermatol* 1988; **19**: 25–31.

90 Viseux V, Schoenlaub P, Cnudde F *et al.* Pigmented purpuric dermatitis preceding the diagnosis of mycosis fungoides by 24 years. *Dermatology* 2003; **207**: 331–2.

91 Bowman PH, Hogan DJ, Sanusi ID. Mycosis fungoides bullosa: report of a case and review of the literature. *J Am Acad Dermatol* 2001; **45**: 934–9.

92 Jakob T, Tiemann M, Kuwert C *et al.* Dyshidrotic cutaneous T-cell lymphoma. *J Am Acad Dermatol* 1996; **34**: 295–7.

93 Soyer HP, Smolle J, Kerl H. Dyshidrotic mycosis fungoides. *J Cutan Pathol* 1987; **14**: 372.

94 Pföhler C, Ugurel S, Seiter S *et al.* Interferon-α-associated development of bullous lesions in mycosis fungoides. *Dermatology* 2000; **200**: 51–3.

95 Ackerman AB, Flaxman BA. Granulomatous mycosis fungoides. *Br J Dermatol* 1970; **82**: 397–401.

96 Scarabello A, Leinweber B, Ardigó M *et al.* Cutaneous lymphomas with prominent granulomatous reaction: a potential pitfall in the histopathologic diagnosis of cutaneous T- and B-cell lymphomas. *Am J Surg Pathol* 2002; **26**: 1259–68.

97 LeBoit PE, Zackheim HS, White CR Jr. Granulomatous variants of cutaneous T-cell lymphoma: the histopathology of granulomatous mycosis fungoides and granulomatous slack skin. *Am J Surg Pathol* 1988; **12**: 83–95.

98 Ackerman AB. Granulomatous slack skin. In: Ackerman AB, ed. *Histologic Diagnosis of Inflammatory Skin Diseases*. Philadelphia: Lea & Febiger, 1978: 483–5.

99 Balus L, Manente L, Remotti D, Grammatico P, Bellocci M. Granulomatous slack skin: report of a case and review of the literature. *Am J Dermatopathol* 1996; **18**: 199–206.

100 LeBoit PE. Granulomatous slack skin. *Dermatol Clin* 1994; **12**: 375–89.

101 Clarijs M, Poot F, Laka A, Pirard C, Bourland A. Granulomatous slack skin: treatment with extensive surgery and review of the literature. *Dermatology* 2003; **206**: 393–7.

102 van Haselen CW, Toonstra J, van der Putte SCJ *et al.* Granulomatous slack skin: report of three patients with an updated review of the literature. *Dermatology* 1998; **196**: 382–91.

103 Flaxmann BA, Koumans JAD, Ackerman AB. Granulomatous mycosis fungoides: a 14-year follow-up of a case. *Am J Dermatopathol* 1983; **5**: 145–51.

104 Gomez de la Fuente E, Ortiz PL, Vanaclocha F, Rodriguez-Peralto JL, Iglesias L. Aggressive granulomatous mycosis fungoides with clinical pulmonary and thyroid involvement. *Br J Dermatol* 2000; **142**: 1026–9.

105 Cerroni L. Cutaneous granulomas and malignant lymphomas. *Dermatology* 2003; **206**: 78–80.

106 Braverman JM, Klein S, Grant A. Electron microscopic and immunolabeling studies of the lesional and normal skin of patients with mycosis fungoides treated by total body electron beam irradiation. *J Am Acad Dermatol* 1987; **16**: 61–74.

107 Bergman R, Cohen A, Harth Y *et al.* Histopathologic findings in the clinically uninvolved skin of patients with mycosis fungoides. *Am J Surg Pathol* 1995; **17**: 452–6.

108 Pujol RM, Gallardo F, Llistosella E *et al.* Invisible mycosis fungoides: a diagnostic challenge. *J Am Acad Dermatol* 2000; **42**: 324–8.

109 Fink-Puches R, Chott A, Ardigo M *et al.* The spectrum of cutaneous lymphomas in patients under 20 years of age. *Pediatr Dermatol* in press.

110 Hickham PR, McBurney EI, Fitzgerald RL. CTCL in patients under 20 years of age: a series of five cases. *Pediatr Dermatol* 1997; **14**: 93–7.

111 Burns MK, Ellis CN, Cooper KD. Mycosis fungoides-type cutaneous T-cell lymphoma arising before 30 years of age: immunophenotypic, immunogenotypic and clinicopathologic analysis of nine cases. *J Am Acad Dermatol* 1992; **27**: 974–8.

112 Neuhaus IM, Ramos-Caro FA, Hassanein AM. Hypopigmented mycosis fungoides in childhood and adolescence. *Pediatr Dermatol* 2000; **17**: 403–6.

113 Peters MS, Thibodeau SN, White JW Jr, Winkelmann RK. Mycosis fungoides in children and adolescents. *J Am Acad Dermatol* 1990; **22**: 1011–8.

114 Quaglino P, Zaccagna A, Verrone A, Dardano F, Bernengo MG. Mycosis fungoides in patients under 20 years of age: report of 7 cases, review of the literature and study of the clinical course. *Dermatology* 1999; **199**: 8–14.

115 Ko JW, Seong JY, Suh KS, Kim ST. Pityriasis lichenoides-like mycosis fungoides in children. *Br J Dermatol* 2000; **142**: 347–52.

116 Whittam LR, Calonje E, Orchard G *et al.* CD-8-positive juvenile onset mycosis fungoides: an immunohistochemical and genotypic analysis of six cases. *Br J Dermatol* 2000; **143**: 1199–204.

117 Ben-Amitai D, David M, Feinmesser M, Hodak E. Juvenile mycosis fungoides diagnosed before 18 years of age. *Acta Derm Venereol (Stockh)* 2003; **83**: 451–6.

118 Zackheim HS, McCalmont TH, Deanovic FW, Odom RB. Mycosis fungoides with onset before 20 years of age. *J Am Acad Dermatol* 1997; **36**: 557–62.

119 Crowley JJ, Nikko A, Varghese A, Hoppe RT, Kim YH. Mycosis fungoides in young patients: clinical characteristics and outcome. *J Am Acad Dermatol* 1998; **38**: 696–701.

120 Wain EM, Orchard GE, Whittaker SJ, Spittle MF, Russell-Jones R. Outcome in 34 patients with juvenile-onset mycosis fungoides. A

clinical, immunophenotypic and molecular study. *Cancer* 2003; **98**: 2282–90.

121 Chiaron-Sileni V, Bononi A, Veller Fornasa C *et al.* Phase II trial of interferon-α2a plus psoralen with ultraviolet light A in patients with cutaneous T-cell lymphoma. *Cancer* 2002; **95**: 569–75.

122 Stadler R, Otte HG, Luger T *et al.* Prospective randomized multicenter clinical trial on the use of interferon-α2a plus acitretin versus interferon-α2a plus PUVA in patients with cutaneous T-cell lymphoma stages I and II. *Blood* 1998; **92**: 3578–81.

123 Diederen PVMM, van Weelden H, Sanders CJG, Toonstra J, van Vloten WA. Narrowband UVB and psoralen-UVA in the treatment of early-stage mycosis fungoides: a retrospective study. *J Am Acad Dermatol* 2003; **48**: 215–9.

124 Kim YH, Martinez G, Varghese A, Hoppe RT. Topical nitrogen mustard in the management of mycosis fungoides. *Arch Dermatol* 2003; **139**: 165–73.

125 Cochran Gathers R, Scherschun L, Malick F, Fivenson DP, Lim HW. Narrowband UVB phototherapy for early-stage mycosis fungoides. *J Am Acad Dermatol* 2002; **47**: 191–7.

126 Hofer A, Cerroni L, Kerl H, Wolf P. Narrowband (311 nm) UV-B therapy for small plaque parapsoriasis and early stage mycosis fungoides. *Arch Dermatol* 1999; **135**: 1377–80.

127 Zackheim HS, Kashani-Sabet M, Amin S. Topical corticosteroids for mycosis fungoides: experience in 79 patients. *Arch Dermatol* 1998; **134**: 949–54.

128 Goldberg DJ, Stampen TM, Schwartz RA. Mycosis fungoides palmaris et plantaris: successful treatment with the carbon dioxide laser. *Br J Dermatol* 1997; **136**: 617–9.

129 Jones GW, Kacinski BM, Wilson LD *et al.* Total skin electron radiation in the management of mycosis fungoides: consensus of the European Organization for Research and Treatment of Cancer (EORTC) Cutaneous Lymphoma Project Group. *J Am Acad Dermatol* 2002; **47**: 364–70.

130 Kaye FJ, Bunn PA Jr, Steinberg SM *et al.* A randomized trial comparing combination electron-beam radiation and chemotherapy with topical therapy in the initial treatment of mycosis fungoides. *N Engl J Med* 1989; **321**: 1784–90.

131 Duvic M, Olsen EA, Omura GA *et al.* A phase III, randomized, double-blind, placebo-controlled study of peldesine (BCX-34) cream as topical therapy for cutaneous T-cell lymphoma. *J Am Acad Dermatol* 2001; **44**: 940–7.

132 Tracey L, Villuendas R, Ortiz P *et al.* Identification of genes involved in resistance to interferon-α in cutaneous T-cell lymphoma. *Am J Pathol* 2002; **161**: 1825–37.

133 Apisarnthanarax N, Talpur R, Duvic M. Treatment of cutaneous T cell lymphoma: current status and future directions. *Am J Clin Dermatol* 2002; **3**: 193–215.

134 Vonderheid EC. Treatment of cutaneous T cell lymphoma 2001. *Recent Results Cancer Res* 2002; **160**: 309–20.

135 Dummer R, Urosevic M, Kempf W, Kazakov D, Burg G. Imiquimod induces complete clearance of a PUVA-resistant plaque in mycosis fungoides. *Dermatology* 2003; **207**: 116–8.

136 Breneman D, Duvic M, Kuzel T *et al.* Phase 1 and 2 trial of bexarotene gel for skin-directed treatment of patients with cutaneous T-cell lymphoma. *Arch Dermatol* 2002; **138**: 325–32.

137 Duvic M, Hymes K, Heald P *et al.* Bexarotene is effective and safe for treatment of refractory advanced-stage cutaneous T-cell lymphoma: multinational phase II–III trial results. *J Clin Oncol* 2001; **19**: 2456–71.

138 Demierre MF, Vachon L, Ho V *et al.* Phase 1/2 pilot study of methotrexate-laurocapram topical gel for the treatment of patients with early-stage mycosis fungoides. *Arch Dermatol* 2003; **139**: 624–8.

139 Wolf P, Fink-Puches R, Cerroni L, Kerl H. Photodynamic therapy for mycosis fungoides after topical photosensitization with 5-aminolevulinic acid. *J Am Acad Dermatol* 1994; **31**: 678–80.

140 Heald P, Mehlmauer M, Martin AG *et al.* Topical bexarotene therapy for patients with refractory or persistent early-stage cutaneous T-cell lymphoma: results of the phase III clinical trial. *J Am Acad Dermatol* 2003; **49**: 801–5.

141 Duvic M, Apisarnthanarax N, Cohen DS *et al.* Analysis of long-term outcomes of combined modality therapy for cutaneous T-cell lymphoma. *J Am Acad Dermatol* 2003; **49**: 35–49.

142 Rubegni P, De Aloe G, Fimiani M. Extracorporeal photochemotherapy in long-term treatment of early stage cutaneous T-cell lymphoma. *Br J Dermatol* 2000; **143**: 894–6.

143 Olavarria E, Child F, Woolford A *et al.* T-cell depletion and autologous stem cell transplantation in the management of tumour stage mycosis · fungoides with peripheral blood involvement. *Br J Haematol* 2001; **114**: 624–31.

144 Soligo D, Ibatici A, Berti E *et al.* Treatment of advanced mycosis fungoides by allogeneic stem-cell transplantation with a non-myeloablative regimen. *Bone Marrow Transplant* 2003; **31**: 663–6.

145 Guitart J, Wickless SC, Oyama Y *et al.* Long-term remission after allogeneic hematopoietic stem cell transplantation for refractory cutaneous T-cell lymphoma. *Arch Dermatol* 2002; **138**: 1359–65.

146 Carretero-Margolis CD, Fivenson DP. A complete and durable response to denileukin diftitox in a patient with mycosis fungoides. *J Am Acad Dermatol* 2003; **48**: 275–6.

147 Lundin J, Hagberg H, Repp R *et al.* Phase 2 study of alemtuzumab (anti-CD52 monoclonal antibody) in patients with advanced mycosis fungoides/Sézary syndrome. *Blood* 2003; **101**: 4267–72.

148 Pangalis GA, Dimopoulou MN, Angelopoulou MK *et al.* Campath-1H (anti-CD52) monoclonal antibody therapy in lymphoproliferative disorders. *Med Oncol* 2001; **18**: 99–107.

149 Scarisbrick JJ, Child FJ, Clift A *et al.* A trial of fludarabine and cyclophosphamide combination chemotherapy in the treatment of advanced refractory primary cutaneous T-cell lymphoma. *Br J Dermatol* 2001; **144**: 1010–5.

150 Zinzani PL, Baliva G, Magagnoli M *et al.* Gemcitabine treatment in pretreated cutaneous T-cell lymphoma: experience in 44 patients. *J Clin Oncol* 2000; **18**: 2603–6.

151 Akpek G, Koh HK, Bogen S, O'Hara C, Foss FM. Chemotherapy with etoposide, vincristine, doxorubicin, bolus cyclophosphamide, and oral prednisone in patients with refractory cutaneous T-cell lymphoma. *Cancer* 1999; **86**: 1368–76.

152 Tsimberidou AM, Giles F, Duvic M, Fayad L, Kurzrock R. Phase II study of pentostatin in advanced T-cell lymphoid malignancies. *Cancer* 2004; **100**: 342–9.

153 Muche JM, Sterry W. Vaccination therapy for cutaneous T-cell lymphoma. *Clin Exp Dermatol* 2002; **27**: 602–7.

154 Maier T, Tun-Kyi A, Tassis A *et al.* Vaccination of patients with cutaneous T-cell lymphoma using intranodal injection of autologous tumor-lysate-pulsed dendritic cells. *Blood* 2003; **102**: 2338–44.

155 Eichmüller S, Usener D, Thiel D, Schadendorf D. Tumor-specific antigens in cutaneous T-cell lymphoma: expression and sero-reactivity. *Int J Cancer* 2003; **104**: 482–7.

156 Weinstock MA, Reynes JF. The changing survival of patients with mycosis fungoides. *Cancer* 1999; **85**: 208–12.

157 van Doorn R, van Haselen CW, van Voorst Vader PC *et al.* Mycosis fungoides: disease evaluation and prognosis of 309 Dutch patients. *Arch Dermatol* 2000; **136**: 504–10.

158 Zackheim HS, Amin S, Kashani-Sabet M, McMillan A. Prognosis in cutaneous T-cell lymphoma by skin stage: long-term survival in 489 patients. *J Am Acad Dermatol* 1999; **40**: 418–25.

159 Kim YH, Liu HL, Mraz-Gernhard S, Varghese A, Hoppe RT. Long-term outcome of 525 patients with mycosis fungoides and Sézary syndrome. *Arch Dermatol* 2003; **139**: 857–66.

160 Fraser-Andrews E, Woolford AJ, Russell-Jones R, Seed PT, Whittaker SJ. Detection of a peripheral blood T cell clone is an independent prognostic marker in mycosis fungoides. *J Invest Dermatol* 2000; **114**: 117–21.

161 Beylot-Barry M, Sibaud V, Thiebaut R *et al.* Evidence that an identical T cell clone in skin and peripheral blood lymphocytes is an independent prognostic factor in primary cutaneous T cell lymphoma. *J Invest Dermatol* 2001; **117**: 920–6.

162 Delfau-Larue MH, Dalac S, Lepage E *et al.* Prognostic significance of a polymerase chain reaction-detectable dominant T-lymphocyte clone in cutaneous lesions of patients with mycosis fungoides. *Blood* 1998; **92**: 3376–80.

163 Guitart J, Camisa C, Ehrlich M, Bergfeld WF. Long-term implications of T-cell receptor gene rearrangement analysis by Southern blot in patients with cutaneous T-cell lymphoma. *J Am Acad Dermatol* 2003; **48**: 775–9.

164 Vega F, Luthra R, Medeiros LJ *et al.* Clonal heterogeneity in mycosis fungoides and its relationship to clinical course. *Blood* 2002; **100**: 3369–73.

165 Sibaud V, Beylot-Barry M, Thiebaut R *et al.* Bone marrow histopathologic and molecular staging in epidermotropic T-cell lymphoma. *Am J Clin Pathol* 2003; **119**: 414–23.

166 Bakels V, van Oostveen JW, Geerts ML *et al.* Diagnostic and prognostic significance of clonal T-cell receptor beta gene rearrangements in lymph nodes of patients with mycosis fungoides. *J Pathol* 1993; **170**: 249–55.

167 Smoller BR, Detwiler SP, Kohler S, Hoppe RT, Kim YH. Role of histology in providing prognostic information in mycosis fungoides. *J Cutan Pathol* 1998; **25**: 311–5.

168 Poszepczynska-Guigne E, Bagot M, Wechsler J *et al.* Minimal residual disease in mycosis fungoides follow-up can be assessed by polymerase chain reaction. *Br J Dermatol* 2003; **148**: 265–71.

Chapter 3 Sézary syndrome

Sézary syndrome is characterized clinically by pruritic erythroderma, generalized lymphadenopathy and the presence of circulating malignant T lymphocytes (Sézary cells) [1–3]. Other typical cutaneous changes include palmoplantar hyperkeratosis, alopecia and onychodystrophy [4]. Differentiation from non-neoplastic erythroderma may be extremely difficult. The main causes of erythroderma, besides cutaneous T-cell lymphoma, are atopic dermatitis, psoriasis and drug reactions [5]. Erythrodermic mycosis fungoides should be distinguished from true Sézary syndrome (see Chapter 2).

One of the major problems in Sézary syndrome is that variable diagnostic criteria have been used in different studies, which hinders comparison of clinicopathological and prognostic data. The presence of a monoclonal population of T lymphocytes within the peripheral blood has been recently proposed by the European Organization for Research and Treatment of Cancer (EORTC) Cutaneous Lymphoma Study Group, by the International Society for Cutaneous Lymphomas and by others as an important criterion for the diagnosis of Sézary syndrome [1,6–10]. Other useful criteria include the presence of more than 1000 circulating Sézary cells/mm [3]; an expanded CD4$^+$ population in the peripheral blood resulting in a markedly increased CD4$^+$: CD8$^+$ ratio (> 10); an increased population of CD4$^+$: CD7$^-$ cells in the peripheral blood; Sézary cells larger than 14 μm in diameter; and Sézary cells representing more than 20% of circulating lymphocytes [1,2,10,11].

Although Sézary syndrome is regarded as the leukaemic variant of cutaneous T-cell lymphoma, involvement of the bone marrow is rare in the early phases but may be found at a later stage [12]. The exact relation to mycosis fungoides is unclear, although some authors consider the two diseases as variations of the same entity (see Chapter 2). In 1975, the term 'cutaneous T-cell lymphoma' was introduced to encompass mycosis fungoides, Sézary syndrome and related disorders [3]. The EORTC classification lists mycosis fungoides and Sézary syndrome as separate entities [1]. By contrast, in the classification of tumours of the haematopoietic system proposed recently by the World Health Organization (WHO), Sézary syndrome, although listed separately, is discussed in a chapter together with mycosis fungoides, mentioning that 'the disease is by tradition regarded as a variant of mycosis fungoides' [2].

Patients usually present with an abrupt onset of erythroderma, or with erythroderma preceded by itching and a nonspecific skin rash. Rarely, a classic Sézary syndrome may develop in patients with preceding mycosis fungoides; it has been suggested to classify these cases as 'Sézary syndrome preceded by mycosis fungoides', as it remains unclear whether the clinical features and prognosis are similar [10]. The presence of neoplastic T cells within the peripheral blood alone should not prompt a diagnosis of Sézary syndrome unless all other main diagnostic criteria are met [10].

The aetiology of Sézary syndrome is unknown. One case with a complex *p53* gene mutation has been observed in a Chernobyl survivor, suggesting a possible relationship with environmental factors [13]. The association with viral infections or previous long-standing dermatoses is unclear [14–16]. Much information on the neoplastic cells has been gathered by studies on tissue samples and cell lines. In most cases, so-called Sézary cells express a predominantly helper T-cell type 2 (Th2) cytokine profile, characterized by expression of interleukin 4 (IL-4), IL-5 and IL-10. Several genetic aberrations as well as aberrant antigen, cytokine or other molecular profiles have been documented in patients with Sézary syndrome, but the diagnostic and therapeutic implications of these findings are still unclear [17–31].

The TNM staging classification used for mycosis fungoides has also been adopted for Sézary syndrome. According to this system, Sézary syndrome is classified as stage III by definition (see p. 10).

Similarly to mycosis fungoides, patients with Sézary syndrome have an increased risk of developing second malignancies [32,33].

Clinical features

Sézary syndrome is a rare malignant T-cell lymphoma affecting elderly adults of both sexes, with a predilection for males.

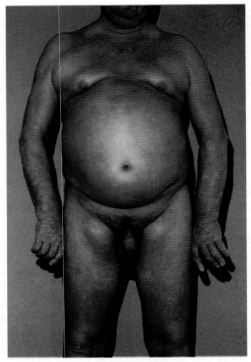

Fig. 3.1 Sézary syndrome. Erythroderma. Note enlarged inguinal lymph nodes.

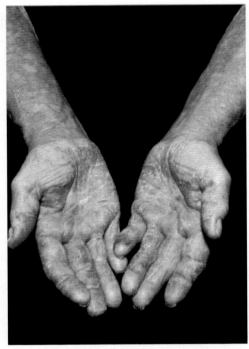

Fig. 3.2 Sézary syndrome. Hyperkeratosis of the palms.

Non-specific skin lesions (eczematous patches) may be present for some time before erythroderma develops. The erythroderma is characterized by intense pruritus and scaling (Fig. 3.1). Common clinical signs are the marked hyperkeratosis of the palms and soles, alopecia and onychodystrophy (Fig. 3.2). Large skin folds (groins, axillae) may be spared. Histopathological analysis of peripheral lymph nodes usually shows evidence of involvement, but differentiation from 'dermatopathic lymphadenopathy' may be very difficult.

As in mycosis fungoides, Sézary syndrome may be associated with follicular mucinosis [34]. Other clinical variants include the presence of diffuse hyperpigmentation as a consequence of melanosis or haemosiderosis (melanoerythroderma) (Fig. 3.3), and of vesiculobullous lesions.

Histopathology, immunophenotype and molecular genetics

Histopathology

The histopathological features of skin lesions in Sézary syndrome are indistinguishable from those of mycosis fungoides [35–37]. Often there is a psoriasiform spongiotic pattern with a variably dense band-like infiltrate of lymphocytes (Fig. 3.4). Epidermotropism is usually less marked than in mycosis fungoides, but typical Darier's nests 'Pautrier's

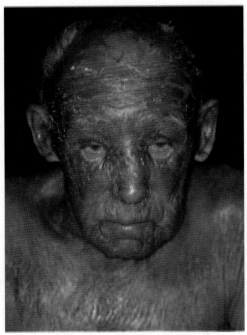

Fig. 3.3 Sézary syndrome. Diffuse hyperpigmentation on the background of erythroderma ('melanoerythroderma'). Note ectropion.

collections' may be observed. Cytomorphology reveals a predominance of small- to medium-sized pleomorphic (cerebriform) lymphocytes, often referred to as 'Sézary cells' (Fig. 3.5). Differential diagnosis from mycosis fungoides can

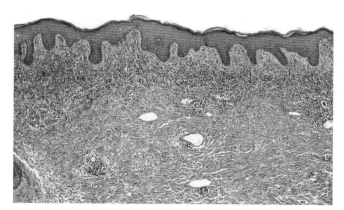

Fig. 3.4 Sézary syndrome. Dense band-like infiltrate of lymphocytes within the superficial dermis. Note psoriasiform hyperplasia of the epidermis.

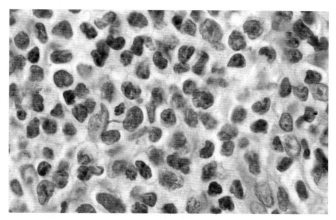

Fig. 3.5 Sézary syndrome. Neoplastic cells are small- to medium-sized pleomorphic ('cerebriform') cells identical to those observed in mycosis fungoides.

be achieved only by correlation of histopathological features with clinical ones.

Histopathological variants of Sézary syndrome include the presence of a prominent granulomatous reaction, deposition of mucin within hair follicles (follicular mucinosis), or large cell transformation [38–43]. Large cell transformation may be detected in skin lesions, lymph nodes, or both, and is indistinguishable from that occurring in advanced mycosis fungoides (see Chapter 2).

The lymph nodes are characterized by monomorphous infiltrates of neoplastic cells, and reveal histopathological differences from lymph nodes involved by cells of mycosis fungoides, suggesting a pathogenetic difference between the two diseases [44].

Immunophenotype

Immunohistology reveals a predominance of T-helper lym-

phocytes (CD3+, CD4+, CD7−, CD8−). The findings are indistinguishable from those observed in mycosis fungoides.

Molecular genetics

Molecular genetic studies show clonal rearrangement of the T-cell receptor (TCR) gene in skin lesions in most cases, but clonality may not be detected in the early stages. Amplification and over-expression of *JUNB* have been observed in some patients in two recent studies [45,46]. A panel of eight genes that can distinguish Sézary syndrome in patients with low numbers of circulating cells has been recently detected by the cDNA microarray technique [46].

Treatment

The therapy of Sézary syndrome remains unsatisfactory. Patients may benefit from total body electron beam therapy, psoralen with UVA treatment (PUVA; alone or associated with etretinate, interferon-α2a, or both), or chlorambucil combined with prednisone (Winkelmann scheme) [1,47–50]. Complete responses have been observed in several patients after extracorporeal photochemotherapy, but recurrence is the rule, and the efficacy has been debated [51–55]. An overall response rate of 62.5% (complete response 18.8%; partial response 43.7%) has been observed with pentostatin therapy in one study [56]. Patients with cutaneous tumours and/or large cell transformation should be treated with systemic chemotherapy or other aggressive treatment modalities.

Recently, new modalities have been introduced in the treatment of patients with Sézary syndrome, including pentostatin, IL-2, bone marrow transplantation, new retinoids such as bexarotene, and new chemotherapeutic agents (see Chapter 2) [57–61]. The association of extracorporeal photopheresis with other treatments has also been tested in a limited number of patients [62]. No single treatment modality revealed clear-cut benefits in comparison to the others, and the management of these patients is still extremely problematic.

Prognosis

The overall survival of patients with Sézary syndrome depends on the criteria adopted for the diagnosis of the disease, and the 5-year survival varies between 11% and almost 50% in different studies, thus clearly showing that different criteria for diagnosis and classification are used in different centres. In this context, it should be emphasized that patients with erythroderma, even if the cause is not Sézary syndrome or mycosis fungoides (non-neoplastic erythroderma), show a decreased survival [5]. If strict criteria are employed (presence of a neoplastic clone in the peripheral blood, $CD4^+ : CD8^+$ ratio > 10), the estimated 5-year survival is approximately 10–15% [1]. The presence of an identical clone in the skin and peripheral blood seems to be an independent prognostic criterion pointing to a worse prognosis [12,63]. Stage at diagnosis, failure to undergo remission after first treatment, age and race also have prognostic value [64]. Elevated lactic dehydrogenase and β_2-microglobulin serum levels and the presence of an elevated tumour burden in the peripheral blood have also been associated with a reduced survival [65–67]. The number of circulating Sézary cells may predict the response to treatment, with higher counts showing better responses. The presence of EBV genome in keratinocytes has been found to worsen the prognosis in one recent study [68].

Recently, a panel of 10 genes that can identify a group of patients with survival shorter than 6 months has been identified by the cDNA microarray technique [46].

RÉSUMÉ

Clinical	Elderly adults. Pruritic erythroderma, generalized lymphadenopathy and circulating Sézary cells. Strict diagnostic criteria include presence of a neoplastic clone and of a CD4+ : CD8+ ratio > 10 in the peripheral blood. Usually aggressive course.
Morphology	Small pleomorphic (cerebriform) cells. During the course of the disease there may be appearance of tumours with large cell morphology (immunoblasts, large cell anaplastic, large cell pleomorphic).
Immunology	CD2, 3, 4, 5 + CD7, 8 –
Genetics	Monoclonal rearrangement of the TCR gene may be absent in early phases. cDNA microarray studies revealed a class of genes that is altered in Sézary syndrome.
Treatment guidelines	PUVA, interferon-α2a, retinoids (alone or in combination); extracorporeal photopheresis; radiotherapy; chlorambucil combined with prednisone (Winkelmann scheme); systemic chemotherapy. *Experimental*: new retinoids, new chemotherapeutic agents, pentostatin, bone marrow transplantation.

References

1 Willemze R, Kerl H, Sterry W *et al.* EORTC classification for primary cutaneous lymphomas: a proposal from the Cutaneous Lymphoma Study Group of the European Organization for Research and Treatment of Cancer. *Blood* 1997; **90**: 354–71.

2 Ralfkiaer E, Jaffe ES. Mycosis fungoides and Sézary syndrome. In: Jaffe ES, Harris NL, Stein H, Vardiman JW, eds. *World Health Organization Classification of Tumours: Tumours of Haematopoietic and Lymphoid Tissues*. Lyon: IARC Press, 2001: 216–20.

3 Edelson RL. Cutaneous T cell lymphoma: the Sézary syndrome, mycosis fungoides, and related disorders (NIH Conference). *Ann Intern Med* 1975; **83**: 534–52.

4 Kerl H. Das Sézary Syndrom. *Zbl Haut Geschl* 1981; **144**: 359–80.

5 Sigurdsson V, Toonstra J, Hezemans-Boer M, van Vloten WA. Erythroderma: a clinical and follow-up study of 102 patients, with special emphasis on survival. *J Am Acad Dermatol* 1996; **35**: 53–7.

6 Cherny S, Mraz S, Su L, Harvell J, Kohler S. Heteroduplex analysis of T-cell receptor γ gene rearrangement as an adjuvant diagnostic tool in skin biopsies for erythroderma. *J Cutan Pathol* 2001; **28**: 351–5.

7 Delfau-Larue MH, Laroche L, Wechsler J *et al.* Diagnostic value of dominant T-cell clones in peripheral blood in 363 patients presenting consecutively with a suspicion of cutaneous lymphoma. *Blood* 2000; **96**: 2987–92.

8 Fraser-Andrews EA, Russell-Jones R, Woolford AJ *et al.* Diagnostic and prognostic importance of T-cell receptor gene analysis in patients with Sézary syndrome. *Cancer* 2001; **92**: 1745–52.

9 Russell-Jones R, Whittaker S. T-cell receptor gene analysis in the diagnosis of Sézary syndrome. *J Am Acad Dermatol* 1999; **41**: 254–9.

10 Vonderheid EC, Bernengo MG, Burg G *et al.* Update on erythrodermic cutaneous T-cell lymphoma: report of the International Society for Cutaneous Lymphomas. *J Am Acad Dermatol* 2002; **46**: 95–106.

11 Vonderheid EC, Bigler RD, Kotecha A *et al.* Variable CD7 expression on T cells in the leukemic phase of cutaneous T cell lymphoma (Sézary syndrome). *J Invest Dermatol* 2001; **117**: 654–62.

12 Sibaud V, Beylot-Barry M, Thiebaut R *et al.* Bone marrow histopathologic and molecular staging in epidermotropic T-cell lymphoma. *Am J Clin Pathol* 2003; **119**: 414–23.

13 Fraser-Andrews E, McGregor JM, Crook T *et al.* Sézary syndrome with a complex, frameshift *p53* gene mutation in a Chernobyl survivor. *Clin Dermatol* 2001; **26**: 683–5.

14 Herne KL, Talpur R, Breuer-McHam J, Champlin R, Duvic M. Cytomegalovirus seropositivity is significantly associated with mycosis fungoides and Sézary syndrome. *Blood* 2003; **101**: 2132–5.

15 Bazarbachi A, Soriano V, Pawson R *et al.* Mycosis fungoides and Sézary syndrome are not associated with HTLV-I infection: an international study. *Br J Haematol* 1997; **98**: 927–33.

16 van Haselen CW, Toonstra J, Preesman AH *et al.* Sézary syndrome in a young man with severe atopic dermatitis. *Br J Dermatol* 1999; **140**: 704–7.

17 Bernengo MG, Novelli M, Quaglino P *et al.* The relevance of the $CD4^+ CD26^-$ subset in the identification of circulating Sézary cells. *Br J Dermatol* 2001; **144**: 125–35.

18 Ferenczi K, Fuhlbrigge RC, Pinkus JL, Pinkus GS, Kupper TS. Increased CCR4 expression in cutaneous T cell lymphoma. *J Invest Dermatol* 2002; **119**: 1405–10.

19 Hwang ST, Fitzhugh DJ. Aberrant expression of adhesion molecules by Sézary cells: functional consequences under physiologic shear stress conditions. *J Invest Dermatol* 2001; **116**: 466–70.

20 Karenko L, Nevala H, Raatikainen M, Franssila K, Ranki A. Chromosomally clonal T cells in the skin, blood, or lymph nodes of two Sézary syndrome patients express CD45RA, CD45RO, CDw150, and interleukin-4, but no interleukin-2 or interferon-γ. *J Invest Dermatol* 2001; **116**: 188–93.

21 Karenko L, Sarna S, Kähkönen M, Ranki A. Chromosomal abnormalities in relation to clinical disease in patients with cutaneous T-cell lymphoma: a 5-year follow-up study. *Br J Dermatol* 2003; **148**: 55–64.

22 Leroy S, Dubois S, Tenaud I *et al.* Interleukin-15 expression in cutaneous T-cell lymphoma (mycosis fungoides and Sézary syndrome). *Br J Dermatol* 2001; **144**: 1016–21.

23 Mao X, Lillington D, Scarisbrick JJ *et al.* Molecular cytogenetic analysis of cutaneous T-cell lymphomas: identification of common genetic alterations in Sézary syndrome and mycosis fungoides. *Br J Dermatol* 2002; **147**: 464–75.

24 Papadavid E, Economidou J, Psarra A *et al.* The relevance of peripheral blood T-helper 1 and 2 cytokine pattern in the evaluation of patients with mycosis fungoides and Sézary syndrome. *Br J Dermatol* 2003; **148**: 709–18.

25 Qin JZ, Dummer R, Burg G, Döbbeling U. Constitutive and interleukin-7/interleukin-15 stimulated DNA binding of Myc, Jun, and novel Myc-like proteins in cutaneous T-cell lymphoma cells. *Blood* 1999; **93**: 260–7.

26 Scarisbrick JJ, Woolford AJ, Calonje E *et al.* Frequent abnormalities of the *p15* and *p16* genes in mycosis fungoides and Sézary syndrome. *J Invest Dermatol* 2002; **118**: 493–9.

27 Scarisbrick JJ, Woolford AJ, Russell-Jones R, Whittaker SJ. Allelotyping in mycosis fungoides and Sézary syndrome: common regions of allelic loss identified on 9p, 10q, and 17p. *J Invest Dermatol* 2001; **117**: 663–70.

28 Wysocka M, Zaki MH, French LE *et al.* Sézary syndrome patients demonstrate a defect in dendritic cell populations: effects of CD40 ligand and treatment with GM-CSF on dendritic cell numbers and the production of cytokines. *Blood* 2002; **100**: 3287–94.

29 Zaki MH, Shane RB, Geng Y *et al.* Dysregulation of lymphocyte interleukin-12 receptor expression in Sézary syndrome. *J Invest Dermatol* 2001; **117**: 119–27.

30 Brender C, Nielsen M, Kaltoft K *et al.* STAT3-mediated constitutive expression of SOCS-3 in cutaneous T-cell lymphoma. *Blood* 2001; **97**: 1056–62.

31 Magazin M, Poszepczynska-Guigne E, Bagot M *et al.* Sézary syndrome cells, unlike normal circulating T lymphocytes, fail to migrate following engagement of NT$_1$ receptor. *J Invest Dermatol* 2004; **122**: 111–8.

32 Väkevä L, Pukkala E, Ranki A. Increased risk of secondary cancers in patients with primary cutaneous T cell lymphoma. *J Invest Dermatol* 2000; **115**: 62–5.

33 Scarisbrick JJ, Child FJ, Evans AV *et al.* Secondary malignant neoplasms in 71 patients with Sézary syndrome. *Arch Dermatol* 1999; **135**: 1381–5.

34 Cerroni L, Fink-Puches R, Bäck B, Kerl H. Follicular mucinosis: a critical reappraisal of clinicopathologic features and association with mycosis fungoides and Sézary syndrome. *Arch Dermatol* 2002; **138**: 182–9.

35 Kohler S, Kim YH, Smoller BR. Histologic criteria for the diagnosis of erythrodermic mycosis fungoides and Sézary syndrome: a critical reappraisal. *J Cutan Pathol* 1997; **24**: 292–7.

36 Trotter MJ, Whittaker SJ, Orchard GE, Smith NP. Cutaneous histopathology of Sézary syndrome: a study of 41 cases with a proven circulating T-cell clone. *J Cutan Pathol* 1997; **24**: 286–91.

37 Walsh NMG, Prokopetz R, Tron VA *et al.* Histopathology in erythroderma: review of a series of cases by multiple observers. *J Cutan Pathol* 1994; **21**: 419–23.

38 Cerroni L, Rieger E, Hödl S, Kerl H. Clinicopathologic and immunologic features associated with transformation of mycosis fungoides to large-cell lymphoma. *Am J Surg Pathol* 1992; **16**: 543–52.

39 Diamandidou E, Colome-Grimmer MI, Fayad L, Duvic M, Kurzrock R. Transformation of mycosis fungoides/Sézary syndrome: clinical characteristics and prognosis. *Blood* 1998; **92**: 1150–9.

40 Carrozza PM, Kempf W, Kazakov DV, Dummer R, Burg G. A case of Sézary's syndrome associated with granulomatous lesions, myelodysplastic syndrome and transformation into CD30-positive large-cell pleomorphic lymphoma. *Br J Dermatol* 2002; **147**: 582–6.

41 Gregg PJ, Kantor GR, Telang GH *et al.* Sarcoidal tissue reaction in Sézary syndrome. *J Am Acad Dermatol* 2000; **43**: 372–6.

42 So CC, Wong KF, Siu LL, Kwong YL. Large cell transformation of Sézary syndrome: a conventional and molecular cytogenetic study. *Am J Clin Pathol* 2000; **113**: 792–7.

43 Scarabello A, Leinweber B, Ardigó M *et al.* Cutaneous lymphomas with prominent granulomatous reaction: a potential pitfall in the histopathologic diagnosis of cutaneous T- and B-cell lymphomas. *Am J Surg Pathol* 2002; **26**: 1259–68.

44 Scheffer E, Meijer CJLM, Willemze R, van Vloten WA. Lymph node histopathology in mycosis fungoides and Sézary's syndrome. In: Van Vloten WA, Willemze R, Lange Vejlsgaard G, Thomsen K, eds. *Cutaneous Lymphomas and Pseudolymphomas.* Basel: Karger, 1990: 105–13.

45 Mao X, Orchard G, Lillington DM *et al.* Amplification and overexpression of *JUNB* is associated with primary cutaneous T-cell lymphomas. *Blood* 2003; **101**: 1513–9.

46 Kari L, Loboda A, Nebozhyn M *et al.* Classification and prediction of survival in patients with the leukemic phase of cutaneous T cell lymphoma. *J Exp Med* 2003; **197**: 1477–88.

47 Apisarnthanarax N, Talpur R, Duvic M. Treatment of cutaneous T cell lymphoma: current status and future directions. *Am J Clin Dermatol* 2002; **3**: 193–215.

48 Jones GW, Rosenthal D, Wilson LD. Total skin electron radiation for patients with erythrodermic cutaneous T-cell lymphoma (mycosis fungoides and the Sézary syndrome). *Cancer* 1999; **85**: 1985–95.

49 Jumbou O, N'Guyen JM, Tessier MH, Legoux B, Dreno B. Long-term follow-up in 51 patients with mycosis fungoides and Sézary syndrome treated by interferon-α. *Br J Dermatol* 1999; **140**: 427–31.

50 Wilson LD, Jones GW, Kim D *et al.* Experience with total skin electron beam therapy in combination with extracorporeal photopheresis in the management of patients with erythrodermic (T4) mycosis fungoides. *J Am Acad Dermatol* 2000; **43**: 54–60.

51 Heald P, Rook A, Perez M *et al.* Treatment of erythrodermic cutaneous T-cell lymphoma with extracorporeal photochemotherapy. *J Am Acad Dermatol* 1992; **27**: 427–33.

52 Edelson RL. Sézary syndrome, cutaneous T-cell lymphoma, and extracorporeal photopheresis. *Arch Dermatol* 1999; **135**: 600–1.

53 Evans AV, Wood WP, Scarisbrick JJ *et al.* Extracorporeal photopheresis in Sézary syndrome: hematologic parameters as predictors of response. *Blood* 2001; **98**: 1298–301.

54 Fraser-Andrews E, Seed P, Whittaker S, Russell-Jones R. Extracorporeal photopheresis in Sézary syndrome: no significant effect in the survival of 44 patients with a peripheral blood T-cell clone. *Arch Dermatol* 1998; **134**: 1001–5.

55 Ferenczi K, Yawalkar N, Jones D, Kupper TS. Monitoring the decrease of circulating malignant T cells in cutaneous T-cell lymphoma during photopheresis and interferon therapy. *Arch Dermatol* 2003; **139**: 909–13.

56 Dearden C, Matutes E, Catovsky D. Pentostatin treatment of cutaneous T-cell lymphoma. *Oncology* 2000; **14** (Suppl. 2): 37–40.

57 Foss FM. Activity of pentostatin (Nipent) in cutaneous T-cell lymphoma: single-agent and combination studies. *Semin Oncol* 2000; **27** (Suppl. 5): 58–63.

58 Molina A, Nademanee A, Arber DA, Forman SJ. Remission of refractory Sézary syndrome after bone marrow transplantation from a matched unrelated donor. *Biol Blood Marrow Transplant* 1999; **5**: 400–4.

59 Sarris AH, Phan A, Duvic M *et al.* Trimetrexate in relapsed T-cell lymphoma with skin involvement. *J Clin Oncol* 2002; **20**: 2876–80.

60 Scarisbrick JJ, Child FJ, Clift A *et al.* A trial of fludarabine and cyclophosphamide combination chemotherapy in the treatment of advanced refractory primary cutaneous T-cell lymphoma. *Br J Dermatol* 2001; **144**: 1010–5.

61 Shapiro M, Rook AH, Lehrer MS *et al.* Novel multimodality biologic response modifier therapy, including bexarotene and long-wave ultraviolet A, for a patient with refractory stage IVa cutaneous T-cell lymphoma. *J Am Acad Dermatol* 2002; **47**: 956–61.

62 Fritz TM, Kleinhans M, Nestle FO, Burg G, Dummer R. Combination treatment with extracorporeal photopheresis, interferon α and interleukin-2 in a patient with the Sézary syndrome. *Br J Dermatol* 1999; **140**: 1144–7.

63 Beylot-Barry M, Sibaud V, Thiebaut R *et al.* Evidence that an identical T cell clone in skin and peripheral blood lymphocytes is an independent prognostic factor in primary cutaneous T cell lymphoma. *J Invest Dermatol* 2001; **117**: 920–6.

64 Kim YH, Liu HL, Mraz-Gernhard S, Varghese A, Hoppe RT. Long-term outcome of 525 patients with mycosis fungoides and Sézary syndrome. *Arch Dermatol* 2003; **139**: 857–66.

65 Diamandidou E, Colome M, Fayad L, Duvic M, Kurzrock R. Prognostic factor analysis in mycosis fungoides/Sézary syndrome. *J Am Acad Dermatol* 1999; **40**: 914–24.

66 Scarisbrick JJ, Whittaker S, Evans AV *et al.* Prognostic significance of tumor burden in the blood of patients with erythrodermic primary cutaneous T-cell lymphoma. *Blood* 2001; **97**: 624–30.

67 Stevens SR, Baron ED, Masten S, Cooper KD. Circulating CD4$^+$ CD7$^-$ lymphocyte burden and rapidity of response: predictors of outcome in the treatment of Sézary syndrome and erythrodermic mycosis fungoides with extracorporeal photopheresis. *Arch Dermatol* 2002; **138**: 1347–50.

68 Foulc P, N'Guyen JM, Dreno B. Prognostic factors in Sézary syndrome: a study of 28 patients. *Br J Dermatol* 2003; **149**: 1152–8.

Chapter 4 CD30⁺ cutaneous lymphoproliferative disorders

The CD30 antigen is a cytokine receptor belonging to the tumour necrosis factor receptor superfamily. The antigen was initially described within Reed–Sternberg and Hodgkin cells of Hodgkin lymphoma, and subsequently identified within neoplastic cells of a new group of non-Hodgkin lymphomas (anaplastic large cell lymphoma) [1,2]. Soon after the first description, it became clear that anaplastic large cell lymphomas could occur as a primary skin tumour, where they were characterized by a good prognosis [3–8]. The term 'cutaneous CD30⁺ lymphoproliferative disorders' has been subsequently proposed to denote a group of primary cutaneous T-cell lymphomas characterized by expression of the CD30 antigen phenotypically and a favourable prognosis biologically, including lymphomatoid papulosis and primary cutaneous anaplastic large cell lymphoma [9–14]. Cases described in the past as 'regressing atypical histiocytosis' or 'pseudo-Hodgkin disease' are part of the spectrum of primary cutaneous CD30⁺ lymphoproliferative disorders [15,16].

It is important to emphasize that there is no clear-cut boundary between 'classical' lymphomatoid papulosis and primary cutaneous anaplastic large cell lymphoma. The term 'borderline lymphomatoid papulosis–anaplastic large cell lymphoma' has been used by some authors for cases where a definitive diagnosis is not possible based on clinicopathological features. In this group are cases with the clinical aspect of lymphomatoid papulosis and the histopathology of primary cutaneous anaplastic large cell lymphoma and vice versa.

The typical features of cutaneous CD30⁺ lymphoproliferative disorders, including partial or complete spontaneous resolution of the lesions and good prognosis, have been the subject of several studies in an attempt to elucidate the reasons for this peculiar clinical behaviour. In recent years it has been suggested that CD30 and CD30-ligand are involved in the control of apoptosis, and that activation of the CD30 signalling pathway has a role in tumour regression [17–21]. Resistance to CD30-mediated growth inhibition provides a possible mechanism for escape from tumour regression in cases with more aggressive behaviour.

LYMPHOMATOID PAPULOSIS

Lymphomatoid papulosis is defined as a chronic recurrent self-healing eruption of papules and small nodules with the histopathological features of a cutaneous T-cell lymphoma ('rhythmic paradoxical eruption') [22].

Although in the past it has been classified among the cutaneous pseudolymphomas, lymphomatoid papulosis is considered today by most authors to be a low-grade cutaneous T-cell lymphoma, and has been included as such in the European Organization for Research and Treatment of Cancer (EORTC) classification of cutaneous lymphomas, and as a T-cell proliferation of uncertain malignant potential in the World Health Organization (WHO) classification of haematological neoplasms [23,24].

No specific genetic alterations or association with inflammatory skin disorders or viral infections have been consistently demonstrated in lymphomatoid papulosis, and the aetiology of the disease is still unknown. The interchromosomal (2;5) translocation is absent [25,26].

In 10–20% of patients, lymphomatoid papulosis is preceded, concomitant with or followed by another type of lymphoma (usually mycosis fungoides, Hodgkin lymphoma or anaplastic large cell lymphoma, but other malignant haematological disorders have been observed; see Chapter 2) [27–37]. In some of these patients, the same clone of neoplastic T lymphocytes has been identified in lesions of lymphomatoid papulosis and those of the associated lymphomas, raising the question of a possible common origin of the diseases [38–41]. However, their response to treatment is different as the lesions of lymphomatoid papulosis may continue to appear while the second lymphoma is in complete remission [42]. In patients with mycosis fungoides, self-healing papules with CD30⁺ lymphoid infiltrates may develop during the course of the disease, suggesting a diagnosis of lymphomatoid papulosis associated with mycosis fungoides. In these patients it is of crucial importance to rule out large cell transformation of mycosis fungoides. In fact, one case that the authors published in 1991 as 'PUVA-induced lymphomatoid papulosis in a patient with mycosis fungoides' [43] died with large cell transformation of mycosis fungoides 48 months after the onset of the 'lymphomatoid papulosis'.

In addition to these haematological malignancies, patients with lymphomatoid papulosis are also at higher risk of developing non-lymphoid second malignancies [44].

In the absence of specific symptoms of other associated diseases, complete staging investigations are not necessary in patients with classical lymphomatoid papulosis.

Clinical features

Young adults are usually affected, but the disease has been reported in children and in the elderly [23,29,30,45–50]. Clinically, lymphomatoid papulosis presents in most patients as a generalized eruption of reddish brown papules or small nodules on the trunk and proximal extremities, but in some cases only a few lesions may be present (Figs 4.1–4.3). The size of the lesions is variable but usually smaller than 1 cm. In a few patients, large, rapidly growing nodules, sometimes with ulceration, may be the first manifestation of the disease (Fig. 4.4) [9]. The onset of large tumours with

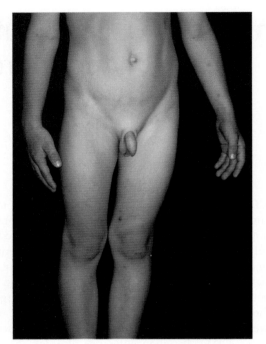

Fig. 4.2 Lymphomatoid papulosis. Few papules and nodules in a 6-year-old child.

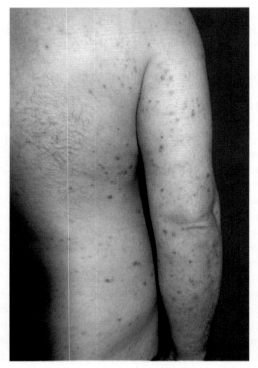

Fig. 4.1 Lymphomatoid papulosis. Generalized eruption of papules and small nodules.

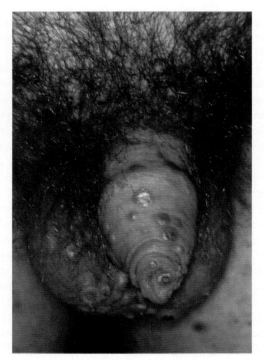

Fig. 4.3 Lymphomatoid papulosis. Multiple papules and small nodules, some ulcerated, on the genital area.

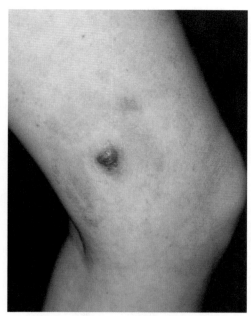

Fig. 4.4 Lymphomatoid papulosis. Nodule on the leg with two small satellite papules at presentation of the disease. The patient then developed a 'conventional' lymphomatoid papulosis.

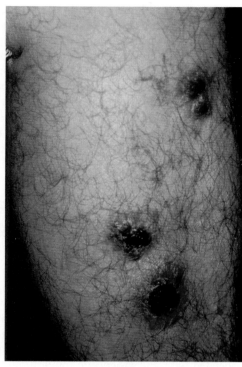

Fig. 4.6 Lymphomatoid papulosis. Ulcerated erythematous nodules.

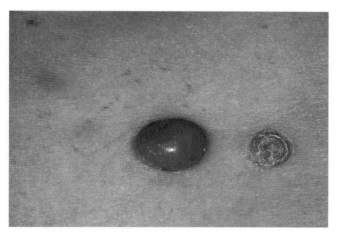

Fig. 4.5 Lymphomatoid papulosis. Small erythematous nodule. Note a resolving lesion on the right side of the nodule.

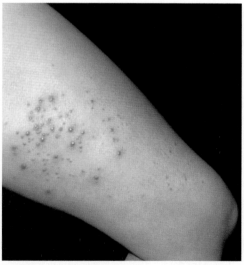

Fig. 4.7 Regional lymphomatoid papulosis. Cluster of erythematous papules restricted to the median aspect of the left thigh.

complete spontaneous resolution has also been observed during the course of the disease but the prognosis seems not to be affected and the disease runs the usual course, suggesting that large tumours may represent a morphological variation of lymphomatoid papulosis rather than transformation into anaplastic large cell lymphoma [9].

The clinical picture is usually polymorphic, because of the presence of lesions in different stages of evolution (Fig. 4.5). Ulceration is common (Fig. 4.6). Spontaneous resolution is observed within a few weeks or, rarely, months. The time interval between two eruptions is variable: some patients may experience several bursts within short periods of time, whereas others may have only a few lesions over several years.

Occasionally, lesions of lymphomatoid papulosis are localized to just one area (regional lymphomatoid papulosis) (Fig. 4.7) [51–53]. In these cases, differentiation from anaplastic large cell lymphoma can be extremely difficult, as this last can present with nodules surrounded by satellite lesions of smaller dimensions simulating clinically lymphomatoid papulosis. Involvement of mucosal regions in lymphomatoid papulosis is possible, but uncommon [54]. Association with pregnancy and with severe hypereosinophilic syndrome has also been reported [55,56]. Other unusual clinical variants of lymphomatoid papulosis include a type characterized by lesions resembling clinically hydroa vacciniformis, and one by the presence of predominant pustular lesions [57,58].

Histopathology, immunophenotype and molecular genetics

Histopathology

The histopathological features of lymphomatoid papulosis are variable. Three main histological subtypes have been described. It is important to recognize that these variants can all be observed in one patient at the same time or during the course of the disease, and that the histopathological picture is not associated with any prognostic implications. Sometimes, single lesions with features of different histological types have been referred to as lymphomatoid papulosis type A/B. We prefer to classify lesions into one of the following three groups according to the predominant histopathological features.

Type A ('histiocytic' type). Characterized by wedge-shaped lesions with the presence of scattered or clustered large atypical cells admixed with small lymphocytes, histiocytes, neutrophils and eosinophils (Figs 4.8 & 4.9). Epidermotropism is variable.

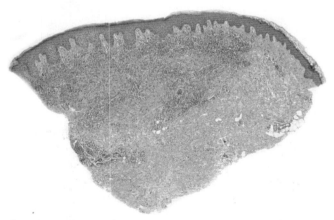

Fig. 4.8 Lymphomatoid papulosis, type A. Wedge-shaped infiltrate in the dermis.

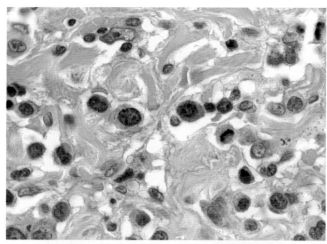

Fig. 4.9 Lymphomatoid papulosis, type A. Detail of atypical cells.

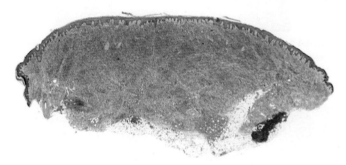

Fig. 4.10 Lymphomatoid papulosis, type B. Wedge-shaped infiltrate of lymphocytes within the entire dermis. Note epidermotropism of solitary lymphocytes aligned along the basal layer.

Type B (mycosis fungoides-like). This is a rare type of lymphomatoid papulosis that reveals a wedge-shaped or, more rarely, band-like infiltrate of small- to medium-sized pleomorphic (cerebriform) cells with epidermotropism (Figs 4.10 & 4.11). It is crucial to understand that the differentiation of lymphomatoid papulosis type B from mycosis fungoides can only be achieved by clinicopathological correlation, and that a diagnosis of lymphomatoid papulosis type B should never be established without a complete clinical history.

Although large atypical cells are the hallmark of lymphomatoid papulosis, and the existence of a 'small cell' variant has been called into question, lymphomatoid papulosis type B composed of small to medium sized cells may be compared to the small to medium cell variant of anaplastic large cell lymphoma, which is now a well-established morphological subtype of that lymphoma.

Type C (anaplastic large cell lymphoma-like). There is a nodular infiltrate characterized by sheets of cohesive large atypical

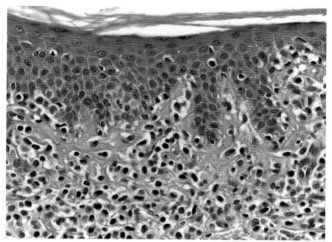

Fig. 4.11 Lymphomatoid papulosis, type B. Note epidermotropism of solitary lymphocytes with small nuclei resembling the histopathological features of mycosis fungoides.

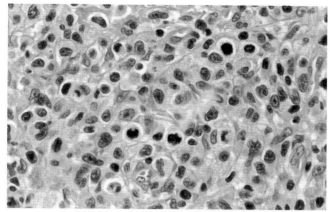

Fig. 4.13 Lymphomatoid papulosis, type C. Detail of the atypical lymphocytes arranged in sheets, simulating the histopathological features of anaplastic large cell lymphoma.

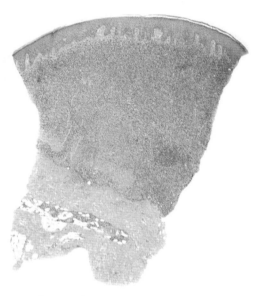

Fig. 4.12 Lymphomatoid papulosis, type C. Dense infiltrate of atypical lymphocytes arranged in sheets.

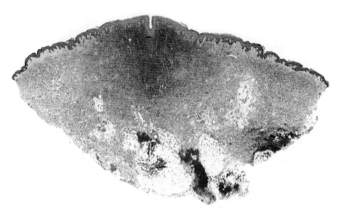

Fig. 4.14 Follicular lymphomatoid papulosis. Note a wedge-shaped infiltrate disposed symmetrically around a hair follicle.

neurotropic infiltrates, follicular mucinosis and subepidermal blisters (Fig. 4.15) [29,62,63]. Rarely, angiocentricity and angiodestruction may be observed.

In some cases of lymphomatoid papulosis, a prominent acanthosis of the epidermis can be observed [64,65]. Rarely, the association with multiple keratoacanthomas has been documented (Fig. 4.16) [66].

Immunophenotype

The hallmark of lymphomatoid papulosis is the expression of CD30 by neoplastic cells (Fig. 4.17) [8,67–69]. Although the infiltrate of type B lymphomatoid papulosis has often been reported as being CD30⁻, many cases do in fact express the antigen (Fig. 4.18) [29]. In this context, care should be taken to avoid misinterpreting the papular variant of mycosis fungoides as type B lymphomatoid papulosis (see Chapter 2). CD30⁺ lymphocytes are often arranged in small clusters (type

cells admixed with a few small lymphocytes, neutrophils and eosinophils (Figs 4.12 & 4.13). The histopathological features are indistinguishable from those of anaplastic large cell lymphoma, and a definitive diagnosis can be achieved only upon clinicopathological correlation.

A variant of lymphomatoid papulosis characterized by lesions centred on a hair follicle has been termed 'follicular lymphomatoid papulosis' (Fig. 4.14) [59–61]. Other unusual histopathological findings in lymphomatoid papulosis include the presence of myxoid changes, eccrinotropic and

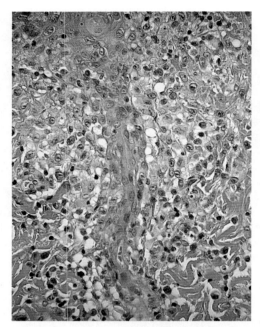

Fig. 4.15 Syringotropic lymphomatoid papulosis. Atypical cells are disposed around an eccrine duct, in part infiltrating it.

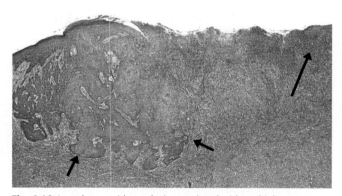

Fig. 4.16 Lymphomatoid papulosis associated with multiple keratoacanthomas. The remnant of a keratoacanthoma is visible on the left side of this lesion (short arrows), whereas most atypical cells of the lymphomatoid papulosis are located on the right part of it (long arrow). The patient, a 79-year-old male, had concomitant typical lesions of keratoacanthoma without infiltrating CD30+ atypical cells, as well as conventional lesions of lymphomatoid papulosis without epidermal hyperplasia.

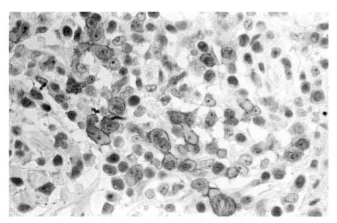

Fig. 4.17 Lymphomatoid papulosis, type A. CD30+ atypical lymphocytes disposed as solitary units and in small clusters.

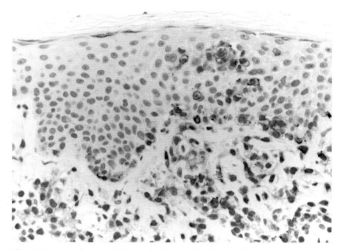

Fig. 4.18 Lymphomatoid papulosis, type B. Intraepidermal lymphocytes positive for CD30.

A) or in sheets (type C), a feature useful in the differential diagnosis of lymphomatoid papulosis from benign inflammatory skin diseases, where CD30+ cells are scattered and isolated (although this can also be observed occasionally in cases of lymphomatoid papulosis). Neoplastic cells express the phenotypical markers of T-helper lymphocytes (CD3+, CD4+, CD8−) in most cases, but a CD8+ phenotype has been observed [29,68–70]. Expression of pan-T-cell antigens may be lost, at least partially, in some cases.

Most cases of lymphomatoid papulosis express cytotoxic markers [71,72]. Expression of CD56 is usually absent, but may be observed in some cases (Fig. 4.19) [29,73–75]. The anaplastic lymphoma kinase (ALK) is not expressed [26,76].

Molecular genetics

There are no specific genetic abnormalities reported for lymphomatoid papulosis. Rearrangement of the T-cell receptor (TCR) gene is found in most lesions [77]. Studies on single cells after microdissection of the specimens showed that the atypical CD30+ large cells have a common clonal origin [78].

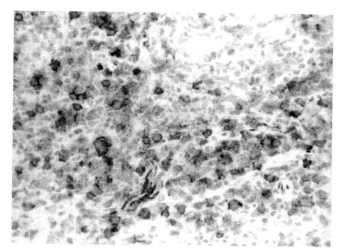

Fig. 4.19 Lymphomatoid papulosis, type A. Large atypical lymphocytes positive for CD56.

Clinicopathological differential diagnosis

Besides anaplastic large cell lymphoma, the differential diagnosis of lymphomatoid papulosis includes mainly papulo-necrotic eruptions such as pityriasis lichenoides et varioliformis acuta (PLEVA). This distinction can be particularly difficult as overlapping clinicopathological features can be seen. However, in the proper clinical background, the presence of large atypical CD30⁺ cells is diagnostic of lymphomatoid papulosis. Cases reported in the past as 'pityriasis lichenoides of childhood with atypical CD30⁺ cells and clonal TCR gene rearrangement' [79] are also most likely to be examples of lymphomatoid papulosis [80].

For a detailed discussion of the differential diagnosis of lymphomatoid papulosis from inflammatory infiltrates of the skin with large atypical CD30⁺ cells, see Chapter 20.

Treatment

As the disease is self-limiting, most patients with lymphomatoid papulosis do not require specific treatment [9]. Therapy should be directed mainly at controlling symptoms in widespread eruptions, or at slowing down the frequency of recurrences [9,23]. Systemic steroids, psoralen with UVA (PUVA), interferon-α2a, interferon-γ and retinoids (alone or in combination) have been used with partial success [9,14,81–85]. Some patients may also benefit from the administration of low-dose methotrexate over a longer period of time [9,86]. Methotrexate has also been administered topically [87]. Recurrences after discontinuation of any type of treatment are the rule.

At present, there are no data to support a preventive effect of any given treatment regimen on the development of a second lymphoma.

Prognosis

Lymphomatoid papulosis is characterized by an excellent prognosis, and the expected 5-year survival is 100% [23,29,30]. Some patients may experience very few recurrences of the disease over the years, whereas others may have lesions appearing almost continuously. At present there are no prognostic features that can help in predicting the course of the disease in a given patient.

The knowledge that 10–20% of patients develop an associated malignant lymphoma means that regular follow-up is required for these patients. Unfortunately, clinicopathological, phenotypical or molecular features provide no clues for the early identification of patients who will progress to a more aggressive lymphoma.

It seems that the occurrence of large CD30⁺ tumours limited to the skin at the onset of lymphomatoid papulosis or during the course of the disease does not worsen the prognosis of these patients [9,28].

RÉSUMÉ

Lymphomatoid papulasis

Clinical	Young adults. Chronic recurrent eruption of papules and nodules that heal within 3–6 weeks without treatment. Excellent prognosis.
Morphology	Three histopathological types: *Type A*: large, atypical, CD30⁺ cells admixed with small lymphocytes, eosinophils and neutrophils. *Type B*: wedge-shaped or band-like infiltrate of small- to medium-sized atypical cells with epidermotropism. CD30±. *Type C*: sheets of large atypical CD30⁺ cells.
Immunology	CD2, 3, 4, 5, 45 + CD30 + CD15 – CD8 – (+) TIA-1 + CD56 – (+)
Genetics	No specific abnormalities. Monoclonal rearrangement of the TCR detected in the majority of cases.
Treatment guidelines	Systemic steroids; PUVA; interferon-α2a (alone or in combination); methotrexate.

ANAPLASTIC LARGE T-CELL LYMPHOMA

Cutaneous anaplastic large cell lymphoma is defined as a CD30⁺ large T-cell lymphoma presenting primarily in the skin and characterized by a good prognosis and response to treatment [23].

The differences in biological behaviour and prognosis between primary cutaneous and nodal anaplastic large cell lymphoma have been known for some time. Although earlier reports suggested that the interchromosomal (2;5) translocation, typical of nodal anaplastic large cell lymphoma, could also be found in cutaneous cases [88,89], it has been subsequently shown that it is absent in most primary cutaneous anaplastic large cell lymphomas, confirming the distinction between the cutaneous and extracutaneous forms of this disease [23–26]. In fact, the WHO classification for haematopoietic neoplasms lists the primary cutaneous form as a distinct entity, separate from the nodal counterpart [24]. Complete staging investigations are mandatory before definitive diagnosis, in order to exclude secondary involvement from nodal disease. The value of sentinel lymph node biopsy as a routine staging procedure has yet to be evaluated in large numbers of patients [90].

It should be emphasized that CD30⁺ tumours with anaplastic large cell morphology may be seen in patients with mycosis fungoides as a consequence of large cell transformation (see Chapter 2). Thus, a diagnosis of primary cutaneous anaplastic large cell lymphoma should be made only when an accurate clinical history and examination exclude the presence of mycosis fungoides. In addition, large ulcerated tumours may be the presenting sign of lymphomatoid papulosis [9], and these lesions should not be misinterpreted as tumours of anaplastic large cell lymphoma. In this context, it should also be noted that expression of CD30 and anaplastic large cell morphology can be observed rarely in diffuse large B-cell lymphomas (see Chapter 12), and that complete phenotypical and genotypical analyses are necessary before classifying any given case.

The association of anaplastic large cell lymphoma and lymphomatoid papulosis has been observed in several instances (see also Lymphomatoid papulosis, page 45) [56,91,92]. Distinction between the two entities may be very difficult as the histological and immunophenotypical features may overlap. In this context, in 1995 LeBoit wrote: 'If one could line up 100 patients with lymphomatoid papulosis, primary cutaneous anaplastic large cell lymphoma, and cutaneous dissemination of Hodgkin's disease, a skilled clinician could more accurately sort the patients into diagnostic groups than a pathologist could by looking only at the immunophenotype of the large atypical cells' [93]. In addition, it seems that progression to an anaplastic large cell lym-

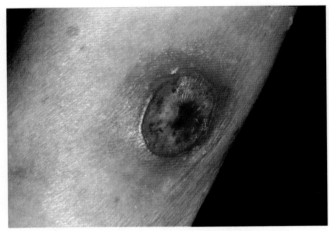

Fig. 4.20 Anaplastic large cell lymphoma. Solitary ulcerated tumour on the arm.

phoma confined to the skin does not affect the favourable prognosis of lymphomatoid papulosis [28].

Cutaneous anaplastic large cell lymphoma has been observed in patients with severe immunodeficiency, brought about both by HIV infection and therapeutic-induced immunosuppression [94–98]. In cases arising in HIV patients, an association with human herpesvirus 8 (HHV-8) infection has been documented [99].

Clinical features

Cutaneous anaplastic large cell lymphomas occur mostly in adults of both sexes, but cases in children have been reported [23,30,100–102]. Clinically, patients present with solitary or localized, often ulcerated, reddish brown tumours (Fig. 4.20). Mucosal regions can be affected. Complete spontaneous regression has been observed in a few cases [103], but regression is more commonly partial (Fig. 4.21).

Clinical variants of the disease include the presence of satellite lesions around the primary tumour, simulating the clinical picture of regional lymphomatoid papulosis. Rarely, a few neoplastic cells can be detected in the peripheral blood in primary cutaneous cases [104].

Histopathology, immunophenotype and molecular genetics

Histopathology

Cutaneous anaplastic large cell lymphoma shows a nodular or diffuse infiltrate within the entire dermis and superficial part of the subcutis, composed of sheets of cohesive large CD30⁺ atypical cells (Fig. 4.22). Most cases are composed of

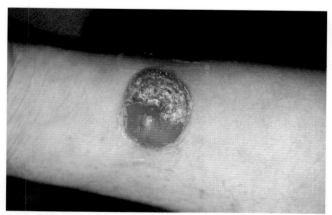

Fig. 4.21 Anaplastic large cell lymphoma. Large tumour on the arm showing partial regression. (Courtesy of I. Höpfel-Kreiner, Linz, Austria.)

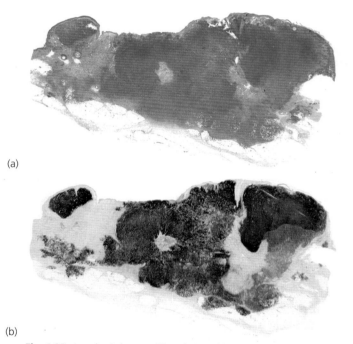

(a)

(b)

Fig. 4.22 Anaplastic large cell lymphoma. (a) Large tumour with sheets of cells infiltrating the entire dermis until the superficial part of the subcutaneous fat. (b) Most cells strongly express CD30. (Courtesy of Esmeralda Vale, Lisboa, Portugal.)

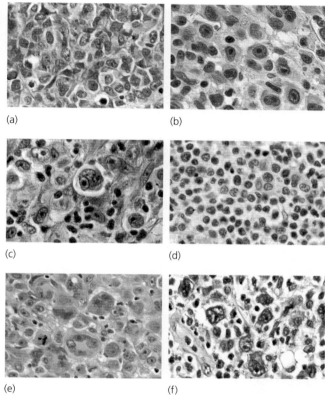

(a)　　　　　(b)

(c)　　　　　(d)

(e)　　　　　(f)

Fig. 4.23 Anaplastic large cell lymphoma. (a) Large pleomorphic and anaplastic cells. (b) Immunoblasts predominate in this case. (c) Presence of multinucleated cells resembling Reed–Sternberg cells of Hodgkin lymphoma. (d) Predominance of small- to medium-sized pleomorphic lymphocytes (so-called 'small cell variant' of anaplastic large cell lymphoma). (e) Predominance of 'epithelioid' cells with abundant eosinophilic cytoplasm. Some multinucleated cells are present. (f) Large anaplastic cells, some multinucleated, admixed with several neutrophils and eosinophils (so-called 'neutrophilic-rich' variant of anaplastic large cell lymphoma).

large anaplastic cells (large rounded or irregularly shaped nuclei with prominent nucleoli and abundant cytoplasm; giant cells with features of Reed–Sternberg cells), but large pleomorphic cells or immunoblasts can also be observed (Fig. 4.23a–c). In addition, cases with a predominant small- to medium-sized pleomorphic cell morphology can be observed occasionally (Fig. 4.23d). Sometimes, anaplastic cells show epithelioid-like cytomorphological features resembling undifferentiated carcinoma (Fig. 4.23e). Epidermotropism may be seen.

Ulcerated lesions usually show epidermal hyperplasia and a prominent reactive infiltrate with small lymphocytes, neutrophils and eosinophils (Fig. 4.23f). These cases may be indistinguishable histologically from lesions of lymphomatoid papulosis, and have been referred to sometimes as the 'inflammatory' type of anaplastic large cell lymphoma. Staining for CD30 may help by highlighting the clusters of CD30+ cells. Cases with prominent neutrophils have been termed 'neutrophil-rich' anaplastic large cell lymphoma [105,106].

Other rare histopathological variants include the presence of prominent involvement of the subcutaneous fat (Fig. 4.24), and of a myxoid stroma resembling a sarcomatous lesion [107,108]. Angiocentricity and angiodestruction, and rarely a signet-ring morphology of the neoplastic cells may be observed (Figs 4.25 & 4.26).

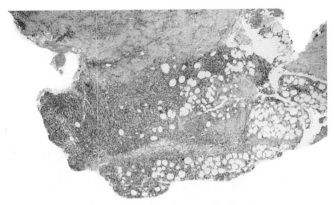

Fig. 4.24 Anaplastic large cell lymphoma confined to the subcutaneous fat.

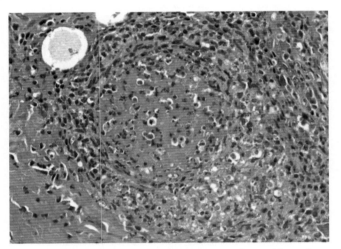

Fig. 4.25 Anaplastic large cell lymphoma. Note angiocentricity and angiodestruction.

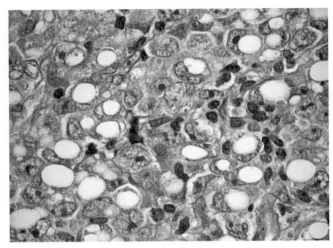

Fig. 4.26 Anaplastic large cell lymphoma with signet-ring cell morphology of neoplastic cells.

Immunophenotype

Most neoplastic cells are CD30+ and generally have a T-helper phenotype (CD3+, CD4+, CD8−) (Fig. 4.22b) [70], although CD8+ cases have been observed [109]. Expression of pan-T-cell antigens may be partially lost. CD15 and epithelial membrane antigen (EMA) are usually negative. Expression of ALK protein is not found in purely cutaneous cases (see Molecular genetics, below) but is present in systemic disease with secondary cutaneous manifestations [76,110,111].

Similarly to lymphomatoid papulosis, most cases of anaplastic large cell lymphoma express a cytotoxic phenotype [72,112,113].

Molecular genetics

Monoclonal rearrangement of the TCR gene is observed in most cases. Single-cell polymerase chain reaction (PCR) analysis has demonstrated that most of the large CD30+ cells are monoclonal [114]. There is good evidence that the inter-chromosomal (2;5) translocation seen in many nodal anaplastic large cell lymphomas is not present in primary cutaneous lesions [23,26].

No specific genetic alterations have been detected repeatably in cutaneous anaplastic large cell lymphoma. Some cases revealed chromosome imbalances by comparative genomic hybridization and cDNA microarray studies [115]. An allelic deletion at the chromosome region 9p21, containing the tumour suppressor gene *p16*, has been shown in some cases [116].

Treatment

Solitary or localized lesions may be treated by surgical excision, radiotherapy, or a combination of the two [9,23,117]. Patients presenting with extracutaneous involvement require systemic chemotherapy. The role of systemic chemotherapy in primary cutaneous lesions has been debated [102,118], but there is a widely accepted view that this treatment can be avoided in most patients with primary skin involvement [9,23].

Complete regression after effective specific antiviral treatment has been observed in patients with HIV-associated primary cutaneous anaplastic large cell lymphoma [119].

Prognosis

Although the morphological features are those of a high-grade non-Hodgkin lymphoma, the prognosis of patients with primary cutaneous anaplastic large cell lymphoma is generally favourable. The estimated 5-year survival is over 90% [23,30,120]. Spontaneous regression and absence of extracutaneous spread have been associated with a better prognosis [121].

It seems that patients presenting with skin tumours and evidence of specific lesions within regional lymph nodes at staging (concomitant cutaneous and nodal anaplastic large cell lymphoma) have a prognosis similar to that of patients with disease confined to the skin [9].

RÉSUMÉ

Anaplastic large T-cell lymphoma

Clinical	Adults and younger patients. Solitary or regionally localized tumours, often ulcerated. Generally favourable prognosis.
Morphology	Nodular infiltrates characterized by cohesive sheets of large CD30⁺ cells. *Cytomorphology*: large anaplastic cells; large pleomorphic cells or immunoblasts; small/medium and signet-ring cell morphology may be observed.
Immunology	CD2, 3, 4, 5 (+) CD30 + CD8 – CD15, EMA – TIA-1 (+) CD56 – (+) ALK-1 –
Genetics	Usually absence of t(2;5). Monoclonal rearrangement of the TCR detected in the majority of cases.
Treatment guidelines	*Solitary or localized lesions*: surgical excision and/or radiotherapy. Systemic chemotherapy should probably be administered only in patients with extracutaneous involvement.

References

1 Stein H, Gerdes J, Schwab U *et al*. Identification of Hodgkin and Sternberg–Reed cells as a unique cell type derived from a newly detected small-cell population. *Int J Cancer* 1982; **30**: 445–59.

2 Stein H, Mason DY, Gerdes J *et al*. The expression of the Hodgkin's disease associated antigen Ki1 in reactive and neoplastic lymphoid tissue: evidence that Reed–Sternberg cells and histiocytic malignancies are derived from activated lymphoid cells. *Blood* 1985; **66**: 848–58.

3 Beljaards RC, Meijer CJLM, Scheffer E *et al*. Prognostic significance of CD30 (Ki-1/Ber-H2) expression in primary cutaneous large-cell lymphomas of T-cell origin. *Am J Pathol* 1989; **135**: 1169–78.

4 Beljaards RC, Kaudewitz P, Berti E *et al*. Primary cutaneous CD30-positive large cell lymphoma: definition of a new type of cutaneous lymphoma with a favorable prognosis. *Cancer* 1993; **71**: 2097–104.

5 Feller AC, Sterry W. Large cell anaplastic lymphoma of the skin. *Br J Dermatol* 1989; **121**: 593–602.

6 Kaudewitz P, Stein H, Dallenbach F *et al*. Primary and secondary cutaneous Ki1⁺ (CD30⁺) anaplastic large cell lymphomas. *Am J Pathol* 1989; **135**: 359–67.

7 Krishnan J, Tomaszewski MM, Kao GF. Primary cutaneous CD30-positive anaplastic large cell lymphoma: report of 27 cases. *J Cutan Pathol* 1993; **20**: 193–202.

8 Ralfkiaer E, Bosq J, Gatter KC *et al*. Expression of Hodgkin and Reed–Sternberg cell associated antigen (Ki1) in cutaneous lymphoid infiltrates. *Arch Dermatol Res* 1987; **279**: 285–92.

9 Bekkenk MW, Geelen FAMJ, van Voorst-Vader PC *et al*. Primary and secondary cutaneous CD30⁺ lymphoproliferative disorders: a report from the Dutch Cutaneous Lymphoma Group on the long-term follow-up data of 219 patients and guidelines for diagnosis and treatment. *Blood* 2000; **95**: 3653–61.

10 Kadin ME. The spectrum of Ki1⁺ cutaneous lymphomas. In: Van Vloten WA, Willemze R, Lange Vejlsgaard G, Thomsen K, eds. *Cutaneous Lymphomas and Pseudolymphomas*. Basel: Karger, 1990: 132–43.

11 Kaudewitz P, Burg G. Lymphomatoid papulosis and Ki1 (CD30) positive cutaneous large cell lymphomas. *Semin Diagn Pathol* 1991; **8**: 117–24.

12 LeBoit PE. Lymphomatoid papulosis and cutaneous CD30⁺ lymphoma. *Am J Dermatopathol* 1996; **18**: 221–35.

13 Paulli M, Berti E, Rosso R *et al*. CD30/Ki-1-positive lymphoproliferative disorders of the skin: clinicopathologic correlation and statistical analysis of 86 cases. A multicentric study from the European Organization for Research and Treatment of Cancer Cutaneous Lymphoma project group. *J Clin Oncol* 1995; **13**: 1343–54.

14 Willemze R, Beljaards RC. The spectrum of primary cutaneous CD30 (Ki-1) positive lymphoproliferative disorders: a proposal for classification and guidelines for management and treatment. *J Am Acad Dermatol* 1993; **28**: 973.

15 Flynn KJ, Dehner LP, Gajl-Peczalska KJ *et al*. Regressing atypical histiocytosis: a cutaneous proliferation of atypical neoplastic histiocytes with unexpectedly indolent biologic behaviour. *Cancer* 1982; **49**: 959–70.

16 Cerio R, Black MM. Regressing atypical histiocytosis and lymphomatoid papulosis: variants of the same disorder? *Br J Dermatol* 1990; **123**: 515–21.

17 Levi E, Wang Z, Petrogiannis-Haliotis T *et al*. Distinct effects of CD30 and Fas signaling in cutaneous anaplastic lymphomas: a possible mechanism for disease progression. *J Invest Dermatol* 2000; **115**: 1034–40.

18 Mori M, Manuelli C, Pimpinelli N *et al*. CD30–CD30 ligand interaction in primary cutaneous CD30⁺ T-cell lymphomas: a clue to the pathophysiology of clinical regression. *Blood* 1999; **94**: 3077–83.

19 Nevala H, Karenko L, Vakeva L, Banki A. Proapoptotic and anti-apoptotic markers in cutaneous T-cell lymphoma skin infiltrates and lymphomatoid papulosis. *Br J Dermatol* 2001; **145**: 928–37.

20 Paulli M, Berti E, Boveri E *et al.* Cutaneous CD30⁺ lymphopro-liferative disorders: expression of bcl-2 and proteins of the tumor necrosis factor receptor superfamily. *Hum Pathol* 1998; **29**: 1223–30.

21 Vermeer MH, de Vries E, van Beek P, Meijer CJLM, Willemze R. Expression of Fas and Fas-ligand in primary cutaneous T-cell lymphoma (CTCL): association between lack of Fas expression and aggressive types of CTCL. *Br J Dermatol* 2000; **143**: 313–9.

22 MacAulay WL. Lymphomatoid papulosis: a continuing self-healing eruption, clinically benign–histologically malignant. *Arch Dermatol* 1968; **97**: 23–30.

23 Willemze R, Kerl H, Sterry W *et al.* EORTC classification for primary cutaneous lymphomas: a proposal from the Cutaneous Lymphoma Study Group of the European Organization for Research and Treatment of Cancer. *Blood* 1997; **90**: 354–71.

24 Ralfkiaer E, Delsol G, Willemze R, Jaffe ES. Primary cutaneous CD30-positive T-cell lymphoproliferative disorders. In: Jaffe ES, Harris NL, Stein H, Vardiman JW, eds. *World Health Organiza-tion Classification of Tumours: Tumours of Haematopoietic and Lymphoid Tissues.* Lyon: IARC Press, 2001: 221–4.

25 Wood GS, Hardman DL, Boni R *et al.* Lack of the t(2;5) or other mutations resulting in expression of anaplastic lymphoma kinase catalytic domain in CD30⁺ primary cutaneous lymphoproliferative disorders and Hodgkin's disease. *Blood* 1996; **88**: 1765–70.

26 DeCoteau JF, Butmarc JR, Kinney MC, Kadin ME. The t(2;5) chromosomal translocation is not a common feature of primary cutaneous CD30⁺ lymphoproliferative disorders: comparison with anaplastic large-cell lymphoma of nodal origin. *Blood* 1996; **87**: 3437–41.

27 Basarab T, Fraser-Andrews EA, Orchard G, Whittaker S, Russell-Jones R. Lymphomatoid papulosis in association with mycosis fungoides: a study of 15 cases. *Br J Dermatol* 1998; **139**: 630–8.

28 Beljaards RC, Willemze R. The prognosis of patients with lymphomatoid papulosis associated with malignant lymphomas. *Br J Dermatol* 1992; **126**: 596–602.

29 El Shabrawi-Caelen L, Kerl H, Cerroni L. Lymphomatoid papulosis: reappraisal of clinicopathologic presentation and classi-fication into subtypes A, B and C. *Arch Dermatol* in press.

30 Fink-Puches R, Zenahlik P, Bäck B *et al.* Primary cutaneous lymphomas: applicability of current classification schemes (Euro-pean Organization for Research and Treatment of Cancer, World Health Organization) based on clinicopathologic features observed in a large group of patients. *Blood* 2002; **99**: 800–5.

31 Harabuchi Y, Kataura A, Kobayashi K *et al.* Lethal midline granuloma (peripheral T-cell lymphoma) after lymphomatoid papulosis. *Cancer* 1992; **70**: 835–9.

32 Karp DL, Horn TD. Lymphomatoid papulosis. *J Am Acad Dermatol* 1994; **30**: 379–95.

33 Kaudewitz P, Stein H, Plewig G *et al.* Hodgkin's disease followed by lymphomatoid papulosis: immunophenotypic evidence for a close relationship between lymphomatoid papulosis and Hodgkin's disease. *J Am Acad Dermatol* 1990; **22**: 999–1006.

34 Thomsen K, Lange Wantzin G. Lymphomatoid papulosis: a follow-up study of 30 patients. *J Am Acad Dermatol* 1987; **17**: 632–6.

35 Weinman VF, Ackerman AB. Lymphomatoid papulosis: a critical review and new findings. *Am J Dermatopathol* 1981; **3**: 129–62.

36 Aronsson A, Jonsson N, Tegner E. Transient lymphomatoid papulosis in mycosis fungoides. *Acta Derm Venereol (Stockh)* 1982; **62**: 529.

37 Lish KM, Ramsay DL, Raphael BG, Jacobson M, Gottesman SRS. Lymphomatoid papulosis followed by acute myeloblastic leukemia. *J Am Acad Dermatol* 1993; **29**: 112–5.

38 Chott A, Vonderheid EC, Olbricht S *et al.* The same dominant T cell clone is present in multiple regressing skin lesions and associated T cell lymphomas of patients with lymphomatoid papulosis. *J Invest Dermatol* 1996; **106**: 696–700.

39 Davis TH, Morton CC, Miller-Cassman R, Balk SP, Kadin ME. Hodgkin's disease, lymphomatoid papulosis, and cutaneous T-cell lymphoma derived from a common T-cell clone. *N Engl J Med* 1992; **326**: 1115–22.

40 Wood GS, Crooks CF, Uluer AZ. Lymphomatoid papulosis and associated cutaneous lymphoproliferative disorders exhibit a common clonal origin. *J Invest Dermatol* 1995; **105**: 51–5.

41 Zackheim HS, Jones C, LeBoit PE *et al.* Lymphomatoid papulosis associated with mycosis fungoides: a study of 21 patients including analyses for clonality. *J Am Acad Dermatol* 2003; **49**: 620–3.

42 Zackheim HS, LeBoit PE, Gordon BI, Glassberg AB. Lymphomatoid papulosis followed by Hodgkin's lymphoma: differential response to therapy. *Arch Dermatol* 1993; **129**: 86–91.

43 Wolf P, Cerroni L, Smolle J, Kerl H. PUVA-induced lymphomatoid papulosis in a patient with mycosis fungoides. *J Am Acad Dermatol* 1991; **25**: 422–6.

44 Wang HH, Myers T, Lach LJ, Hsieh CC, Kadin ME. Increased risk of lymphoid and non-lymphoid malignancies in patients with lymphomatoid papulosis. *Cancer* 1999; **86**: 1240–5.

45 Aoki E, Aoki M, Kono M, Kawana S. Two cases of lymphomatoid papulosis in children. *Pediatr Dermatol* 2003; **20**: 146–9.

46 el-Azhary RA, Gibson LE, Kurtin PJ, Pittelkow MR, Muller SA. Lymphomatoid papulosis: a clinical and histopathologic review of 53 cases with leukocyte immunophenotyping, DNA flow cytometry, and T-cell receptor gene rearrangement studies. *J Am Acad Dermatol* 1994; **30**: 210–8.

47 Rogers M, de Launey J, Kemp A, Bishop A. Lymphomatoid papulosis in an 11-month-old infant. *Pediatr Dermatol* 1984; **2**: 124–30.

48 Sanchez NP, Pittelkow MR, Muller SA, Banks PM, Winkelmann RK. The clinicopathologic spectrum of lymphomatoid papulosis: study of 31 cases. *J Am Acad Dermatol* 1983; **8**: 81–94.

49 van Neer FJMA, Toonstra J, van Voorst Vader PC, Willemze R, van Vloten WA. Lymphomatoid papulosis in children: a study of 10 children registered by the Dutch cutaneous lymphoma working group. *Br J Dermatol* 2001; **144**: 351–4.

50 Willemze R, Meijer CJLM, van Vloten WA, Scheffer E. The clinical and histological spectrum of lymphomatoid papulosis. *Br J Dermatol* 1982; **107**: 131–44.

51 Kagaya M, Kondo S, Kamada A *et al.* Localized lymphomatoid papulosis. *Dermatology* 2002; **204**: 72–4.

52 Scarisbrick JJ, Evans AV, Woolford AJ, Black MM, Russell-Jones R. Regional lymphomatoid papulosis: a report of four cases. *Br J Dermatol* 1999; **141**: 1125–8.

53 Thomas GJ, Conejo-Mir JS, Ruiz AP, Barrios ML, Navarrete M. Lymphomatoid papulosis in childhood with exclusive acral involvement. *Pediatr Dermatol* 1998; **15**: 146–7.

54 Kato N, Tomita Y, Yoshida K, Hisai H. Involvement of the tongue by lymphomatoid papulosis. *Am J Dermatopathol* 1998; **20**: 522–6.

55 Yamamoto O, Tajiri M, Asahi M. Lymphomatoid papulosis associated with pregnancy. *Clin Exp Dermatol* 1997; **22**: 141–3.

56 Granel B, Serratrice J, Swiader L et al. Lymphomatoid papulosis associated with both severe hypereosinophilic syndrome and CD30 positive large T-cell lymphoma: a case report. *Cancer* 2000; **89**: 2138–43.

57 Tabata N, Aiba S, Ichinohazama R et al. Hydroa vacciniforme-like lymphomatoid papulosis in a Japanese child: a new subset. *J Am Acad Dermatol* 1995; **32**: 378–81.

58 Barnadas MA, Lopez D, Pujol RM et al. Pustular lymphomatoid papulosis in childhood. *J Am Acad Dermatol* 1992; **27**: 627.

59 Kato N, Matsue K. Follicular lymphomatoid papulosis. *Am J Dermatopathol* 1997; **19**: 189–96.

60 Pierard GE, Ackerman AB, Lapiere CM. Follicular lymphomatoid papulosis. *Am J Dermatopathol* 1980; **2**: 173–80.

61 Requena L, Sanchez M, Coca S, Sanchez Yus E. Follicular lymphomatoid papulosis. *Am J Dermatopathol* 1990; **12**: 67–75.

62 Atkins KA, Dahlem MM, Kohler S. A case of lymphomatoid papulosis with prominent myxoid change resembling a mesenchymal neoplasm. *Am J Dermatopathol* 2003; **25**: 62–5.

63 Baschinsky D, Magro CM, Kovatich A, Crowson AN. Eccrinotropic and neurotropic lymphomatoid papulosis (LyP): a novel variant. *Mod Pathol* 2001; **14**: 65.

64 Cespedes YP, Rockley PF, Flores F et al. Is there a special relationship between CD30-positive lymphoproliferative disorders and epidermal proliferation? *J Cutan Pathol* 2000; **27**: 271–5.

65 Scarisbrick JJ, Calonje E, Orchard G, Child FJ, Russell-Jones R. Pseudocarcinomatous change in lymphomatoid papulosis and primary cutaneous CD30⁺ lymphoma: a clinicopathologic and immunohistochemical study of 6 patients. *J Am Acad Dermatol* 2001; **44**: 239–47.

66 Guitart J, Gordon K. Keratoacanthomas and lymphomatoid papulosis. *Am J Dermatopathol* 1998; **20**: 430–2.

67 Kaudewitz P, Stein H, Burg G, Mason DY, Braun-Falco O. Atypical cells in lymphomatoid papulosis express the Hodgkin cell-associated antigen Ki-1. *J Invest Dermatol* 1986; **86**: 350–4.

68 Kadin ME. Characteristic immunologic profile of large atypical cells in lymphomatoid papulosis. *Arch Dermatol* 1986; **122**: 1388–90.

69 Kadin ME, Nasu K, Sako D, Said J, Vonderheid EC. Lymphomatoid papulosis: a cutaneous proliferation of activated helper T cells expressing Hodgkin's disease-associated antigens. *Am J Pathol* 1985; **119**: 315–25.

70 Kummer JA, Vermeer MH, Dukers D, Meijer CJLM, Willemze R. Most primary cutaneous CD30-positive lymphoproliferative disorders have a CD4-positive cytotoxic T-cell phenotype. *J Invest Dermatol* 1997; **109**: 636–40.

71 Jang KA, Choi JC, Choi JH. Expression of cutaneous lymphocyte-associated antigen and TIA-1 by lymphocytes in pityriasis lichenoides et varioliformis acuta and lymphomatoid papulosis: immunohistochemical study. *J Cutan Pathol* 2001; **28**: 453–9.

72 Boulland ML, Wechsler J, Bagot M et al. Primary CD30-positive cutaneous T-cell lymphomas and lymphomatoid papulosis frequently express cytotoxic proteins. *Histopathology* 2000; **36**: 136–44.

73 Harvell JD, Vaseghi M, Natkunam Y, Kohler S, Kim Y. Large atypical cells of lymphomatoid papulosis are CD56-negative: a study of 18 cases. *J Cutan Pathol* 2002; **29**: 88–92.

74 Bekkenk MW, Kluin PM, Jansen PM, Meijer CJLM, Willemze R. Lymphomatoid papulosis with a natural killer-cell phenotype. *Br J Dermatol* 2001; **145**: 318–22.

75 Natkunam Y, Warnke RA, Haghighi B et al. Co-expression of CD56 and CD30 in lymphomas with primary presentation in the skin: clinicopathologic, immunohistochemical and molecular analyses of seven cases. *J Cutan Pathol* 2000; **27**: 392–9.

76 Herbst H, Sander C, Tronnier M et al. Absence of anaplastic lymphoma kinase (ALK) and Epstein–Barr virus gene products in primary cutaneous anaplastic large cell lymphoma and lymphomatoid papulosis. *Br J Dermatol* 1997; **137**: 680–6.

77 Weiss LM, Wood GS, Trela M, Warnke RA, Sklar JL. Clonal T-cell populations in lymphomatoid papulosis: evidence for a lymphoproliferative origin for a clinically benign disease. *N Engl J Med* 1986; **315**: 475–9.

78 Steinhoff M, Hummel M, Anagnostopoulos I et al. Single-cell analysis of CD30⁺ cells in lymphomatoid papulosis demonstrates a common clonal T-cell origin. *Blood* 2002; **100**: 578–84.

79 Panhans A, Bodemer C, Macinthyre E et al. Pityriasis lichenoides of childhood with atypical CD30-positive cells and clonal T-cell receptor gene rearrangements. *J Am Acad Dermatol* 1996; **35**: 489–90.

80 Cerroni L. Lymphomatoid papulosis, pityriasis lichenoides et varioliformis acuta, and anaplastic large cell (Ki-1⁺) lymphoma. *J Am Acad Dermatol* 1997; **37**: 287.

81 Proctor SJ, Jackson GH, Lennard AL, Marks J. Lymphomatoid papulosis: response to treatment with recombinant interferon α-2b. *J Clin Oncol* 1992; **10**: 270.

82 Schmuth M, Topar G, Illersperger B et al. Therapeutic use of interferon-α for lymphomatoid papulosis. *Cancer* 2000; **89**: 1603–10.

83 Volkenandt M, Kerscher M, Sander CA, Meurer M, Rocken M. PUVA-bath photochemotherapy resulting in rapid clearance of lymphomatoid papulosis in a child. *Arch Dermatol* 1995; **131**: 1094.

84 Wyss M, Dummer R, Dommann SN et al. Lymphomatoid papulosis: treatment with recombinant interferon α-2a and etretinate. *Dermatology* 1995; **190**: 288–91.

85 Yagi H, Tokura Y, Furukawa F, Takigawa M. Th2 cytokine mRNA expression in primary cutaneous CD30-positive lymphoproliferative disorders: successful treatment with recombinant interferon-γ. *J Invest Dermatol* 1996; **107**: 827–32.

86 Vonderheid EC, Sajjadian A, Kadin ME. Methotrexate is effective therapy for lymphomatoid papulosis and other primary cutaneous CD30-positive lymphoproliferative disorders. *J Am Acad Dermatol* 1996; **34**: 470–81.

87 Bergstrom JS, Jaworsky C. Topical methotrexate for lymphomatoid papulosis. *J Am Acad Dermatol* 2003; **49**: 937–9.

88 Beylot-Barry M, Lamant L, Vergier B et al. Detection of t(2;5)(p23;q35) translocation by reverse transcriptase polymerase chain reaction and *in situ* hybridization in CD30-positive primary cutaneous lymphoma and lymphomatoid papulosis. *Am J Pathol* 1996; **149**: 483–92.

89 Beylot-Barry M, Groppi A, Vergier B, Pulford K, Merlio JP. Characterization of t(2;5) reciprocal transcripts and genomic breakpoints in CD30⁺ cutaneous lymphoproliferations. *Blood* 1998; **91**: 4668–76.

90 Krämer KU, Starz H, Balda BR. Primary cutaneous CD30-positive large T-cell lymphoma with secondary lymph node involvement

detected by sentinel lymphonodectomy. *Acta Derm Venereol (Stockh)* 2002; **82**: 73–4.

91 McCarty MJ, Vukelja SJ, Sausville EA *et al.* Lymphomatoid papulosis associated with Ki-1-positive anaplastic large cell lymphoma: a report of two cases and a review of the literature. *Cancer* 1994; **74**: 3051–8.

92 Aoki M, Nhmi Y, Takezaki S *et al.* CD30⁺ lymphoproliferative disorder: primary cutaneous anaplastic large cell lymphoma followed by lymphomatoid papulosis. *Br J Dermatol* 2001; **145**: 123–6.

93 LeBoit PE. Hodgkin's disease, anaplastic large cell lymphoma, and lymphomatoid papulosis: another scalpel blunted. *Am J Clin Pathol* 1995; **104**: 3–4.

94 Corazza M, Zampino MR, Montanari A, Altieri E, Virgili A. Primary cutaneous CD30⁺ large T-cell lymphoma in a patient with psoriasis treated with cyclosporine. *Dermatology* 2003; **206**: 330–3.

95 Kirby B, Owen CM, Blewitt RW, Yates VM. Cutaneous T-cell lymphoma developing in a patient on cyclosporin therapy. *J Am Acad Dermatol* 2002; **47**: S165–7.

96 Beylot-Barry M, Vergier B, Masquelier B *et al.* The spectrum of cutaneous lymphomas in HIV infection: a study of 21 cases. *Am J Surg Pathol* 1999; **23**: 1208–16.

97 Chadburn A, Cesarman E, Jagirdar J *et al.* CD30 (Ki-1) positive anaplastic large cell lymphomas in individuals infected with the human immunodeficiency virus. *Cancer* 1993; **72**: 3078–90.

98 Jhala DN, Medeiros LJ, Lopez-Terrada D *et al.* Neutrophil-rich anaplastic large cell lymphoma of T-cell lineage: a report of two cases arising in HIV-positive patients. *Am J Clin Pathol* 2000; **114**: 478–82.

99 Katano H, Suda T, Morishita Y *et al.* Human herpesvirus 8-associated solid lymphomas that occur in AIDS patients take anaplastic large cell morphology. *Mod Pathol* 2000; **13**: 77–85.

100 Gould JW, Eppes RB, Gilliam AC *et al.* Solitary primary cutaneous CD30⁺ large cell lymphoma of natural killer cell phenotype bearing the t(2;5)(p23;q35) translocation and presenting in a child. *Am J Dermatopathol* 2000; **22**: 422–8.

101 Meier F, Schaumburg-Lever G, Kaiserling E, Scheel-Walter H, Scherwitz C. Primary cutaneous large-cell anaplastic (Ki-1) lymphoma in a child. *J Am Acad Dermatol* 1992; **26**: 813–7.

102 Tomaszewski MM, Moad JC, Lupton GP. Primary cutaneous Ki-1 (CD30) positive anaplastic large cell lymphoma in childhood. *J Am Acad Dermatol* 1999; **40**: 857–61.

103 Bernier M, Bagot M, Broyer M *et al.* Distinctive clinicopathologic features associated with regressive primary CD30 positive cutaneous lymphomas: analysis of 6 cases. *J Cutan Pathol* 1997; **24**: 157–63.

104 Dereure O, Portales P, Balavoine M *et al.* Rare occurrence of CD30⁺ circulating cells in patients with cutaneous CD30⁺ anaplastic large cell lymphoma: a study of nine patients. *Br J Dermatol* 2003; **148**: 246–51.

105 Burg G, Kempf W, Kazakov DV *et al.* Pyogenic lymphoma of the skin: a peculiar variant of primary cutaneous neutrophil-rich CD30⁺ anaplastic large-cell lymphoma—clinicopathological study of four cases and review of the literature. *Br J Dermatol* 2003; **148**: 580–6.

106 Kato N, Mizuno O, Ito K, Kimura K, Shibata M. Neutrophil-rich anaplastic large cell lymphoma presenting in the skin. *Am J Dermatopathol* 2003; **25**: 142–7.

107 Monterroso V, Bujan W, Jaramillo O, Medeiros LJ. Subcutaneous tissue involvement by T-cell lymphoma: a report of 2 cases. *Arch Dermatol* 1996; **132**: 1345–50.

108 Chan JKC, Buchanan R, Fletcher CDM. Sarcomatoid variant of anaplastic large cell Ki1 lymphoma. *Am J Surg Pathol* 1990; **14**: 983–8.

109 Kikuchi A, Sakuraoka K, Kurihara S *et al.* CD8⁺ cutaneous anaplastic large cell-lymphoma: report of two cases with immunophenotyping, T-cell receptor gene rearrangement and electron microscopic studies. *Br J Dermatol* 1992; **126**: 404–8.

110 Su LD, Schnitzer B, Ross CW *et al.* The t(2;5)-associated p80 NPM/ALK fusion protein in nodal and cutaneous CD30⁺ lymphoproliferative disorders. *J Cutan Pathol* 1997; **24**: 597–603.

111 ten Berge RL, Oudejans JJ, Ossenkoppele GJ *et al.* ALK expression in extranodal anaplastic large cell lymphoma favours systemic disease with (primary) nodal involvement and a good prognosis and occurs before dissemination. *J Clin Pathol* 2000; **53**: 445–50.

112 Stein H, Foss HD, Dürkop H *et al.* CD30⁺ anaplastic large cell lymphoma: a review of its histopathologic, genetic, and clinical features. *Blood* 2000; **96**: 3681–95.

113 Felgar RE, Salhany KE, MacOn WR, Pietra GG, Kinney MC. The expression of TIA-1⁺ cytolytic type granules and other cytolytic lymphocyte-associated markers in CD30⁺ anaplastic large cell lymphomas (ALCL): correlation with morphology, immunophenotype, ultrastructure, and clinical features. *Hum Pathol* 1999; **30**: 228–36.

114 Gellrich S, Wilks A, Lukowsky A *et al.* T cell receptor-γ gene analysis of CD30⁺ large atypical individual cells in CD30⁺ large primary cutaneous T cell lymphomas. *J Invest Dermatol* 2003; **120**: 670–5.

115 Mao X, Orchard G, Lillington DM *et al.* Genetic alterations in primary cutaneous CD30⁺ anaplastic large cell lymphoma. *Genes Chromosomes Cancer* 2003; **37**: 176–85.

116 Böni R, Xin H, Kamarashev J *et al.* Allelic deletion at 9p21-22 in primary cutaneous CD30⁺ large cell lymphoma. *J Invest Dermatol* 2000; **115**: 1104–7.

117 Piccinno R, Caccialanza M, Berti E, Beretta M, Gnecchi L. Radiotherapy of primary cutaneous CD30-positive large cell lymphoma: a preliminary study of eight patients. *J Dermatol Treat* 1996; **7**: 183–5.

118 Vermeer MH, Bekkenk MW, Willemze R. Should primary cutaneous Ki-1 (CD30) -positive anaplastic large cell lymphoma in childhood be treated with multiple-agent chemotherapy? *J Am Acad Dermatol* 2001; **45**: 638–9.

119 Fatkenheuer G, Hell K, Roers A, Diehl V, Salzberger B. Spontaneous regression of HIV associated T-cell non-Hodgkin's lymphoma with highly active antiretroviral therapy. *Eur J Med Res* 2000; **5**: 236–40.

120 Liu HL, Hoppe RT, Kohler S *et al.* CD30⁺ cutaneous lymphoproliferative disorders: the Stanford experience in lymphomatoid papulosis and primary cutaneous anaplastic large cell lymphoma. *J Am Acad Dermatol* 2003; **49**: 1049–58.

121 Vergier B, Beylot-Barry M, Pulford K *et al.* Statistical evaluation of diagnostic and prognostic features of CD30⁺ cutaneous lymphoproliferative disorders: a clinicopathologic study of 56 cases. *Am J Surg Pathol* 1998; **22**: 1192–202.

Chapter 5 Subcutaneous T-cell lymphoma

A degree of involvement of subcutaneous fat by neoplastic lymphocytes is common in many primary or secondary cutaneous T- and B-cell lymphomas. One particular variant of T-cell lymphoma presents with predominant or exclusive involvement of the subcutaneous tissues and has been termed subcutaneous 'panniculitis-like' T-cell lymphoma in recent years [1,2]. In our view, the term 'panniculitis-like' is redundant and we will refer to this entity henceforth as 'subcutaneous T-cell lymphoma'. Subcutaneous T-cell lymphoma has been included as a provisional entity in the European Organization for Research and Treatment of Cancer (EORTC) classification of cutaneous lymphomas, and as a distinct entity in the World Health Organization (WHO) classification of haematopoietic neoplasms [1,2].

Some cases of subcutaneous T-cell lymphoma were classified in the past as malignant histiocytosis or histiocytic cytophagic panniculitis [3–13]. Soon after the first description, it became clear that many cases of histiocytic cytophagic panniculitis showed a monoclonal population of T lymphocytes, proving the lymphoid origin of the disease [10]. It subsequently became clear that histiocytic cytophagic panniculitis was not always fatal, as previously thought, and that cases with a good prognosis could be observed [7,11,14,15]. Not all cases of histiocytic cytophagic panniculitis are examples of subcutaneous T-cell lymphoma and some probably represent examples of γ/δ T-cell lymphoma or Epstein–Barr virus (EBV)-associated NK/T-cell lymphoma of nasal type. In fact, involvement of the subcutis is common in these types of lymphoma (see Chapter 6) [16–20]. It has also been demonstrated that some cases classified in the past as Weber–Christian panniculitis are examples of subcutaneous T-cell lymphoma [21,22].

It seems likely that at least some of the cases diagnosed in the past as lupus panniculitis (lupus erythematosus profundus) or 'benign panniculitis evolving into overt lymphoma' represent examples of subcutaneous T-cell lymphoma with a slow progression [22]. In this context, it has been proposed recently that lupus panniculitis and subcutaneous T-cell lymphoma represent two ends of a spectrum of the same entity [23]. However, we have never observed progression from true lupus panniculitis to subcutaneous T-cell lymphoma and strongly believe that these two entities are completely distinct (see also Chapter 20). Cases showing 'progression' were most likely examples of subcutaneous T-cell lymphoma from the outset.

The literature on subcutaneous T-cell lymphoma is confusing. In the past, based only on the involvement of the subcutis, many different types of lymphoma with different clinicopathological features and prognostic behaviour have been lumped together in this group, and the exact definition and diagnostic criteria remain unclear [18–20,22,24–38]. Moreover, any review of the literature is hindered by the fact that complete phenotypical investigations were not carried out in many of the cases described in the past (and even in recent years) and thus rely only on the involvement of the subcutis for diagnosis and classification. Association with EBV infection, too, has been observed irregularly. However, many overlapping features can be observed in the group of so-called 'cytotoxic lymphomas' (see Chapter 6), including subcutaneous involvement by neoplastic lymphocytes, and multiple parameters are required to classify a given case into a precise category [39]. In this chapter, we restrict the use of the term subcutaneous T-cell lymphoma to a malignant T-cell lymphoma characterized by *exclusive* involvement of the subcutaneous fat (no dermal and/or epidermal involvement), absence of EBV in neoplastic cells and T-$\alpha/\beta^+/CD8^+$ phenotype. In this way, a group of patients with relatively homogeneous clinicopathological, phenotypical and prognostic features can be identified.

It should be remembered that lesions with exclusive subcutaneous involvement have been observed in patients with mycosis fungoides [40]. An accurate clinical history should always be obtained in patients with a putative subcutaneous T-cell lymphoma, and any skin lesions clinically suspicious of mycosis fungoides should be biopsied. It must also be emphasized that a purely subcutaneous pattern ('lobular panniculitis-like') can be observed rarely in other cutaneous lymphomas of T- and B-cell phenotype and that a prominent involvement of the subcutis *per se* is not a sufficient criterion for the diagnosis of subcutaneous T-cell lymphoma [41,42].

Transmission of subcutaneous T-cell lymphoma by allogeneic bone marrow transplantation has been documented in a single case [43], and interferon-γ production by the neoplastic cells has been observed in a case with a γ/δ phenotype [24].

Clinical features

Exact characterization of the clinicopathological features of subcutaneous T-cell lymphoma is hindered by the different criteria used in the past for the diagnosis and classification of this disease.

Patients are adults of both sexes [1,2,44]. Reports in children exist but phenotypical data in some cases are incomplete [45,46]. A long history of 'benign panniculitis' is often present [22]. Clinically, patients present with solitary or multiple erythematous tumours or plaques, which are usually not ulcerated and are located most commonly on the extremities, especially the lower ones (Figs 5.1 & 5.2) [1,2,44]. Other sites of the body, including the head, may be affected (Fig. 5.3) [22,47]. Skin lesions are non-specific and may simulate erythema nodosum, lupus panniculitis or other panniculitic diseases. One patient with alopecic lesions on the scalp has also been described [48]. Spontaneous resolution of some of the

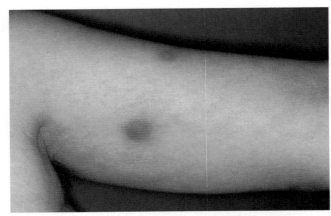

Fig. 5.2 Subcutaneous T-cell lymphoma. Erythematous nodule ('erythema nodosum-like') on the arm.

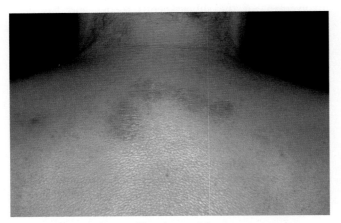

Fig. 5.3 Subcutaneous T-cell lymphoma. Subcutaneous tumour on the back.

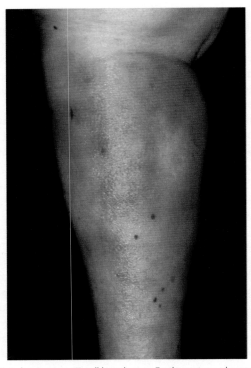

Fig. 5.1 Subcutaneous T-cell lymphoma. Erythematous plaques ('panniculitis-like') on the leg.

lesions may be observed [20,33]. In one patient, neoplastic T-lymphocytes have been detected in the peripheral blood [49].

In a subset of patients (probably a small minority) there are accompanying symptoms such as fever, malaise, fatigue and weight loss. A haemophagocytic syndrome may be seen in advanced stages, and can be the cause of death in these patients. The haemophagocytic syndrome is probably more common in the aggressive lymphomas with a γ/δ T-cell or NK-cell phenotype (see Chapter 6).

Histopathology, immunophenotype and molecular genetics

Histopathology

Histopathology reveals a dense, nodular or diffuse infiltrate of small, medium and large pleomorphic cells confined to the subcutaneous fat (Figs. 5.4 & 5.5). Perivascular aggregates of

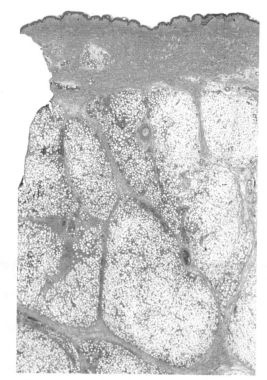

Fig. 5.4 Subcutaneous T-cell lymphoma. Dense infiltrate showing prominent involvement of the subcutaneous fat, mimicking the histopathological picture of a lobular panniculitis.

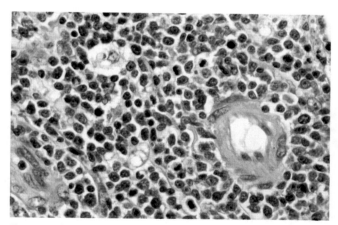

Fig. 5.5 Subcutaneous T-cell lymphoma. Infiltration of subcutaneous fat by small- to medium-sized pleomorphic lymphocytes.

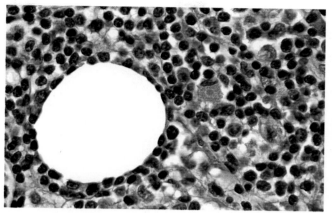

Fig. 5.6 Subcutaneous T-cell lymphoma. Note 'rimming' of an adipocyte by neoplastic lymphocytes. (Reprinted with permission from *The American Journal of Surgical Pathology*, in press.)

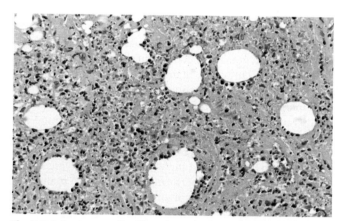

Fig. 5.7 Subcutaneous T-cell lymphoma. Prominent necrosis with several atypical lymphocytes left within the infiltrate.

non-neoplastic cells may be located within the reticular dermis, but clusters of neoplastic T lymphocytes are almost never situated outside the subcutaneous tissues. The epidermis is spared as a rule. Neoplastic cells within the subcutaneous fat are arranged in small clusters or as solitary units around the single adipocytes (so-called 'rimming' of the adipocytes) (Fig. 5.6). Necrosis is often a prominent feature,

and may completely mask the specific histopathological features (Fig. 5.7). A histiocytic infiltrate, often with the formation of granulomas, is also common [50,51]. In addition, reactive small lymphocytes can be admixed with the neoplastic cells but plasma cells and eosinophils are rare. Membranocystic (lipomembranous) lesions have been described in some cases [52,53].

In some lesions, the specific findings are confined to a small portion of the subcutaneous fat, thus rendering the examination of small biopsies (punch biopsies) problematic or even impossible (Fig. 5.8). In this context, it must be underlined that a diagnosis of subcutaneous T-cell lymphoma can only be made when large deep biopsies are available.

Immunophenotype

Immunohistological analysis shows an α/β T-suppressor phenotype (βF1+, CD3+, CD4−, CD8+) of neoplastic cells

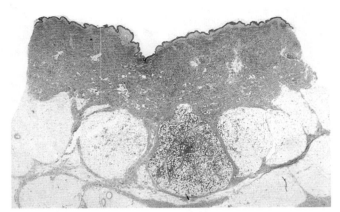

Fig. 5.8 Subcutaneous T-cell lymphoma. Focal involvement of the fat restricted to one lobule of adipocytes. According to the patient, this lesion was only a few days old; clinically, the overlying epidermis was normal but one could detect a subcutaneous induration.

(Fig. 5.9a) [37,54,55]. Cytotoxic markers are always expressed (TIA-1, granzyme B, perforin) [56], but CD56 is negative in $\alpha/\beta^+/CD8^+$ cases. Staining for CD30 is consistently negative in true subcutaneous T-cell lymphoma. Proliferation markers (MIB-1) highlight a characteristic pattern of proliferating cells arranged in small clusters and around the adipocytes (Fig. 5.9b) [55]. *In situ* hybridization for EBV is negative.

It should be emphasized that complete phenotypical analyses should always be performed in cases of malignant lymphoma with prominent involvement of the subcutis, and that only examination of a broad panel of antibodies allows a proper classification of the lesions. In fact, it is not uncommon to observe cases of B-cell lymphoma with the neoplastic infiltrate confined to the subcutaneous fat or cases of other T-cell lymphomas with similar architectural features (mycosis fungoides, anaplastic large cell lymphoma, cutaneous γ/δ T-cell lymphoma, nasal-type NK/T-cell lymphoma). Cases of T-cell lymphoma with involvement of the subcutaneous tissue and positive for γ/δ T-cell markers or for CD30, or with a positive signal for EBV by *in situ* hybridization, should be more appropriately classified as γ/δ cutaneous T-cell lymphoma, cutaneous anaplastic large cell lymphoma and nasal-type NK/T-cell lymphoma, respectively.

Molecular genetics

Molecular analysis of the T-cell receptor (TCR) genes shows a monoclonal rearrangement in the majority of cases [1,2,57]. Specific genetic features have not been identified.

Differential diagnosis

Subcutaneous T-cell lymphoma should be distinguished from other cutaneous NK/T-cell lymphomas with prominent involvement of the subcutaneous tissue. Rare cases of mycosis fungoides presenting with subcutaneous lesions can only be excluded by an accurate clinical history and clinicopathological correlation. In addition, mycosis fungoides usually shows a $CD4^+$ phenotype, in contrast to the $CD8^+$

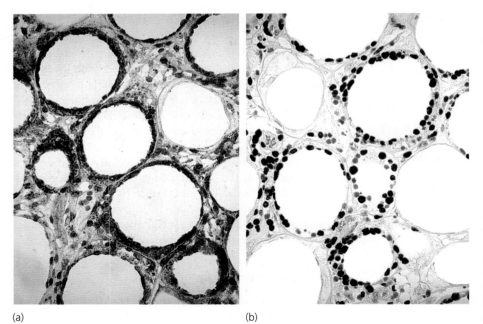

(a)　　　　　　　　　(b)

Fig. 5.9 Subcutaneous T-cell lymphoma. (a) Staining for CD8 demonstrates positivity of neoplastic lymphocytes around the adipocytes. (b) Staining for proliferating cells (MIB-1) is a helpful diagnostic tool, highlighting proliferating neoplastic lymphocytes around the adipocytes.

of subcutaneous T-cell lymphoma. The following features favour a diagnosis of cutaneous γ/δ T-cell lymphoma:
• Involvement of the dermis and/or the epidermis (often with marked epidermotropism) in the same biopsy or in sequential biopsies taken at the same time or over time.
• Negativity for α/β T-cell markers (markers for γ/δ T cells are available at present only for investigation of frozen sections of tissue).
• Positivity for CD56.

Features that favour the diagnosis of nasal-type NK/T-cell lymphoma are:
• Marked involvement of the dermis, more rarely also of the epidermis, in the same biopsy or in sequential biopsies taken at the same time or over time.
• Positivity for CD56.
• Positivity of *in situ* hybridization for EBV.
• Lack of monoclonal rearrangement of the TCR gene.

Treatment

Evaluation of different treatment schemes reported in the literature reflects the confusion concerning the classification of these cases. The extremely aggressive treatment modalities reported in some cases [58] are probably not necessary for patients with subcutaneous T-cell lymphoma as defined in this chapter. Systemic chemotherapy (CHOP or other schemes) and radiotherapy have been used in many instances [20,33,37,47,59]. Many patients can be controlled for long periods of time with systemic steroids [22]. Denileukin diftitox (Ontak, DAB_{389}–IL-2 fusion protein) has been used in one case, but phenotypical data were unavailable [60]. Complete remission has been achieved in one of two children with subcutaneous T-cell lymphoma treated by cyclosporine followed by chemotherapy [46]. The role of other treatment options (interferon, retinoids, low-dose methotrexate) has not been fully evaluated.

Prognosis

In the past it was believed that in most patients the course of subcutaneous T-cell lymphoma was rapidly fatal (we too stated this in the first edition of this book). Recent experience contradicts this and shows that many patients follow a protracted course with recurrent subcutaneous lesions but without extracutaneous spread or haemophagocytic syndrome, indicating that at least two groups of patients with different prognostic features can be identified [22,61]. Once more, exact appreciation of the prognosis of subcutaneous T-cell lymphoma is hindered by the confusion existent in the literature, and by the lack of proper phenotypical investigations

performed in many of the reported cases. Applying strictly the diagnostic criteria referred to in this chapter, the estimated 5-year survival is probably over 80%.

The onset of a haemophagocytic syndrome is a bad prognostic sign. In the literature, a worse prognosis has been observed in cases characterized by a γ/δ T-cell phenotype or associated with EBV infection [14,22,25,28,35,62]. We believe that these cases are better classified as cutaneous γ/δ T-cell lymphoma and nasal-type NK/T-cell lymphoma, respectively.

RÉSUMÉ

Clinical	Adults. Localized subcutaneous erythematous plaques and tumours arising preferentially on the lower extremities. Usually protracted course. In some patients a haemophagocytic syndrome occurs.
Morphology	Dense, nodular or diffuse infiltrates within the subcutaneous fat. 'Rimming' of adipocytes by neoplastic lymphocytes. Cytomorphology characterized by small- to medium-sized and large pleomorphic cells admixed with variable numbers of macrophages. Necrosis prominent.
Immunology	CD2, 3, 5 + CD8 + βF1 + CD4, 30, 56 – TIA-1 +
Genetics	Monoclonal rearrangement of the TCR genes detected in the majority of cases. No specific genetic alteration.
Treatment guidelines	Systemic steroids may be efficacious; systemic chemotherapy; radiotherapy.

References

1 Willemze R, Kerl H, Sterry W *et al.* EORTC classification for primary cutaneous lymphomas: a proposal from the Cutaneous Lymphoma Study Group of the European Organization for Research and Treatment of Cancer. *Blood* 1997; **90**: 354–71.

2 Jaffe ES, Ralfkiaer E. Subcutaneous panniculitis-like T-cell lymphoma. In: Jaffe ES, Harris NL, Stein H, Vardiman JW, eds. *World Health Organization Classification of Tumours: Tumours of Haematopoietic and Lymphoid Tissues.* Lyon: IARC Press, 2001: 212–5.

3 Winkelmann RK, Bowie EJW. Hemorrhagic diathesis associated with benign histiocytic, cytophagic panniculitis and systemic histiocytosis. *Arch Intern Med* 1980; **140**: 1460–3.

4 Alegre VA, Winkelmann RK. Histiocytic cytophagic panniculitis. *J Am Acad Dermatol* 1989; **20**: 177–85.

5 Aronson IK, West DP, Variakojis D *et al.* Panniculitis associated with cutaneous T-cell lymphoma and cytophagocytic histiocytosis. *Br J Dermatol* 1985; **112**: 87–96.

6 Barron DR, Davis BR, Pomeranz JR, Hines JD, Park CH. Cytophagic histiocytic panniculitis: a variant of malignant histiocytosis. *Cancer* 1985; **55**: 2538–42.

7 Craig AJ, Cualing H, Thomas G, Lamerson C, Smith R. Cytophagic histiocytic panniculitis: a syndrome associated with benign and malignant panniculitis—case comparison and review of the literature. *J Am Acad Dermatol* 1998; **39**: 721–36.

8 Crotty CP, Winkelmann RK. Cytophagic histiocytic panniculitis with fever, cytopenia, liver failure, and terminal hemorrhagic diathesis. *J Am Acad Dermatol* 1981; **4**: 181–94.

9 Huilgol SC, Fenton D, Pambakian H *et al.* Fatal cytophagic panniculitis and haemophagocytic syndrome. *Clin Exp Dermatol* 1998; **23**: 51–5.

10 Hytiroglou P, Phelps RG, Wattenberg DJ, Strauchen JA. Histiocytic cytophagic panniculitis: molecular evidence for a clonal T-cell disorder. *J Am Acad Dermatol* 1992; **27**: 333–6.

11 Willis SM, Opal SM, Fitzpatrick JE. Cytophagic histiocytic panniculitis: systemic histiocytosis presenting as chronic, non-healing, ulcerative skin lesions. *Arch Dermatol* 1985; **121**: 910–3.

12 Wick MR, Patterson JW. Cytophagic histiocytic panniculitis: a critical reappraisal. *Arch Dermatol* 2000; **136**: 922–4.

13 Wick MR, Sanchez NP, Crotty CP, Winkelmann RK. Cutaneous malignant histiocytosis: a clinical and histopathologic study of eight cases, with immunohistochemical analysis. *J Am Acad Dermatol* 1999; **8**: 50–62.

14 Iwatsuki K, Harada H, Ohtsuka M, Han G, Kaneko F. Latent Epstein–Barr virus infection is frequently detected in subcutaneous lymphoma associated with hemophagocytosis but not in non-fatal cytophagic histiocytic panniculitis. *Arch Dermatol* 1997; **133**: 787–8.

15 White JW Jr, Winkelmann RK. Cytophagic histiocytic panniculitis is not always fatal. *J Cutan Pathol* 1989; **16**: 137–44.

16 Arnulf B, Copie-Bergman C, Delfau-Larue MH *et al.* Non-hepatosplenic γ/δ T-cell lymphoma: a subset of cytotoxic lymphomas with mucosal or skin localization. *Blood* 1998; **91**: 1723–31.

17 Chan JKC. Peripheral T-cell and NK-cell neoplasms: an integrated approach to diagnosis. *Mod Pathol* 1999; **12**: 177–99.

18 Kim YC, Kim SC, Yang WI, Go JH, Vandersteen DP. Extranodal NK/T-cell lymphoma with extensive subcutaneous involvement, mimicking subcutaneous panniculitis-like T cell lymphoma. *Int J Dermatol* 2002; **41**: 919–21.

19 Munn SE, McGregor JM, Jones A *et al.* Clinical and pathological heterogeneity in cutaneous γ/δ T-cell lymphoma: a report of three cases and a review of the literature. *Br J Dermatol* 1996; **135**: 976–81.

20 Santucci M, Pimpinelli N, Massi D *et al.* Cytotoxic/natural killer cell cutaneous lymphomas: report of the EORTC cutaneous lymphoma task force workshop. *Cancer* 2003; **97**: 610–27.

21 White JW Jr, Winkelmann RK. Weber–Christian panniculitis: a review of 30 cases with this diagnosis. *J Am Acad Dermatol* 1998; **39**: 56–62.

22 Hoque SR, Child FJ, Whittaker SJ *et al.* Subcutaneous panniculitis-like T-cell lymphoma: a clinicopathological, immunophenotypic and molecular analysis of six patients. *Br J Dermatol* 2003; **148**: 516–25.

23 Magro CM, Crowson AN, Kovatich AJ, Burns F. Lupus profundus, indeterminate lymphocytic lobular panniculitis and subcutaneous T-cell lymphoma: a spectrum of subcuticular T-cell lymphoid dyscrasia. *J Cutan Pathol* 2001; **28**: 235–47.

24 Burg G, Dummer R, Wilhelm M *et al.* A subcutaneous δ-positive T cell lymphoma that produces interferon γ. *N Engl J Med* 1991; **325**: 1078–81.

25 Chang SE, Huh J, Choi JH *et al.* Clinicopathological features of CD56+ nasal-type T/natural killer cell lymphomas with lobular panniculitis. *Br J Dermatol* 2000; **142**: 924–30.

26 Dargent JL, Roufosse C, Delville JP *et al.* Subcutaneous panniculitis-like T-cell lymphoma: further evidence for a distinct neoplasm originating from large granular lymphocytes of T/NK phenotype. *J Cutan Pathol* 1998; **25**: 394–400.

27 Gonzalez CL, Medeiros LJ, Braziel RM, Jaffe ES. T-cell lymphoma involving subcutaneous tissue: a clinicopathologic entity commonly associated with hemophagocytic syndrome. *Am J Surg Pathol* 1991; **15**: 17–27.

28 Avinoach I, Halevy S, Argov S, Sacks M. γ/δ T-cell lymphoma involving the subcutaneous tissue and associated with a hemophagocytic syndrome. *Am J Dermatopathol* 1994; **16**: 426–33.

29 Jang KA, Choi JH, Sung KJ *et al.* Primary CD56+ nasal-type T/natural killer-cell subcutaneous panniculitic lymphoma: presentation as haemophagocytic syndrome. *Br J Dermatol* 1999; **141**: 706–9.

30 Kumar S, Krenacs L, Medeiros J *et al.* Subcutaneous panniculitic T-cell lymphoma is a tumor of cytotoxic T lymphocytes. *Hum Pathol* 1998; **29**: 397–403.

31 Mehregan DA, Su WPD, Kurtin PJ. Subcutaneous T-cell lymphoma: a clinical, histopathologic, and immunohistochemical study of six cases. *J Cutan Pathol* 1994; **21**: 110–7.

32 Monterroso V, Bujan W, Jaramillo O, Medeiros LJ. Subcutaneous tissue involvement by T-cell lymphoma: a report of 2 cases. *Arch Dermatol* 1996; **132**: 1345–50.

33 Perniciaro C, Zalla MJ, White JW Jr, Menke DM. Subcutaneous T cell lymphoma: report of two additional cases and further observations. *Arch Dermatol* 1993; **129**: 1171–6.

34 Romero LS, Goltz RW, Nagi C, Shin SS, Ho AD. Subcutaneous T-cell lymphoma with associated hemophagocytic syndrome and terminal leukemic transformation. *J Am Acad Dermatol* 1996; **34**: 904–10.

35 Salhany KE, MacOn WR, Choi JK *et al.* Subcutaneous panniculitis-like T-cell lymphoma: clinicopathologic, immunophenotypic, and genotypic analysis of α/β and γ/δ subtypes. *Am J Surg Pathol* 1998; **22**: 881–93.

36 von den Driesch P, Staib G, Simon M Jr, Sterry W. Subcutaneous T-cell lymphoma. *J Am Acad Dermatol* 1997; **36**: 285–9.

37 Wang CY, Su WP, Kurtin PJ. Subcutaneous panniculitic T-cell lymphoma. *Int J Dermatol* 1996; **35**: 1–8.

38 Marzano AV, Berti E, Paulli M, Caputo R. Cytophagic histiocytic panniculitis and subcutaneous panniculitis-like T-cell lymphoma. *Arch Dermatol* 2000; **136**: 889–96.

39 Kinney MC. The role of morphologic features, phenotype, genotype, and anatomic site in defining extranodal T-cell or NK-cell neoplasms. *Am J Clin Pathol* 1999; **111**: S104–18.

40 Proctor MS, Price NM, Cox AJ, Hoppe RT. Subcutaneous mycosis fungoides. *Arch Dermatol* 1978; **114**: 1326–8.

41 Cerroni L. Subcutaneous immunocytoma. *Dermatopathol Pract Concept* 2000; **6**: 87–8.

42 Marzano AV, Alessi E, Berti E. CD30-positive multilobated peripheral T-cell lymphoma primarily involving the subcutaneous tissue. *Am J Dermatopathol* 1997; **19**: 284–8.

43 Berg KD, Brinster NK, Huhn KM *et al.* Transmission of a T-cell lymphoma by allogeneic bone marrow transplantation. *N Engl J Med* 2001; **345**: 1458–63.

44 Fink-Puches R, Zenahlik P, Bäck B *et al.* Primary cutaneous lymphomas: applicability of current classification schemes (European Organization for Research and Treatment of Cancer, World Health Organization) based on clinicopathologic features observed in a large group of patients. *Blood* 2002; **99**: 800–5.

45 Taniguchi S, Kono T. Subcutaneous T-cell lymphoma in a child with eosinophilia. *Br J Dermatol* 2000; **142**: 183–4.

46 Shani-Adir A, Lucky AW, Prendiville J *et al.* Subcutaneous panniculitic T-cell lymphoma in children: response to combination therapy with cyclosporine and chemotherapy. *J Am Acad Dermatol* 2004; **50**: S18–22.

47 Au WY, Ng WM, Choy C, Kwong YL. Aggressive subcutaneous panniculitis-like T-cell lymphoma: complete remission with fludarabine, mitoxantrone and dexamethasone. *Br J Dermatol* 2000; **143**: 408–10.

48 Török L, Gurbity TP, Kirschner A, Krenacs L. Panniculitis-like T-cell lymphoma clinically manifested as alopecia. *Br J Dermatol* 2002; **147**: 785–8.

49 Nishie W, Yokota K, Sawamura D *et al.* Detection of circulating lymphoma cells in subcutaneous panniculitis-like T-cell lymphoma. *Br J Dermatol* 2003; **149**: 1081–2.

50 Scarabello A, Leinweber B, Ardigó M *et al.* Cutaneous lymphomas with prominent granulomatous reaction: a potential pitfall in the histopathologic diagnosis of cutaneous T- and B-cell lymphomas. *Am J Surg Pathol* 2002; **26**: 1259–68.

51 Prescott RJ, Banerjee SS, Cross PA. Subcutaneous T-cell lymphoma with florid granulomatous panniculitis. *Histopathology* 1992; **20**: 535–7.

52 Ohtake N, Shimada S, Mizoguchi S, Setoyama M, Kanzaki T. Membranocystic lesions in a patient with cytophagic histiocytic panniculitis associated with subcutaneous T-cell lymphoma. *Am J Dermatopathol* 1998; **20**: 276–80.

53 Weenig RH, Ng CS, Perniciaro C. Subcutaneous panniculitis-like T-cell lymphoma: an elusive case presenting as lipomembranous panniculitis and a review of 72 cases in the literature. *Am J Dermatopathol* 2001; **23**: 206–15.

54 El-Shabrawi-Caelen L, Cerroni L, Kerl H. The clinicopathologic spectrum of cytotoxic lymphomas of the skin. *Semin Cutan Med Surg* 2000; **19**: 118–23.

55 Cerroni L, Kerl H. Diagnostic immunohistology: cutaneous lymphomas and pseudolymphomas. *Semin Cutan Med Surg* 1999; **18**: 64–70.

56 Felgar RE, MacOn WR, Kinney MC *et al.* TIA-1 expression in lymphoid neoplasms: identification of subsets with cytotoxic T lymphocyte or natural killer cell differentiation. *Am J Pathol* 1997; **150**: 1893–900.

57 Kadin ME. Genetic and molecular genetic studies in the diagnosis of T-cell malignancies. *Hum Pathol* 2003; **34**: 322–9.

58 Haycox CL, Back AL, Raugi GJ, Piepkorn M. Subcutaneous T-cell lymphoma treated with systemic chemotherapy, autologous stem cell support, and limb amputation. *J Am Acad Dermatol* 1997; **37**: 832–5.

59 McGinnis KS, Shapiro M, Junkins-Hopkins JM *et al.* Denileukin diftitox for the treatment of panniculitic lymphoma. *Arch Dermatol* 2002; **138**: 740–2.

60 Cho KH, Oh JK, Kim CW, Heo DS, Kim ST. Peripheral T-cell lymphoma involving subcutaneous tissue. *Br J Dermatol* 1995; **132**: 290–5.

61 Burg G, Dummer R, Nestle F. Distinct subtypes of subcutaneous T-cell lymphoma. *Arch Dermatol* 1994; **130**: 1073.

62 Abe Y, Muta K, Ohshima K *et al.* Subcutaneous panniculitis by Epstein–Barr virus-infected natural killer (NK) cell proliferation terminating in aggressive subcutaneous NK cell lymphoma. *Am J Hematol* 2000; **64**: 221–5.

Chapter 6 Other cutaneous cytotoxic lymphomas

Cytotoxic lymphomas are tumours derived from T or natural killer (NK) lymphocytes with a cytotoxic phenotype. Neoplastic cells typically express at least one cytotoxic protein such as T-cell intracellular antigen-1 (TIA-1), granzyme B or perforin, and show a variable expression of CD56 [1–8]. Although cytotoxic NK/T-cell lymphomas are commonly described as aggressive neoplasms, the expression of cytotoxic proteins themselves is not restricted to a specific group of lymphomas, as they can be observed in cases of mycosis fungoides (rarely in early lesions, more commonly in late stages of the disease; see Chapter 2), and commonly in the so-called CD30+ cutaneous lymphoproliferative disorders (see Chapter 4). Expression of cytotoxic proteins is also the rule in cases of subcutaneous T-cell lymphoma (see Chapter 5). In short, cytotoxic proteins do not have any diagnostic or prognostic value *per se*, and their expression should be evaluated in the context of the clinicopathological and molecular features of the lesions. It has been shown recently that the expression of cytotoxic proteins and inhibitory receptors varies in different types of cytotoxic lymphomas, suggesting that they may differ with regard to their functional profiles [9].

We would also like to stress that these lymphomas show many overlapping clinicopathological features and that classification may be subjective in some cases. In particular, distinction from mycosis fungoides and from subcutaneous T-cell lymphoma can be difficult (see Chapters 2 and 5). Moreover, in spite of extensive phenotypical and genotypical studies, a few cases defy precise classification [8,10].

It is important to emphasize that for most of these lymphomas, cytomorphological features are variable and are not associated with prognostic features. In addition, cytomorphology is similar in all of these entities, and may be characterized by predominance of small-, medium- or large-sized cells (usually with pleomorphic nuclei). Thus, cytomorphological aspects are neither useful for a specific diagnosis and classification of the lymphoma, nor are a feature associated with the biological behaviour, and should always be analysed together with all other clinical, histopathological, phenotypical and molecular genetic features.

Finally, it should be emphasized that distinguishing between primary and secondary cutaneous involvement is less important for this group of tumours than for most other skin lymphomas [8,11]. In fact, cases with a primary cutaneous presentation usually develop extracutaneous dissemination within a short period of time, and the prognosis is usually very poor, regardless of the results of staging investigations at presentation.

EPIDERMOTROPIC CD8+ CUTANEOUS T-CELL LYMPHOMA

Epidermotropic CD8+ cutaneous T-cell lymphoma is a disease characterized by aggressive behaviour clinically, and proliferation of epidermotropic CD8+ T lymphocytes histopathologically [12]. Distinction from the rare cases of CD8+ mycosis fungoides (see Chapter 2) is made exclusively on the basis of the clinical presentation and behaviour. In contrast to mycosis fungoides, patients with epidermotropic CD8+ cutaneous T-cell lymphoma present with plaques and tumours, often ulcerated, at the onset of their disease [12–14].

In the past, cases of epidermotropic CD8+ cutaneous T-cell lymphoma were classified as either aggressive mycosis fungoides or generalized pagetoid reticulosis (Ketron–Goodman type), or mycosis fungoides 'a tumeur d'emblee'. In the European Organization for Research and Treatment of Cancer (EORTC) and the World Health Organization (WHO) classifications, epidermotropic CD8+ cutaneous T-cell lymphoma is not listed as a specific entity. In the EORTC classification, depending on the size of the tumour cells, it would be classified either as a cutaneous CD30− large T-cell lymphoma or as a small–medium pleomorphic T-cell lymphoma [15]; in the WHO classification, it would be classified as a peripheral T-cell lymphoma, unspecified [6].

Clinical features

Patients are usually adults of both sexes, possibly with a small male predominance [5,12]. They present with generalized

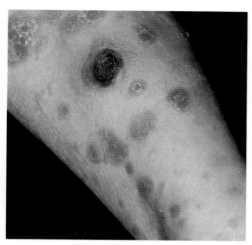

Fig. 6.1 Epidermotropic CD8+ cutaneous T-cell lymphoma. Multiple plaques and ulcerated tumours on the arm. (Reprinted with permission from *The American Journal of Surgical Pathology*, in press.)

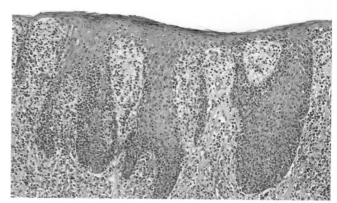

Fig. 6.3 Epidermotropic CD8+ cutaneous T-cell lymphoma. Hyperplastic epidermis with many epidermotropic lymphocytes. (Reprinted with permission from *The American Journal of Surgical Pathology*, in press.)

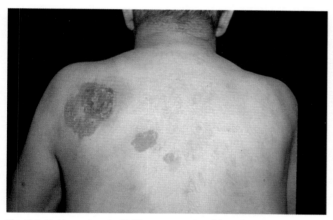

Fig. 6.2 Epidermotropic CD8+ cutaneous T-cell lymphoma. Multiple plaques and flat tumours with large erosions. The clinical presentation is identical to that described in the past as generalized pagetoid reticulosis (Ketron–Goodman type).

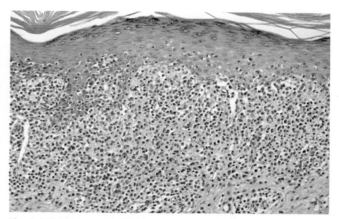

Fig. 6.4 Epidermotropic CD8+ cutaneous T-cell lymphoma. Epidermotropism is less marked in this case.

Histopathology, immunophenotype and molecular genetics

Histopathology

patches, plaques and tumours, almost invariably with ulceration (Figs 6.1 & 6.2). The clinical features are indistinguishable from those observed in patients with cutaneous γ/δ-positive T-cell lymphoma, and are identical to those of generalized pagetoid reticulosis (and of advanced mycosis fungoides). Involvement of the mucosal regions is common [12,16].

A rare clinical presentation with hydroa vacciniformis-like lesions has been described in paediatric patients [17–19].

For a diagnosis of epidermotropic CD8+ cutaneous T-cell lymphoma, it is crucial to exclude a history of mycosis fungoides. Lesions of lymphomatoid papulosis with a CD8+ phenotype should also be ruled out (see Chapter 4).

Histology reveals a nodular or diffuse proliferation of lymphocytes, usually with marked epidermotropism (Fig. 6.3). In spite of the name of this lymphoma, the epidermotropism may be less pronounced in some lesions, especially in advanced stages (Fig. 6.4). As in all aggressive cutaneous lymphomas, invasion and destruction of adnexal skin structures are common (Fig. 6.5). Cytomorphology is variable and can be characterized by small-, medium- or large-sized pleomorphic cells (Fig. 6.6). Some cases may show a predominance of immunoblasts. Intraepidermal vesiculation and necrosis can be seen. Angiocentricity and angiodestruction are uncommon.

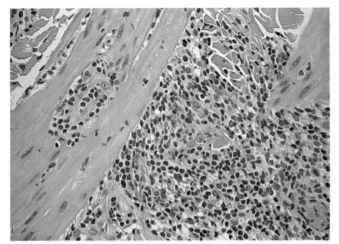

Fig. 6.5 Epidermotropic CD8⁺ cutaneous T-cell lymphoma. Pleomorphic lymphocytes predominate. Note invasion of a smooth muscle.

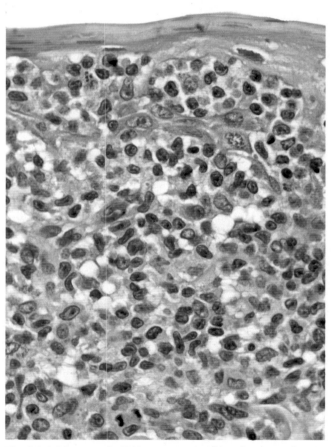

Fig. 6.6 Epidermotropic CD8⁺ cutaneous T-cell lymphoma. Medium–large pleomorphic lymphocytes with epidermotropism.

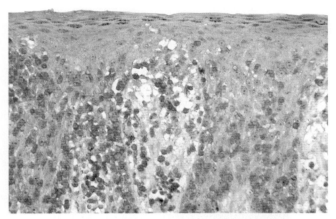

Fig. 6.7 Epidermotropic CD8⁺ cutaneous T-cell lymphoma. Staining for CD8 highlights the epidermotropic lymphocytes.

Cases of CD8⁺ T-cell lymphoma with exclusive involvement of the subcutis should be classified as subcutaneous T-cell lymphomas (see Chapter 5).

Distinction of epidermotropic CD8⁺ cutaneous T-cell lymphomas from cutaneous γ/δ T-cell lymphomas is difficult and often determined on an arbitrary basis. We prefer to classify those cases with a γ/δ phenotype independently as they usually show a more prominent involvement of the subcutaneous fat than cases of epidermotropic CD8⁺ cutaneous T-cell lymphoma. Another differential feature is the presence of a marked interface dermatitis in many cases of cutaneous γ/δ T-cell lymphoma. However, it remains to be determined whether or not these two diseases represent phenotypical variations of the same entity.

Immunophenotype

Immunohistology reveals a characteristic phenotypical profile of neoplastic lymphocytes (βF1⁺, CD3⁺, CD4⁻, CD7⁺, CD8⁺, TIA-1⁺, CD45RA⁺, CD45RO⁻) (Fig. 6.7) [12]. Some pan-T-cell markers may be lost. In the original description by Berti *et al.*, CD56 was consistently negative [12], but CD56⁺ cases classified as epidermotropic CD8⁺ cutaneous T-cell lymphoma have been described recently by Santucci *et al.* [2]. However, in this last paper, cutaneous γ/δ T-cell lymphoma was not included as a specific category, and it may be that these cases represented examples of this type of lymphoma.

The Epstein–Barr virus (EBV) is not detectable in neoplastic cells.

Molecular genetics

Molecular biology shows a monoclonal rearrangement of the T-cell receptor (TCR) gene. No specific genetic alterations have been described.

Treatment

The treatment of choice is systemic chemotherapy.

Prognosis

The prognosis of patients with epidermotropic CD8+ cutaneous T-cell lymphoma is poor, and the estimated 5-year survival is 0% [5,12]. The disease often metastasizes to unusual sites such as the lung, testis and central nervous system.

RÉSUMÉ

Epidermotropic CD8+ cutaneous T-cell lymphoma

Clinical	Adults. Generalized plaques and tumours, commonly ulcerated. Aggressive course. Involvement of mucosal sites. No previous history of mycosis fungoides.
Morphology	Nodular or diffuse infiltrates characterized by small-, medium- or large-sized pleomorphic cells or immunoblasts. Prominent epidermotropism.
Immunology	CD3, 7, 8, 45RA + βF1 + CD4, 30 – CD56 – TIA-1 +
Genetics	Monoclonal rearrangement of the TCR genes detected in the majority of cases. No specific genetic alteration.
Treatment guidelines	Systemic chemotherapy.

CUTANEOUS γ/δ T-CELL LYMPHOMA

Cutaneous γ/δ T-cell lymphoma is a tumour of γ/δ T lymphocytes with specific tropism for the skin [20–25]. The precise definition and characterization of this lymphoma are hindered by the overlapping features with many other cutaneous lymphoma entities, especially with subcutaneous T-cell lymphoma and epidermotropic CD8+ cutaneous T-cell lymphoma (see Chapter 5 and Epidermotropic CD8+ cutaneous T-cell lymphoma, above). Even the existence of cutaneous γ/δ T-cell lymphoma as a specific entity is debated [26–28]. In the EORTC classification, depending on the size of the tumour cells and the distribution of the infiltrate, these cases would be classified as CD30− large T-cell lymphoma, subcutaneous 'panniculitis-like' T-cell lymphoma or small–medium pleomorphic T-cell lymphoma [15]. In the WHO classification they would be classified as peripheral T-cell lymphoma, unspecified, or subcutaneous 'panniculitis-like' T-cell lymphoma [6].

In the past, cases of cutaneous γ/δ T-cell lymphoma were classified as either aggressive mycosis fungoides or generalized pagetoid reticulosis (Ketron–Goodman type), or mycosis fungoides 'a tumeur d'emblee' [8,29]. Distinction from classical mycosis fungoides with a rare γ/δ T-cell phenotype (see Chapter 2) is made exclusively on the basis of the clinical presentation and behaviour. In contrast to 'classic' mycosis fungoides, patients with cutaneous γ/δ T-cell lymphoma present at the onset with rapidly growing, disseminated patches, plaques and tumours, which are often ulcerated. For cutaneous γ/δ T-cell lymphoma, as for CD8+ cutaneous T-cell lymphomas, two main subtypes have been identified in the literature: the first characterized by rapidly progressive disease and poor prognosis (representing true cutaneous γ/δ T-cell lymphoma), the second showing a chronic course and better prognosis (this last representing mycosis fungoides) [28]. It must be stressed that the importance of an α/β vs. a γ/δ T-cell subset antigen expression in the classification of peripheral T-cell lymphomas is still unclear.

Because of the frequent prominent involvement of subcutaneous tissues, many cases of cutaneous γ/δ T-cell lymphoma are classified as subcutaneous T-cell lymphomas (see Chapter 5). However, γ/δ T-cell lymphoma almost invariably shows prominent involvement of the epidermis, either in the same biopsy specimen or in other biopsies taken at the same time or during the course of the disease. A typical example is represented by the patient pictured in Fig. 6.8, who was included in the chapter on subcutaneous T-cell lymphomas in the first edition of this book (see Figs 7.1 & 7.2 of that edition). The same patient was included as an example of 'malignant histiocytosis' in the book on cutaneous lymphomas by Burg and Braun-Falco in 1983 [30]; this case clearly shows how these unusual lymphomas are reclassified over time, thanks to new phenotypical and molecular studies that allow us to define more specific categories and to classify the cases more precisely. As already stated in Chapter 5, these authors believe that cutaneous γ/δ T-cell lymphoma should be distinguished and separated from the less aggressive subcutaneous T-cell lymphoma.

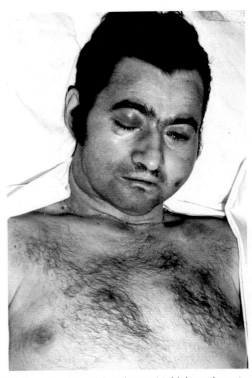

Fig. 6.8 Cutaneous γ/δ T-cell lymphoma. Multiple erythematous plaques and tumours on the trunk and face. Histopathological features of two lesions from this patient are depicted in Figs 6.12 and 6.13. This patient was included within the 'subcutaneous T-cell lymphomas' in the first edition of our book (Figs 7.1 & 7.2 of that edition), but upon reclassification of skin biopsies revealed the typical features of cutaneous γ/δ T-cell lymphoma.

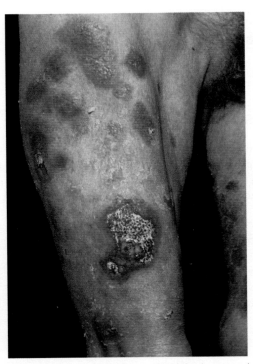

Fig. 6.9 Cutaneous γ/δ T-cell lymphoma. Multiple plaques and tumours, some ulcerated, on the leg.

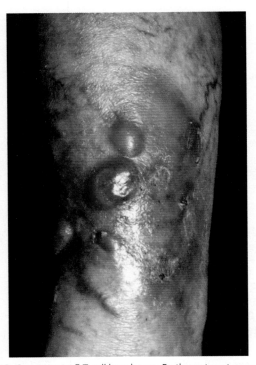

Fig. 6.10 Cutaneous γ/δ T-cell lymphoma. Erythematous tumours surrounded by red–brownish flat lesions resembling clinically lesions of severe interface dermatitis.

Clinical features

Patients are adults, with an equal distribution of males and females. They present with generalized patches, plaques and tumours, which are often ulcerated (Figs 6.8 & 6.9). Large solitary tumours may also be seen. The clinical features are similar to those observed in patients with epidermotropic CD8+ cutaneous T-cell lymphoma or with generalized page-toid reticulosis. The patches of the disease, unlike the common patches of mycosis fungoides, reveal the clinical features of severe interface dermatitis with a red–brown aspect and small superficial erosions (Fig. 6.10). Involvement of the mucosal regions and other locations unusual for mycosis fungoides is common (Fig. 6.11). Haemophagocytic syndrome is a frequent complication.

For a diagnosis of cutaneous γ/δ T-cell lymphoma, it is crucial to exclude a history of mycosis fungoides.

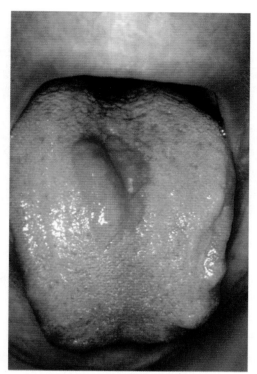

Fig. 6.11 Cutaneous γ/δ T-cell lymphoma. Large tumour on the tongue.

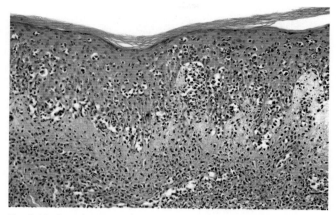

Fig. 6.12 Cutaneous γ/δ T-cell lymphoma. Markedly epidermotropic infiltrate. Note oedema of the papillary dermis (same patient as Figs 6.8 and 6.13).

Histopathology, immunophenotype and molecular genetics

Histopathology

Histology reveals a proliferation of lymphocytes, usually with both marked epidermotropism and involvement of the subcutaneous tissues (Figs 6.12 & 6.13). Cytomorphology is variable and can be characterized by small-, medium- or large-sized pleomorphic cells (Fig. 6.14). Intraepidermal vesiculation and necrosis can be seen. Angiocentricity and/or angiodestruction are commonly seen (Fig. 6.15). The presence of large macrophages engulfing neoplastic lymphocytes or other blood cells can be seen in cases with a haemophagocytic syndrome (Fig. 6.16).

Although epidermotropic lesions may resemble those observed in mycosis fungoides, unlike mycosis fungoides cutaneous γ/δ T-cell lymphoma is often characterized by the presence within the papillary dermis of prominent oedema rather than of fibrosis and coarse bundles of collagen (Fig. 6.12), probably reflecting the different biology of the lesions (acute rapid onset in cutaneous γ/δ T-cell lymphoma, chronic lesions in mycosis fungoides).

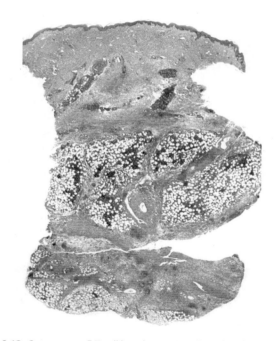

Fig. 6.13 Cutaneous γ/δ T-cell lymphoma. Prominent involvement of the subcutaneous fat (same patient as Figs 6.8 and 6.12).

The distinction of cutaneous γ/δ T-cell lymphoma from epidermotropic CD8+ cutaneous T-cell lymphoma is difficult, and can be subjective (see above). We prefer to classify lesions with γ/δ T-cell phenotype as cutaneous γ/δ T-cell lymphoma; these cases usually show a more prominent involvement of the subcutaneous fat than those of epidermotropic CD8+ cutaneous T-cell lymphoma. Another differential feature is the presence of a marked interface dermatitis in many

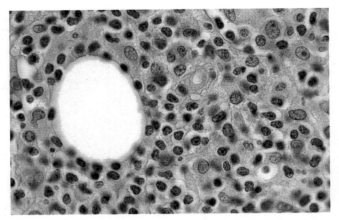

Fig. 6.14 Cutaneous γ/δ T-cell lymphoma. Predominance of medium- and large-sized lymphocytes.

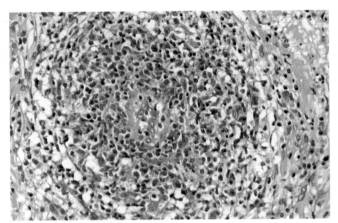

Fig. 6.15 Cutaneous γ/δ T-cell lymphoma. Prominent angiocentricity with early angiodestruction. Note pleomorphic lymphocytes.

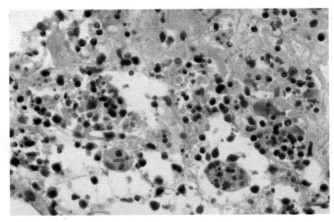

Fig. 6.16 Cutaneous γ/δ T-cell lymphoma. Haemophagocytosis characterized by large histiocytes engulfing leucocytes. This histopathological feature may be associated with overt haemophagocytic syndrome.

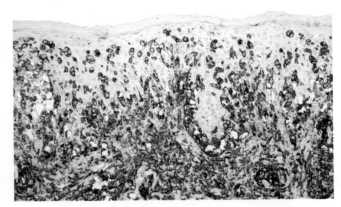

Fig. 6.17 Cutaneous γ/δ T-cell lymphoma. Strong positivity of neoplastic cells for CD56.

cases of cutaneous γ/δ T-cell lymphoma, but not in those of epidermotropic CD8⁺ cutaneous T-cell lymphoma.

Immunophenotype

Immunohistology reveals a characteristic phenotypical profile of neoplastic lymphocytes (βF1⁻, CD3⁺, TIA-1⁺, CD56⁺, CD57⁻) (Fig. 6.17). CD4 is absent, although CD8 may be expressed in some cases. Immunohistology on frozen sections reveals positivity for δ1. Some pan-T-cell markers may be lost.

EBV is not present in the neoplastic cells.

Molecular genetics

Molecular biology shows a monoclonal rearrangement of the TCR genes. No specific genetic alterations have been described.

Treatment

The treatment of choice is systemic chemotherapy.

Prognosis

The prognosis of patients with cutaneous γ/δ T-cell lymphoma is poor. It has been shown that expression of the γ/δ phenotype is a bad prognostic indicator in cutaneous T-cell lymphomas, irrespective of the classification (mycosis fungoides, subcutaneous T-cell lymphoma, epidermotropic CD8⁺ T-cell lymphoma) [31]. In patients with cutaneous γ/δ T-cell lymphoma, involvement of the subcutaneous fat tissues seems to be a bad prognostic factor [31].

Recently it has been proposed that expression of human leucocyte antigen G (HLA-G) and interleukin 10 (IL-10) may be one of the factors accounting for evosion of immuno-surveillance by neoplastic cells in CD8+ and CD56+ cutaneous T-cell lymphomas, thus contributing to their aggressive behavior [32].

RÉSUMÉ

Cutaneous γ/δ T-cell lymphoma

Clinical	Adults, rarely children. Generalized plaques and tumours, commonly ulcerated. Aggressive course. No previous history of mycosis fungoides.
Morphology	Nodular or diffuse infiltrates characterized by small- to medium- or large-sized pleomorphic cells. Subcutaneous fat commonly involved. Prominent epidermotropism.
Immunology	CD3, 5 + δ1 (frozen) + βF1 − CD4, 30 − CD8 − (+) TIA-1 +
Genetics	Monoclonal rearrangement of the TCR-γ gene detected in the majority of cases. No specific genetic alteration.
Treatment guidelines	Systemic chemotherapy.

EXTRANODAL NK/T-CELL LYMPHOMA, NASAL TYPE

Extranodal NK/T-cell lymphoma, nasal type, is a well-defined cytotoxic lymphoma [6]. This lymphoma is commonly located in the upper respiratory tract, especially the nasal cavity, but involvement of other organs can be observed, particularly the skin. The disease may be primary cutaneous: that is, staging investigations can be negative at presentation [2,8,33,34]. This lymphoma is not recognized in the EORTC classification where, depending on the size of neoplastic cells, cases would be classified as CD30− large T-cell lymphomas or small- to medium-sized pleomorphic T-cell lymphomas [15]. The WHO classification recognizes extranodal NK/T-cell lymphoma, nasal type, as a distinct entity [35]. The dis-

ease is more common in particular areas such as Asia, Mexico, and Central and South America.

In the past, similar cases were reported as 'lethal midline granuloma' or 'granuloma gangrenescens' [36–39]. Over many years, it has become recognized that lethal midline granuloma is a term encompassing various diseases with different aetiologies and pathogeneses, and that the majority of cases are associated with EBV, have a lymphoid differentiation and an aggressive course [40–44]. Lethal midline granuloma represents direct extension of the lymphoma from the nasal cavity to the overlying skin, with destruction of the bone and soft tissues. Some cases of extranodal NK/T-cell lymphoma, nasal type, were also included in the groups of angiocentric lymphoma and polymorphic reticulosis [6,45,46].

As for all lymphomas listed in this chapter, overlapping clinicopathological features are common and classification can be arbitrary. Most cases have an NK phenotype and are associated with EBV infection [6]. Negativity for T-cell markers and germline rearrangement of T lymphocytes, together with positivity for EBV in neoplastic cells, should be interpreted as a strong hint towards a diagnosis of extranodal NK/T-cell lymphoma, nasal type.

Clinical features

Patients are adults, with a predominance of males. Children are rarely affected. The skin lesions are erythematous or violaceous plaques and tumours, which are sometimes ulcerated (Fig. 6.18). The oral cavity and upper respiratory tract should

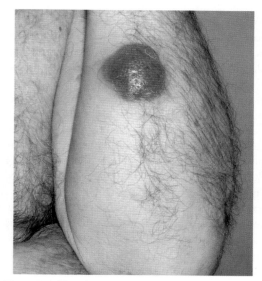

Fig. 6.18 NK/T-cell lymphoma, nasal type. Erythematous tumour on the arm. The patient had more tumours on the upper and lower extremities. (Courtesy of Esmeralda Vale, Lisboa, Portugal.)

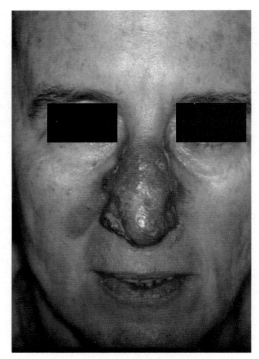

Fig. 6.19 NK/T-cell lymphoma, nasal type. Erythematous, partly crusted plaques on the nose and cheek (so-called 'lethal midline granuloma', early lesion).

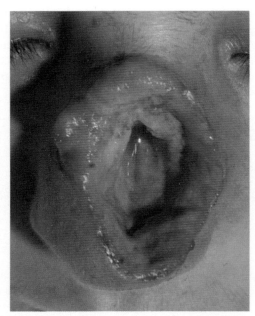

Fig. 6.20 NK/T-cell lymphoma, nasal type. Large ulcerated tumour on the nose in a 15-year-old girl (so-called 'lethal midline granuloma', late lesion).

be checked carefully at presentation and during follow-up, as involvement of these regions is common. Symptoms of nasal obstruction and/or epistaxis should be thoroughly investigated for evidence of nasal lymphoma. The variant described in the past as lethal midline granuloma is associated with large ulcers of the nose and adjacent tissues (Figs 6.19 & 6.20). Haemophagocytic syndrome is a possible complication.

In some cases of extranodal NK/T-cell lymphoma, nasal type, the clinical features of cutaneous manifestations can be similar to those seen in mycosis fungoides, and only phenotypical and molecular analyses allow these cases to be classified correctly. An accurate clinical history to rule out mycosis fungoides is mandatory before establishing the diagnosis.

A case of 'lethal midline granuloma' in a patient with lymphomatoid papulosis has been described [47]. In this case, the nasal lesion had a CD30+ phenotype and showed the same monoclonal rearrangement of the TCR gene as the skin lesions of the lymphomatoid papulosis. This probably represented progression of the lymphomatoid papulosis to an anaplastic large cell lymphoma rather than to a true nasal-type NK/T-cell lymphoma. In this context, it should be remembered that lymphoma types of both B- and T-cell origin other than the nasal-type NK/T-cell lymphoma can develop in the mucosa of the nasal and upper respiratory tract.

Histopathology, immunophenotype and molecular genetics

Histopathology

Histology reveals a diffuse proliferation of lymphocytes involving the dermis and, often, the subcutaneous tissues (Fig. 6.21). Epidermotropism may be present (Fig. 6.22), being a possible source of mistake in the differential diagnosis with mycosis fungoides. Usually there is prominent angiocentricity and/or angiodestruction; necrosis may also be found [48]. The cytomorphological features are variable: some cases show a predominance of small pleomorphic, some of medium-sized pleomorphic, and some of large pleomorphic lymphocytes (Fig. 6.23) [48]. Azurophilic granules are commonly observed in Giemsa-stained sections of tissue. In some cases, a prominent involvement of the subcutaneous tissues can be observed, resembling the morphological picture of subcutaneous T-cell lymphoma [49,50]. However, the same biopsy or other biopsies show invariably involvement of the dermis, and sometimes of the epidermis too.

Reactive cells, including small lymphocytes, histiocytes and eosinophils, are admixed with the neoplastic lymphocytes in some cases. A granulomatous reaction may also be present, as well as pseudoepitheliomatous epidermal hyperplasia.

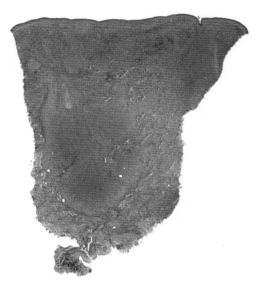

Fig. 6.21 NK/T-cell lymphoma, nasal type. Dense infiltrate of lymphocytes within the entire dermis. (Reprinted with permission from *The American Journal of Surgical Pathology*, in press.)

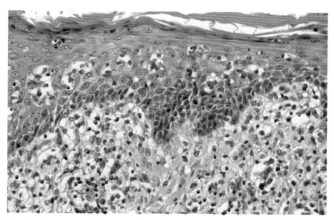

Fig. 6.22 NK/T-cell lymphoma, nasal type. Epidermotropism of small-sized lymphocytes, mimicking the histopathological picture of mycosis fungoides.

Immunophenotype

Neoplastic cells are characterized in the great majority of cases by negativity for T-cell markers such as TCRβ, TCRδ, CD3, CD4, CD5, CD7 and CD8. The ε chain of the CD3 molecule is usually expressed intracytoplasmically [51]. CD2, CD56 and TIA-1 are positive in practically all cases, but CD57 is negative (Fig. 6.24a). Aberrant expression of B-cell markers (CD79a) has been detected in one case, underlying the need for complete phenotypical investigations [52].

EBV can be demonstrated in practically all cases in the majority of the neoplastic cells (Fig. 6.24b).

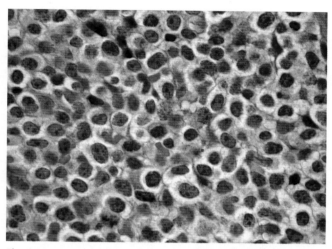

Fig. 6.23 NK/T-cell lymphoma, nasal type. Predominance of medium- and large-sized pleomorphic lymphocytes. (Reprinted with permission from *The American Journal of Surgical Pathology*, in press.)

Molecular genetics

Molecular analyses reveal a germline configuration of the TCR genes in most cases. A restricted killer cell immunoglobulin-like receptor repertoire has been found by the reverse transcriptase polymerase chain reaction (RT-PCR) technique, indicating the presence of a monoclonal or possibly oligoclonal NK-cell proliferation [53]. Rare cases of extranodal NK/T-cell lymphoma, nasal type, show a true T-cell phenotype with a monoclonal TCR gene rearrangement.

Mutations of the *Fas* gene have been described in nasal-type extranodal NK/T-cell lymphoma [54]. Oncogene copy number gains and other chromosomal alterations have also been detected in a few cases [55].

Treatment

Cases with involvement limited to the skin should be treated like those with extracutaneous involvement. The therapy of choice is systemic chemotherapy.

Prognosis

The prognosis of extranodal NK/T-cell lymphoma, nasal type, is poor, and most patients die a few months after the diagnosis [5,48]. The estimated 5-year survival is 0% [5]. Patients reported to have better prognosis and coexpression of CD30 and CD56 probably had examples of CD30+ anaplastic large cell lymphoma [56].

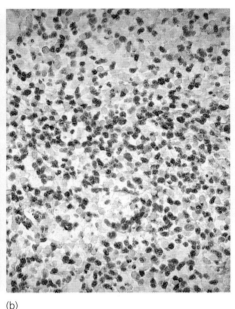

(a)   (b)

Fig. 6.24 NK/T-cell lymphoma, nasal type. (a) Positivity of neoplastic cells for the cytotoxic marker TIA-1. (b) Positive signal within neoplastic cells after *in situ* hybridization for the Epstein–Barr virus (EBER-1).

RÉSUMÉ

Extranodal NK/T-cell lymphoma, nasal type

Clinical	Adults. Solitary, regionally localized or generalized plaques and tumours, sometimes ulcerated. Aggressive course. No previous history of mycosis fungoides.
Morphology	Nodular or diffuse infiltrates characterized by small-, medium- or large-sized pleomorphic cells.
Immunology	CD2, 3ε, 56 + CD3, 4, 5, 8 – (some cases CD3+) CD30 – TIA-1 + EBER-1 +
Genetics	TCR genes in germline in the majority of cases. No specific genetic alteration.
Treatment guidelines	Systemic chemotherapy.

CD30⁻ PLEOMORPHIC LARGE T-CELL LYMPHOMA

CD30⁻ pleomorphic medium–large T-cell lymphomas arising primarily in the skin have been described rarely in the past [57–59]. It seems likely that many of these cases represent in truth one or another of the newly characterized cytotoxic lymphomas of the skin (see previous sections), or rarely so-called blastic NK-cell lymphoma (see Chapter 16). However, even after complete phenotypical and genotypical investigations, a small group of cases of cutaneous CD30⁻ medium–large T-cell lymphoma that do not fit into one of the categories mentioned above can be identified [8]. These patients do not have a clinical history of mycosis fungoides, nor do they have lesions suspicious of mycosis fungoides clinically. The phenotype of the tumour cells is βF1⁺, CD4±, CD8⁻, CD56⁻, and cytotoxic proteins are expressed in the majority of cases. They are classifed as cutaneous CD30⁻ large T-cell lymphoma in the EORTC classification, and as peripheral T-cell lymphoma, unspecified, in the WHO classification [6,15].

It is important to emphasize that the diagnosis of cutaneous CD30⁻ large T-cell lymphoma is one of exclusion, and that large cell transformation of mycosis fungoides or Sézary syndrome can show identical features to those observed in these patients, thus implying that an accurate clinical history is crucial for the diagnosis [60]. In the past, the majority of these cases were designated as mycosis fungoides 'a tumeur d'emblee'.

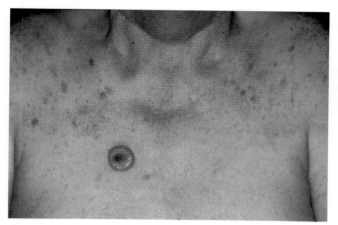

Fig. 6.25 CD30⁻ pleomorphic large T-cell lymphoma. Large erythematous tumour on the chest. The small crust in the centre represents the site of a punch biopsy.

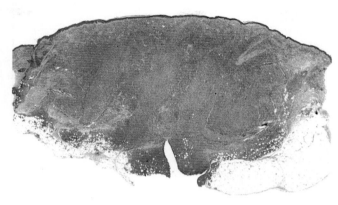

Fig. 6.26 CD30⁻ pleomorphic large T-cell lymphoma. Dense nodules of lymphocytes within the entire dermis involving the subcutaneous fat.

Clinical features

Patients are adults of both sexes. Clinically, they present with solitary, regionally localized or generalized reddish to brown–purplish plaques and tumours, often ulcerated (Fig. 6.25). The clinical features are similar to those observed in other high-grade lymphomas of the skin.

Histopathology, immunophenotype and molecular genetics

Histopathology

Histology shows nodular or diffuse infiltrates involving the entire dermis and subcutaneous fat, characterized by the predominance of medium- and large-sized pleomorphic cells or immunoblasts (Figs 6.26 & 6.27). Epidermotropism is infrequent. There is a high mitotic rate. Prominent necrosis, presence of angiocentricity and/or angiodestruction and predominant involvement of the subcutaneous tissues are uncommon.

Immunophenotype

Immunohistology reveals a characteristic phenotype of the neoplastic cells (βF1⁺, CD4±, CD8⁻, CD56⁻), commonly with the loss of one or more pan-T-cell antigens. CD30 and anaplastic lymphoma kinase (ALK) are negative. Cytotoxic proteins are expressed in the great majority of cases, demonstrating that these lesions belong to the group of so-called cytotoxic lymphomas [8].

There is no association with EBV infection.

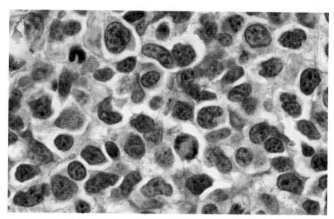

Fig. 6.27 CD30⁻ pleomorphic large T-cell lymphoma. Medium- and large-sized pleomorphic lymphocytes.

Molecular genetics

Molecular analysis of the TCR gene reveals a monoclonal rearrangement in most cases. At present no specific genetic features associated with this type of lymphoma have been detected.

Treatment

The treatment of choice is systemic chemotherapy using regimens for high-grade T-cell non-Hodgkin lymphoma.

Prognosis

The prognosis of cutaneous CD30⁻ large T-cell lymphoma is very poor, and most patients die within a few months from the onset of the disease. The estimated 5-year survival is 0% [5].

RÉSUMÉ

CD30⁻ pleomorphic large T-cell lymphoma

Clinical	Adults. Solitary, regionally localized or generalized plaques and tumours, sometimes ulcerated. Aggressive course. No previous history of mycosis fungoides.
Morphology	Nodular or diffuse infiltrates characterized by medium- and large-sized pleomorphic cells or immunoblasts.
Immunology	CD2, 3, 5 + CD4 + (−) βF1 + CD30 − CD8 − TIA-1 +
Genetics	Monoclonal rearrangement of the TCR genes detected in the majority of cases. No specific genetic alteration.
Treatment guidelines	Systemic chemotherapy.

References

1 Chan JKC. Peripheral T-cell and NK-cell neoplasms: an integrated approach to diagnosis. *Mod Pathol* 1999; **12**: 177–99.

2 Santucci M, Pimpinelli N, Massi D *et al.* Cytotoxic/natural killer cell cutaneous lymphomas: report of the EORTC cutaneous lymphoma task force workshop. *Cancer* 2003; **97**: 610–27.

3 Cerroni L, Kerl H. Diagnostic immunohistology: cutaneous lymphomas and pseudolymphomas. *Semin Cutan Med Surg* 1999; **18**: 64–70.

4 El-Shabrawi-Caelen L, Cerroni L, Kerl H. The clinicopathologic spectrum of cytotoxic lymphomas of the skin. *Semin Cutan Med Surg* 2000; **19**: 118–23.

5 Fink-Puches R, Zenahlik P, Bäck B *et al.* Primary cutaneous lymphomas: applicability of current classification schemes (European Organization for Research and Treatment of Cancer, World Health Organization) based on clinicopathologic features observed in a large group of patients. *Blood* 2002; **99**: 800–5.

6 Ralfkiaer E, Müller-Hermelink HK, Jaffe ES. Peripheral T-cell lymphoma, unspecified. In: Jaffe ES, Harris NL, Stein H, Vardiman JW, eds. *World Health Organization Classification of Tumours: Tumours of haematopoietic and lymphoid tissues.* Lyon: IARC press, 2001: 227–9.

7 Kluin PM, Feller A, Gaulard P *et al.* Peripheral T/NK-cell lymphoma: a report of the IXth Workshop of the European Association for Haematopathology. *Histopathology* 2001; **38**: 250–70.

8 Massone C, Chott A, Metze D *et al.* Subcutaneous, blastic natural killer (NK) NK/T-cell and other cytotoxic lymphomas of the skin: a morphologic, immunophenotypic and molecular study of 50 patients. *Am J Surg Pathol* in press.

9 Kamarashev J, Burg G, Mingari MC *et al.* Differential expression of cytotoxic molecules and killer cell inhibitory receptors in CD8⁺ and CD56⁺ cutaneous lymphomas. *Am J Pathol* 2001; **158**: 1593–8.

10 Tao J, Shelat SG, Jaffe ES, Bagg A. Aggressive Epstein–Barr virus-associated, CD8⁺, CD30⁺, CD56⁺, surface CD3⁻ natural killer (NK)-like cytotoxic T-cell lymphoma. *Am J Surg Pathol* 2002; **26**: 111–8.

11 Bekkenk MW, Vermeer MH, Jansen PM *et al.* Peripheral T-cell lymphomas unspecified presenting in the skin: analysis of prognostic factors in a group of 82 patients. *Blood* 2003; **102**: 2213–9.

12 Berti E, Tomasini D, Vermeer MH *et al.* Primary cutaneous CD8-positive epidermotropic cytotoxic T cell lymphomas: a distinct clinicopathological entity with an aggressive clinical behaviour. *Am J Pathol* 1999; **155**: 483–92.

13 Agnarsson BA, Vonderheid EC, Kadin ME. Cutaneous T-cell lymphoma with suppressor/cytotoxic (CD8) phenotype: identification of rapidly progressive and chronic subtypes. *J Am Acad Dermatol* 1990; **22**: 569–77.

14 Lu D, Patel KA, Duvic M, Jones D. Clinical and pathological spectrum of CD8-positive cutaneous T-cell lymphomas. *J Cutan Pathol* 2002; **29**: 465–72.

15 Willemze R, Kerl H, Sterry W *et al.* EORTC classification for primary cutaneous lymphomas: a proposal from the Cutaneous Lymphoma Study Group of the European Organization for Research and Treatment of Cancer. *Blood* 1997; **90**: 354–71.

16 Quarterman MJ, Lesher JL Jr, Davis LS, Pantazis CG, Mullins S. Rapidly progressive CD8-positive cutaneous T-cell lymphoma with tongue involvement. *Am J Dermatopathol* 1995; **17**: 287–91.

17 Barrionuevo C, Anderson VM, Zevallos-Giampietri E *et al.* Hydroa-like cutaneous T-cell lymphoma: a clinicopathologic and molecular genetic study of 16 pediatric cases from Peru. *Appl Immunohistochem Mol Morphol* 2002; **10**: 7–14.

18 Chen HH, Hsiao CH, Chiu HC. Hydroa vacciniforme-like primary cutaneous CD8-positive T-cell lymphoma. *Br J Dermatol* 2002; **147**: 587–91.

19 Magana M, Sangueza P, Gil-Beristain J *et al.* Angiocentric cutaneous T-cell lymphoma of childhood (hydroa-like lymphoma): a distinctive type of cutaneous T-cell lymphoma. *J Am Acad Dermatol* 1998; **38**: 574–9.

20 Arnulf B, Copie-Bergman C, Delfau-Larue MH *et al.* Non-hepatosplenic γ/δ T-cell lymphoma: a subset of cytotoxic lymphomas with mucosal or skin localization. *Blood* 1998; **91**: 1723–31.

21 Heald P, Buckley P, Gilliam A *et al.* Correlations of unique clinical, immunotypic, and histologic findings in a cutaneous γ/δ T-cell lymphoma. *J Am Acad Dermatol* 1992; **26**: 865–70.

22 Jones D, Vega F, Sarris AH, Medeiros LJ. CD4⁻ CD8⁻ 'double-negative' cutaneous T-cell lymphomas share common histologic features and an aggressive clinical course. *Am J Surg Pathol* 2002; **26**: 225–31.

23 Kadin ME. Cutaneous γ/δ T-cell lymphomas: how and why should they be recognized? *Arch Dermatol* 2000; **136**: 1052–4.

24 Ralfkiaer E, Wolff-Sneedorff A, Thomsen K, Geisler C, Lange Vejlsgaard G. T-cell receptor γ/δ-positive peripheral T-cell lymphomas presenting in the skin: a clinical, histological and immunophenotypic study. *Exp Dermatol* 1992; **1**: 31–6.

25 Toro JR, Beaty M, Sorbara L *et al.* γδ T-cell lymphoma of the skin: a clinical, microscopic, and molecular study. *Arch Dermatol* 2000; **136**: 1024–32.

26 de Wolf-Peeters C, Achten R. γ/δ T-cell lymphomas: a homogeneous entity? *Histopathology* 2000; **36**: 294–305.

27 Kinney MC. The role of morphologic features, phenotype, genotype, and anatomic site in defining extranodal T-cell or NK-cell neoplasms. *Am J Clin Pathol* 1999; **111**: S104–18.

28 Munn SE, McGregor JM, Jones A *et al.* Clinical and pathological heterogeneity in cutaneous γ/δ T-cell lymphoma: a report of three cases and a review of the literature. *Br J Dermatol* 1996; **135**: 976–81.

29 Berti E, Cerri A, Cavicchini S *et al.* Primary cutaneous γ/δ T-cell lymphoma presenting as disseminated pagetoid reticulosis. *J Invest Dermatol* 1991; **96**: 718–23.

30 Burg G, Braun-Falco O. *Cutaneous Lymphomas*. Berlin: Springer Verlag, 1983: 391–2.

31 Toro JR, Liewehr DJ, Pabby N *et al.* γ/δ T-cell phenotype is associated with significantly decreased survival in cutaneous T-cell lymphoma. *Blood* 2003; **101**: 3407–12.

32 Urosevic M, Kamarashev J, Burg G, Dummer R. Primary cutaneous CD8+ and CD56+ T-cell lymphomas express HLA-G and killer-cell inhibitory ligand, ILT2. *Blood* 2004; **103**: 1796–8.

33 Miyamoto T, Yoshino T, Takehisa T, Hagari Y, Mihara M. Cutaneous presentation of nasal/nasal type T/NK cell lymphoma: clinicopathological findings of four cases. *Br J Dermatol* 1998; **139**: 481–7.

34 Natkunam Y, Smoller BR, Zehnder JL, Dorfman RF, Warnke RA. Aggressive cutaneous NK and NK-like T-cell lymphomas: clinicopathologic, immunohistochemical, and molecular analyses of 12 cases. *Am J Surg Pathol* 1999; **23**: 571–81.

35 Chan JKC, Jaffe ES, Ralfkiaer E. Extranodal NK/T-cell lymphoma, nasal type. In: Jaffe ES, Harris NL, Stein H, Vardiman JW, eds. *World Health Organization Classification of Tumours: Tumours of haematopoietic and lymphoid tissues*. Lyon: IARC press, 2001, pp. 204–7.

36 Schafer RJ, Schuster HH. Granuloma gangraenescens als maligne Retikulose. *Zentralbl Allg Pathol* 1975; **119**: 111–5.

37 Chott A, Rappersberger K, Schlossarek W, Radaszkiewicz T. Peripheral T-cell lymphoma presenting primarily as lethal midline granuloma. *Hum Pathol* 1988; **19**: 1093–101.

38 Kassel SH, Echevarria RA, Guzzo FP. Midline malignant reticulosis (so-called lethal midline granuloma). *Cancer* 1969; **23**: 920–35.

39 Fechner RE, Lamppin DW. Midline malignant reticulosis: a clinicopathologic entity. *Arch Otolaryngol* 1972; **95**: 467–76.

40 Gaulard P, Henni T, Marolleau JP *et al.* Lethal midline granuloma (polymorphic reticulosis) and lymphomatoid granulomatosis: evidence for a monoclonal T-cell lymphoproliferative disorder. *Cancer* 1988; **62**: 705–10.

41 Eichel BS, Harrison EG Jr, Devine KD, Scanlon PW, Brown HA. Primary lymphoma of the nose including a relationship to lethal midline granuloma. *Am J Surg* 1966; **112**: 597–605.

42 Ishii Y, Yamanaka N, Ogawa K *et al.* Nasal T-cell lymphoma as a type of so-called 'lethal midline granuloma'. *Cancer* 1982; **50**: 2336–44.

43 Harabuchi Y, Yamanaka N, Kataura A *et al.* Epstein–Barr virus in nasal T-cell lymphomas in patients with lethal midline granuloma. *Lancet* 1990; **335**: 128–30.

44 Vilde JL, Perronne C, Huchon A *et al.* Association of Epstein–Barr virus with lethal midline granuloma. *N Engl J Med* 1985; **313**: 1161.

45 Aozasa K, Ohsawa M, Tomita Y, Tagawa S, Yamamura T. Polymorphic reticulosis is a neoplasm of large granular lymphocytes with CD3+ phenotype. *Cancer* 1995; **75**: 894–901.

46 Strickler JG, Meneses MF, Habermann TM *et al.* Polymorphic reticulosis: a reappraisal. *Hum Pathol* 1994; **25**: 659–65.

47 Harabuchi Y, Kataura A, Kobayashi K *et al.* Lethal midline granuloma (peripheral T-cell lymphoma) after lymphomatoid papulosis. *Cancer* 1992; **70**: 835–9.

48 Chan JKC, Sin VC, Wong KF *et al.* Non-nasal lymphoma expressing the natural killer marker CD56: a clinicopathologic study of 49 cases of an uncommon aggressive neoplasm. *Blood* 1997; **89**: 4501–13.

49 Jang KA, Choi JH, Sung KJ *et al.* Primary CD56+ nasal-type T/natural killer-cell subcutaneous panniculitic lymphoma: presentation as haemophagocytic syndrome. *Br J Dermatol* 1999; **141**: 706–9.

50 Chang SE, Huh J, Choi JH *et al.* Clinicopathological features of CD56+ nasal-type T/natural killer cell lymphomas with lobular panniculitis. *Br J Dermatol* 2000; **142**: 924–30.

51 Ohno T, Yamaguchi M, Oka K *et al.* Frequent expression of CD3 epsilon in CD3 (Leu 4)-negative nasal T-cell lymphomas. *Leukemia* 1995; **9**: 44–52.

52 Blakolmer K, Vesely M, Kummer JA *et al.* Immunoreactivity of B-cell markers (CD79a, L26) in rare cases of extranodal cytotoxic peripheral T (NK/T-) cell lymphomas. *Mod Pathol* 2000; **13**: 766–72.

53 Lin CW, Lee WH, Chang CL, Yang SY, Hsu SM. Restricted killer cell immunoglobulin-like receptor repertoire without T-cell receptor γ rearrangement supports a true natural killer-cell lineage in a subset of sinonasal lymphomas. *Am J Pathol* 2001; **159**: 1671–9.

54 Takakuwa T, Dong Z, Nakatsuka S *et al.* Frequent mutations of Fas gene in nasal NK/T-cell lymphoma. *Oncogene* 2002; **21**: 4702–5.

55 Mao X, Onadim Z, Price EA *et al.* Genomic alterations in blastic natural killer/extranodal natural killer-like T cell lymphoma with cutaneous involvement. *J Invest Dermatol* 2003; **121**: 618–27.

56 Mraz-Gernhard S, Natkunam Y, Hoppe RT *et al.* Natural killer/natural killer-like T-cell lymphoma, CD56+, presenting in the skin: an increasingly recognized entity with an aggressive course. *J Clin Oncol* 2001; **19**: 2179–88.

57 Beljaards RC, Meijer CJLM, van der Putte SCJ *et al.* Primary cutaneous T-cell lymphoma: clinicopathological features and prognostic parameters of 35 cases other than mycosis fungoides and CD30-positive large cell lymphoma. *J Pathol* 1994; **172**: 53–60.

58 Joly P, Vasseur E, Esteve E *et al.* Primary cutaneous medium and large cell lymphomas other than mycosis fungoides: an immunohistological and follow-up study on 54 cases. *Br J Dermatol* 1995; **132**: 506–12.

59 Sterry W, Siebel A, Mielke V. HTLV-I-negative pleomorphic T-cell lymphoma of the skin: the clinicopathological correlations and natural history of 15 patients. *Br J Dermatol* 1992; **126**: 456–62.

60 Cerroni L, Rieger E, Hödl S, Kerl H. Clinicopathologic and immunologic features associated with transformation of mycosis fungoides to large-cell lymphoma. *Am J Surg Pathol* 1992; **16**: 543–52.

Chapter 7 Small–medium pleomorphic T-cell lymphoma

The existence of a primary cutaneous small–medium pleomorphic T-cell lymphoma distinct from mycosis fungoides and Sézary syndrome has been postulated in recent years [1–4]. This lymphoma has been listed as a provisional entity in the European Organization for Research and Treatment of Cancer (EORTC) classification scheme [5]. There is no specific category for cutaneous small–medium pleomorphic T-cell lymphoma in the World Health Organization (WHO) classification of haematopoietic neoplasms, and these cases would be classified as peripheral T-cell lymphomas, not otherwise specified, according to that scheme [6].

Because mycosis fungoides and Sézary syndrome are also cutaneous T-cell lymphomas characterized by the predominance of small–medium pleomorphic T lymphocytes, the diagnosis of cutaneous small–medium pleomorphic T-cell lymphoma can only be accepted if they are excluded by a complete clinical examination [7,8]. In fact, a careful re-examination of the clinical pictures of some of the cases reported previously as small–medium pleomorphic T-cell lymphoma suggests that at least some of these were actually examples of mycosis fungoides.

There is still no consensus on the existence, definition and classification of small–medium pleomorphic T-cell lymphomas as a distinct entity, nor is there agreement on the diagnosis of cases classified as such in the literature. Cases similar on clinical and histopathological grounds have been reported in the past under different diagnoses, including 'idiopathic pseudo-T-cell lymphoma', 'pseudolymphomatous folliculitis', 'unilesional mycosis fungoides', 'mycosis fungoides à tumeur d'emblée' and 'monoclonal atypical T-cell hyperplasia', among others [9–11]. In addition, some cases of so-called aggressive CD8+ epidermotropic T-cell lymphoma and anaplastic large cell lymphoma may show a small–medium pleomorphic cytomorphology [12], generating more disarray in an already confused field. The diagnosis of small–medium pleomorphic T-cell lymphoma should probably be restricted to those cases characterized by the following features:

1 Absence of other lesions and/or a clinical history of mycosis fungoides.

2 Nodular or diffuse infiltrates of small–medium pleomorphic (monoclonal) T lymphocytes admixed with many reactive cells.
3 Absence of marked epidermotropism of neoplastic cells.
4 α/β phenotype.
5 Absence of CD30 expression.

The presence of Epstein–Barr virus DNA has been detected by polymerase chain reaction (PCR) techniques in small–medium pleomorphic T-cell lymphomas, but the exact role (if any) of this virus in the pathogenesis of the disease is unclear [13].

Clinical features

Patients are adults or elderly, without a clear-cut gender predilection. They present usually with solitary tumours, commonly located on the face and neck or upper trunk, but multiple tumours may be seen (Fig. 7.1). The surface of the tumours is erythematous or purplish; ulceration can be seen but is uncommon (Fig. 7.2).

Histopathology, immunophenotype and molecular genetics

Histopathology

Histology reveals dense, nodular or diffuse lymphoid infiltrates within the entire dermis, often involving the superficial part of the subcutaneous fat (Fig. 7.3). Cytomorphology shows a predominance of small- to medium-sized lymphocytes (Fig. 7.4). Large cells, when present, should not exceed 30% of the neoplastic infiltrate [14]. Epidermotropism is usually completely absent or present only focally. Many reactive cells are commonly found admixed with the neoplastic ones. A granulomatous reaction can be observed in a proportion of cases, and may sometimes cause diagnostic problems [15,16].

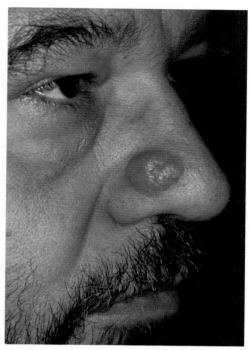

Fig. 7.1 Small–medium pleomorphic T-cell lymphoma. Solitary tumour on the nose.

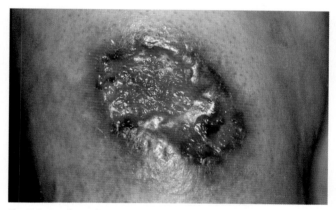

Fig. 7.2 Small–medium pleomorphic T-cell lymphoma. Large ulcerated tumour on the thigh.

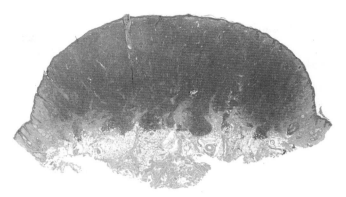

Fig. 7.3 Small–medium pleomorphic T-cell lymphoma. Dense infiltrate of lymphocytes extending throughout the dermis into the superficial part of the subcutaneous fat.

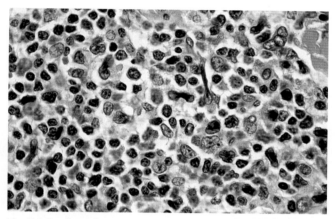

Fig. 7.4 Small–medium pleomorphic T-cell lymphoma. Small- and medium-sized pleomorphic lymphocytes predominate, admixed with a few larger cells.

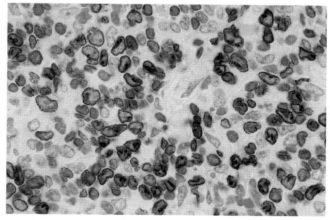

Fig. 7.5 Small–medium pleomorphic T-cell lymphoma. Staining for CD3 confirms the lineage of the lymphocytes and helps by highlighting the pleomorphic morphology of the nuclei.

Immunophenotype

The neoplastic cells often show a T-helper phenotype, sometimes with the loss of pan-T-cell antigens. Immunohistochemical staining may help in highlighting the pleomorphic morphology of the cells (Fig. 7.5). CD30 is not expressed by the neoplastic cells. A reactive infiltrate of B lymphocytes is commonly found. Although cases with a CD8$^+$ phenotype have been reported, care should be taken to distinguish small–medium pleomorphic T-cell lymphoma from aggressive CD8$^+$ epidermotropic T-cell lymphoma, as they represent two completely distinct entities with different clinical presentations and behaviour.

Molecular genetics

Molecular analysis of the T-cell receptor (TCR) gene rearrangement shows monoclonality of the T lymphocytes in the majority of cases.

Treatment

Most patients present with solitary tumours which can be treated by surgical excision alone, local radiotherapy, or a combination of the two [5]. In one study, cyclophosphamide or interferon-α has been used for patients with generalized skin lesions [1].

Prognosis

The potential of small–medium pleomorphic T-cell lymphomas to disseminate is unclear, and evaluation of prognosis has been hindered by the difficulties in diagnosis and classification referred to above. Provisionally, it seems that the prognosis is good, with an estimated 5-year survival of approximately 80% [4,17]. Patients with solitary tumours may be compared conceptually to those with solitary lesions in mycosis fungoides, and probably have a better prognosis.

References

RÉSUMÉ

Clinical	Adults and elderly adults. Localized or, less commonly, multiple tumours. Preferential locations: head and neck, upper trunk. Usually non-aggressive course.
Morphology	Small–medium pleomorphic cells.
Immunology	CD2, 3, 4, 5 + βF1 + CD7, 8, 30 –
Genetics	No specific abnormalities. Monoclonal rearrangement of the TCR is present in most cases.
Treatment guidelines	*Solitary tumours:* surgical excision, local radiotherapy, or a combination of the two. *Multiple lesions:* cyclophosphamide, interferon-α

1 Friedmann D, Wechsler J, Delfan MH *et al.* Primary cutaneous pleomorphic small T-cell lymphoma: a review of 11 cases. *Arch Dermatol* 1995; **131**: 1009–15.

2 Kim YC, Vandersteen DP. Primary cutaneous pleomorphic small/medium-sized T-cell lymphoma in a young man. *Br J Dermatol* 2001; **144**: 903–5.

3 von den Driesch P, Coors EA. Localized cutaneous small to medium-sized pleomorphic T-cell lymphoma: a report of 3 cases stable for years. *J Am Acad Dermatol* 2002; **46**: 531–5.

4 Sterry W, Siebel A, Mielke V. HTLV-I-negative pleomorphic T-cell lymphoma of the skin: the clinicopathological correlations and natural history of 15 patients. *Br J Dermatol* 1992; **126**: 456–62.

5 Willemze R, Kerl H, Sterry W *et al.* EORTC classification for primary cutaneous lymphomas: a proposal from the Cutaneous Lymphoma Study Group of the European Organization for Research and Treatment of Cancer. *Blood* 1997; **90**: 354–71.

6 Ralfkiaer E, Müller-Hermelink HK, Jaffe ES. Peripheral T-cell lymphoma, unspecified. In: Jaffe ES, Harris NL, Stein H, Vardiman JW, eds. *World Health Organization Classification of Tumours: Tumours of Haematopoietic and Lymphoid Tissues.* Lyon: IARC Press, 2001.

7 Kerl H, Cerroni L. Controversies in cutaneous lymphomas. *Semin Cutan Med Surg* 2000; **19**: 157–60.

8 Kerl H, Cerroni L. Is small/medium-sized pleomorphic T-cell lymphoma a distinct cutaneous lymphoma? *Dermatopathol Pract Concept* 2000; **6**: 298–300.

9 Arai E, Okubo H, Tsuchida T, Kitamura K, Katayama I. Pseudolymphomatous folliculitis: a clinicopathologic study of 15 cases of cutaneous pseudolymphoma with follicular invasion. *Am J Surg Pathol* 1999; **23**: 1313–9.

10 Oliver GF, Winkelmann RK. Unilesional mycosis fungoides: a distinct entity. *J Am Acad Dermatol* 1989; **20**: 63–70.

11 Rijlaarsdam JU, Willemze R. Cutaneous pseudo-T-cell lymphomas. *Semin Diagn Pathol* 1991; **8**: 102–8.

12 Berti E, Tomasini D, Vermeer MH *et al.* Primary cutaneous CD8-positive epidermotropic cytotoxic T-cell lymphomas: a distinct clinicopathological entity with an aggressive clinical behaviour. *Am J Pathol* 1999; **155**: 483–92.

13 Nagore E, Ledesma E, Collado C *et al.* Detection of Epstein–Barr virus and human herpesvirus 7 and 8 genomes in primary cutaneous T- and B-cell lymphomas. *Br J Dermatol* 2000; **143**: 320–3.

14 Beljaards RC, Meijer CJLM, van der Putte SCJ *et al.* Primary cutaneous T-cell lymphoma: clinicopathological features and prognostic parameters of 35 cases other than mycosis fungoides and CD30-positive large cell lymphoma. *J Pathol* 1994; **172**: 53–60.

15 Scarabello A, Leinweber B, Ardigó M *et al.* Cutaneous lymphomas with prominent granulomatous reaction: a potential pitfall in the histopathologic diagnosis of cutaneous T- and B-cell lymphomas. *Am J Surg Pathol* 2002; **26**: 1259–68.

16 Blechet C, Pasquier Y, Maitre F, Esteve E. Lymphome cutane T pleomorphe simulant une sarcoidose. *Les Nouvelles Dermatologiques* 2000; **19**: 212–3.

17 Fink-Puches R, Zenahlik P, Bäck B *et al.* Primary cutaneous lymphomas: applicability of current classification schemes (European Organization for Research and Treatment of Cancer, World Health Organization) based on clinicopathologic features observed in a large group of patients. *Blood* 2002; **99**: 800–5.

Chapter 8 Other cutaneous T-cell lymphomas

Several other types of T-cell lymphoma have been described at cutaneous sites, including cases arising both primarily and secondarily in the skin. The following text summarizes the entities that have been best characterized.

ADULT T-CELL LEUKAEMIA–LYMPHOMA

Adult T-cell leukaemia–lymphoma (ATLL) is a malignant lymphoproliferative disease associated with a retrovirus infection caused by the human T-cell lymphotrophic virus I (HTLV-I). The disease is endemic in the south of Japan and in the Caribbean Islands but is rare in other regions. It is not included in the European Organization for Research and Treatment of Cancer (EORTC) classification, but is included as a specific entity in the World Health Organization (WHO) classification [1,2]. Five variants of ATLL are recognized: acute and chronic leukaemic, lymphomatous, smoldering and crisis types.

Clinical features

Specific skin manifestations can be observed in approximately half of patients, especially those presenting with indolent forms of the disease [3–5]. Primary cutaneous involvement may also be seen [5]. Elderly men are affected more frequently. Anti-HTLV-I antibodies can be demonstrated in the serum of affected individuals. The clinical presentation resembles mycosis fungoides. Cutaneous lesions are localized or generalized macules and papules, plaques and tumours [3,4]. Erythroderma may also develop. A leukaemic blood picture and involvement of the bone marrow are found in more than half of patients. Spontaneous regression of skin lesions has been observed rarely [6].

Histopathology, immunophenotype and molecular genetics

Histology shows an infiltrate of small–medium- or medium–large-sized pleomorphic lymphocytes with prominent epidermotropism [3,4]. The histopathological picture is often indistinguishable from that of mycosis fungoides. Variants of ATLL with angiocentricity and/or angiodestruction or with bullous lesions have been observed [7,8]. Immunohistology usually reveals a T-helper (CD3+, CD4+, CD8−) phenotype. Molecular analyses show a monoclonal rearrangement of the T-cell receptor (TCR) gene as well as the presence of the integrated genome of HTLV-I [9].

In this context, it should be underlined that several investigators have looked for the presence of HTLV-I DNA in cases of 'classic' mycosis fungoides and Sézary syndrome prompted by the clinicopathological similarities to ATLL. So far, there is no convincing evidence of the involvement of HTLV-I in these diseases (see Chapter 2). Demonstration of monoclonal integration of HTLV-I DNA in neoplastic cells may therefore be used as a reliable means to distinguish ATLL from mycosis fungoides.

RÉSUMÉ

Adult T-cell leukaemia–lymphoma

Clinical	Adults. Five variants recognized: acute and chronic leukaemic, lymphomatous, smoldering and crisis types. Primary cutaneous involvement may be seen.
Morphology	Histopathological features similar to those observed in mycosis fungoides.
Immunology	CD3, 4 + CD8 −
Genetics	Monoclonal integration of HTLV-I DNA.
Treatment guidelines	Systemic chemotherapy. PUVA may be used for cases restricted to the skin.

Treatment and prognosis

The prognosis is generally poor, but indolent variants have been described. The treatment of choice is usually systemic chemotherapy, but less aggressive therapeutic options such as psoralen with UVA (PUVA) may be used for cases with an indolent behaviour and restricted to the skin [3,4,10,11].

INTRAVASCULAR LARGE T-CELL LYMPHOMA

Intravascular large cell lymphoma (angiotrophic lymphoma) is a rare type of non-Hodgkin lymphoma, usually showing a B-cell phenotype (see Chapter 15). Rarely, cases of cutaneous intravascular large cell lymphoma may show a T-cell phenotype (Fig. 8.1) [12–14]. One case with a CD56+ phenotype has also been reported [15]. Intravascular large T-cell lymphoma is included as a provisional entity together with the more frequent B-cell type in the EORTC and WHO classifications [2,16].

Patients are usually elderly adults, although a congenital case has been reported [17]. The clinical presentation and histopathological picture are similar to those seen in the more common B-cell variant. Association with virus infection (Epstein–Barr virus [EBV], HTLV) has been postulated in some cases [18,19].

The prognosis and treatment of intravascular large T-cell lymphoma do not seem to differ from those of the B-cell type of the disease.

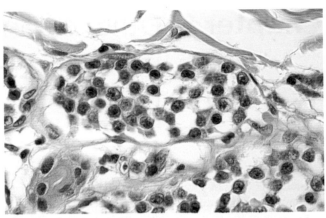

Fig. 8.1 Cutaneous intravascular large T-cell lymphoma. Intravascular cluster of large pleomorphic lymphocytes.

T-CELL PROLYMPHOCYTIC LEUKAEMIA

T-cell prolymphocytic leukaemia (T-PLL) is a rare haematological disease. Cutaneous involvement occurs in up to one-third of patients and is characterized by papules, plaques or tumours, often indistinguishable from those of mycosis fungoides and Sézary syndrome. Erythroderma may develop (Fig. 8.2). Skin manifestations may be the first sign of the disease [20]. Histology reveals a monomorphous infiltrate of small lymphocytes, sometimes with epidermotropism (Fig. 8.3). Immunohistology shows a T-helper phenotype (CD3+, CD4+, CD8−) in the majority of lesions, but coexpression of CD4 and CD8 is found in a small number of cases. The TCR genes are monoclonally rearranged. The most frequent chromosomal aberration is inversion of chromosome 14 with breakpoints in the long arm at q11 and q32 [1]. The disease usually runs an aggressive course and the prognosis is poor. Recently, treatment with anti-CD52 antibody (Campath) showed promising results [21].

Differentiation of cutaneous manifestations of T-PLL from Sézary syndrome may be extremely difficult on clinicopathological grounds alone.

PRECURSOR T-LYMPHOBLASTIC LEUKAEMIA–LYMPHOBLASTIC LYMPHOMA

Precursor T-lymphoblastic leukaemia–lymphoblastic lymphoma is a malignant proliferation of precursor T lymphocytes. The exact incidence of specific skin involvement in these patients is not known. It must be stressed that histological features alone do not allow the differentiation of lym-

RÉSUMÉ

Intravascular large T-cell lymphoma

Clinical	Very rare variant of intravascular large cell lymphoma. Adults. Solitary or multiple indurated patches and plaques.
Morphology	Intravascular proliferation of large atypical lymphoid cells.
Immunology	CD3, 5 + CD20, 79a −
Genetics	Monoclonal rearrangement of the TCR genes.
Treatment guidelines	Systemic chemotherapy.

RÉSUMÉ

T-cell prolymphocytic leukaemia

Clinical	Adults. Generalized papules, plaques and tumours. Erythroderma may develop.
Morphology	Histopathological features similar to those of mycosis fungoides/Sézary syndrome.
Immunology	CD3, 4, 5 + βF1 + CD8 –
Genetics	Monoclonal rearrangement of the TCR genes detected in the majority of cases. Inversion of chromosome 14 with breakpoints in the long arm at q11 and q32.
Treatment guidelines	Systemic chemotherapy; Campath.

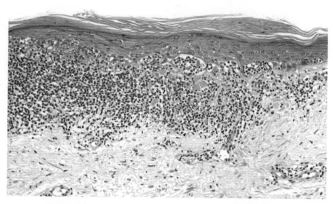

Fig. 8.3 Cutaneous involvement in T-cell prolymphocytic leukaemia. Dense band-like infiltrate of lymphocytes with epidermotropism. The histopathological features are indistinguishable from those of mycosis fungoides and Sézary syndrome.

phoblastic lymphomas of T phenotype from those of B-cell lineage [1,22]. In the skin, lymphoblastic T-cell lymphoma almost always represents a secondary manifestation of a primary extracutaneous disease [22,23].

Clinical features

Although precursor T-lymphoblastic leukaemia–lymphoblastic lymphoma is observed mainly in children and adolescents, reports of cutaneous involvement are mainly in adult patients [22,24]. Clinically, patients present with localized or generalized large cutaneous–subcutaneous tumours (Fig. 8.4) [22,24]. Involvement of the central nervous system may be observed.

Histopathology, immunophenotype and molecular genetics

Histology reveals a monomorphous proliferation of medium-sized cells, with round or convoluted nuclei with finely dispersed chromatin and scanty cytoplasm (Fig. 8.5). A 'starry sky' pattern is often observed at low magnification because of the presence of macrophages with inclusion bodies. There are abundant mitoses and necrotic ('apoptotic') cells. The immunophenotype of neoplastic cells is characterized by positivity for TdT, CD1a, cytoplasmic CD3, and CD7, and in some cases for CD99 and CD34 (Fig. 8.6). Both CD4 and CD8 can be positive or negative. Molecular genetics usually shows monoclonally rearranged TCR and germline J_H genes, but both a TCR^-/J_H^- and a TCR^+/J_H^+ pattern can be observed.

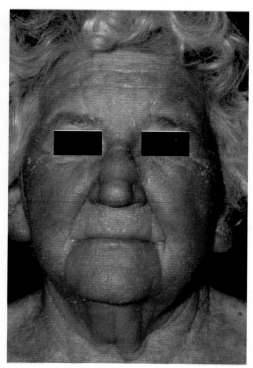

Fig. 8.2 Cutaneous involvement in T-cell prolymphocytic leukaemia. Erythematous scaly lesions on the face in a patient with erythroderma.

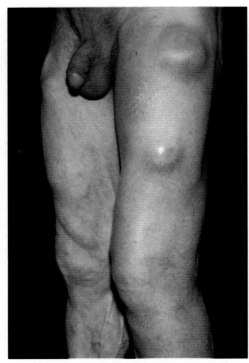

Fig. 8.4 Cutaneous T-lymphoblastic lymphoma. Subcutaneous tumours on the leg.

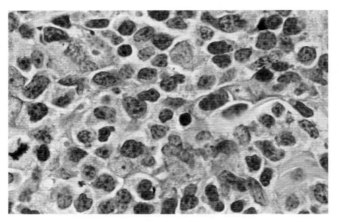

Fig. 8.5 Cutaneous T-lymphoblastic lymphoma. Medium-sized cells, some with convoluted nuclei, with finely dispersed chromatin. Note several mitoses.

Treatment and prognosis

The treatment of choice is systemic chemotherapy. Patients are treated with regimens similar to those for other types of acute lymphoblastic leukaemia–lymphoma.

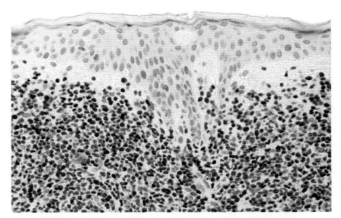

Fig. 8.6 Cutaneous T-lymphoblastic lymphoma. Positive nuclear staining for TdT.

RÉSUMÉ

Precursor T-lymphoblastic leukaemia–lymphoblastic lymphoma

Clinical	Skin involvement mainly in adults. Localized or generalized large cutaneous or subcutaneous tumours.
Morphology	Monomorphous proliferation of medium-sized cells, with round or convoluted nuclei with finely dispersed chromatin and scanty cytoplasm.
Immunology	CD1a, 3, 7 + TδT + CD34 + (–) CD99 +
Genetics	Monoclonal rearrangement of the TCR genes detected in the majority of cases.
Treatment guidelines	Systemic chemotherapy.

ANGIOIMMUNOBLASTIC T-CELL LYMPHOMA

Angioimmunoblastic T-cell lymphoma, formerly called angioimmunoblastic lymphadenopathy, is considered to be a peripheral T-cell lymphoma with a peculiar proliferation of so-called high endothelial venules. It is recognized as a distinct entity in the WHO classification [25]. Non-specific skin manifestations have been described in several patients, including maculopapular eruptions, purpura and erythroderma. Specific skin involvement is uncommon.

Patients are elderly adults, although cutaneous involvement in children has been reported [1,26]. Restriction to the skin is rare but cutaneous lesions may be the first manifestation of the disease [27]. Cutaneous involvement in angioimmunoblastic T-cell lymphoma is characterized by erythematous papules, plaques and tumours consisting of an infiltrate of small- to medium-sized pleomorphic lymphocytes intermingled with plasma cells, eosinophils, histiocytes and immunoblasts. Increased numbers of venules with a prominent endothelial lining are typically found ('high endothelial venules') [28,29]. Clusters of CD21$^+$ cells (variably interpreted as follicular dendritic cells or fibroblastic reticulum cells) can be observed, especially around the high endothelial venules. Immunohistology reveals a T-helper phenotype (CD3$^+$, CD4$^+$, CD8$^-$) of neoplastic cells. Clusters of polyclonal B lymphocytes are commonly present. EBV can be demonstrated often within these B lymphocytes (development of a second EBV-associated B-cell lymphoma has been observed) [30]. Molecular genetics shows a monoclonal rearrangement of TCR genes, and usually a polyclonal pattern of J_H genes. Recently, in a case with cutaneous involvement, DNA microarrays have revealed the expression of secondary lymphoid tissue chemokines, including tumour necrosis factor-β, and of an apoptosis–inhibitory protein in the affected lymph nodes [31].

There are only limited data on the prognosis and treatment of patients with specific skin involvement of angioimmunoblastic T-cell lymphoma. The prognosis is generally poor. Systemic treatment options include glucocorticoids, interferon-α and chemotherapy. Commencing therapy at an early stage of the disease may give better results in terms of survival.

RÉSUMÉ

Angioimmunoblastic T-cell lymphoma

Clinical	Elderly adults. Cutaneous lesions may be the first manifestation of the disease.
Morphology	Small- to medium-sized pleomorphic lymphocytes intermingled with plasma cells, eosinophils, histiocytes and immunoblasts.
Immunology	CD3, 4, 5 + CD8 − EBV$^+$/CD20$^+$ cells (non-neoplastic) CD21$^+$ cells in clusters (non-neoplastic)
Genetics	Monoclonal rearrangement of the TCR genes.
Treatment guidelines	Glucocorticoids; interferon-α; systemic chemotherapy.

References

1 Kikuchi M, Jaffe ES, Ralfkiaer E. Adult T-cell leukaemia/lymphoma. In: Jaffe ES, Harris NL, Stein H, Vardiman JW, eds. *World Health Organization Classification of Tumours: Tumours of Haematopoietic and Lymphoid Tissues.* Lyon: IARC Press, 2001: 200–3.

2 Willemze R, Kerl H, Sterry W *et al.* EORTC classification for primary cutaneous lymphomas: a proposal from the Cutaneous Lymphoma Study Group of the European Organization for Research and Treatment of Cancer. *Blood* 1997; **90**: 354–71.

3 DiCaudo DJ, Perniciaro C, Worrell JT, White JW Jr, Cockerell CJ. Clinical and histologic spectrum of human T-cell lymphotropic virus type I-associated lymphoma involving the skin. *J Am Acad Dermatol* 1996; **34**: 69–76.

4 Nagatani T, Miyazawa M, Matsuzaki T *et al.* Adult T-cell leukemia–lymphoma (ATLL): clinical, histopathological, immunological and immunohistochemical characteristics. *Exp Dermatol* 1992; **1**: 248–52.

5 Shimoyama M. Diagnostic criteria and classification of clinical subtypes of adult T-cell leukaemia–lymphoma: a report from the Lymphoma Study Group (1984–87). *Br J Haematol* 1991; **79**: 428–37.

6 Kawabata H, Setoyama M, Fukushige T, Kanzaki T. Spontaneous regression of cutaneous lesions in adult T-cell leukaemia–lymphoma. *Br J Dermatol* 2001; **144**: 434–5.

7 Manabe T, Hirokawa M, Sugihara K, Kohda M. Angiocentric and angiodestructive infiltration of adult T cell leukemia–lymphoma (ATLL) in the skin: report of two cases. *Am J Dermatopathol* 1988; **10**: 487–96.

8 Michael EJ, Shaffer JJ, Collins HE, Grossman ME. Bullous adult T-cell lymphoma–leukemia and human T-cell lymphotropic virus-1 associated myelopathy in a 60-year-old man. *J Am Acad Dermatol* 2002; **46**: S137–41.

9 Kato N, Sugawara H, Aoyagi S, Mayuzumi M. Lymphoma-type adult T-cell leukemia–lymphoma with a bulky cutaneous tumour showing multiple human T-lymphotropic virus-1 DNA integration. *Br J Dermatol* 2001; **144**: 1244–8.

10 Chan EF, Dowdy YG, Lee B *et al.* A novel chemotherapeutic regimen (interferon-α, zidovudine, and etretinate) for adult T-cell lymphoma resulting in rapid tumor destruction. *J Am Acad Dermatol* 1999; **40**: 116–21.

11 Takemori N, Hirai K, Onodera R *et al.* Satisfactory remission achieved by PUVA therapy in a case of crisis-type adult T-cell leukemia–lymphoma with generalized cutaneous leukaemic cell infiltration. *Br J Dermatol* 1995; **133**: 955–60.

12 Sangueza O, Hyder DM, Sangueza P. Intravascular lymphomatosis:

report of an unusual case with T-cell phenotype occurring in an adolescent male. *J Cutan Pathol* 1992; **19**: 226–31.

13 Sepp N, Schuler G, Romani N *et al.* Intravascular lymphomatosis (angioendotheliomatosis): evidence for a T-cell origin in two cases. *Hum Pathol* 1990; **21**: 1051–8.

14 Yegappan S, Coupland R, Arber DA *et al.* Angiotropic lymphoma: an immunophenotypically and clinically heterogeneous lymphoma. *Mod Pathol* 2001; **14**: 1147–56.

15 Santucci M, Pimpinelli N, Massi D *et al.* Cytotoxic/natural killer cell cutaneous lymphomas: Report of the EORTC cutaneous lymphoma task force workshop. *Cancer* 2003; **97**: 610–27.

16 Gatter KC, Warnke RA. Intravascular large B-cell lymphoma. In: Jaffe ES, Harris NL, Stein H, Vardiman JW, eds. *World Health Organization Classification of Tumours: Tumours of haematopoietic and lymphoid tissues.* Lyon: IARC press, 2001: 177–8.

17 Tateyama H, Eimoto T, Tada T *et al.* Congenital angiotropic lymphoma (intravascular lymphomatosis) of the T-cell type. *Cancer* 1991; **67**: 2131–6.

18 Shimokawa I, Higami Y, Sakai H *et al.* Intravascular malignant lymphomatosis: a case of T-cell lymphoma probably associated with human T-cell lymphotropic virus. *Hum Pathol* 1991; **22**: 200–2.

19 Au WY, Shek WH, Nicholls J *et al.* T-cell intravascular lymphomatosis (angiotropic large cell lymphoma): association with Epstein–Barr viral infection. *Histopathology* 1997; **31**: 563–7.

20 Serra A, Estrach MT, Marti R, Villamor N, Rafel M. Cutaneous involvement as the first manifestation in a case of T-cell prolymphocytic leukaemia. *Acta Derm Venereol (Stockh)* 1998; **78**: 198–200.

21 Pawson R, Dyer MJ, Barge R *et al.* Treatment of T-cell prolymphocytic leukemia with human CD52 antibody. *J Clin Oncol* 1997; **15**: 2667–72.

22 Chimenti S, Fink-Puches R, Peris K *et al.* Cutaneous involvement in lymphoblastic lymphoma. *J Cutan Pathol* 1999; **26**: 379–85.

23 van Zuuren EJ, Wintzen M, Jansen PM, Willemze R. Aleukaemic leukaemia cutis in a patient with acute T-cell lymphoblastic leukaemia. *Clin Exp Dermatol* 2003; **28**: 330–2.

24 Sander CA, Medeiros LJ, Abruzzo LV, Horak ID, Jaffe ES. Lymphoblastic lymphoma presenting in cutaneous sites: a clinicopathologic analysis of six cases. *J Am Acad Dermatol* 1991; **25**: 1023–31.

25 Jaffe ES, Ralfkiaer E. Angioimmunoblastic T-cell lymphoma. In: Jaffe ES, Harris NL, Stein H, Vardiman JW, eds. *World Health Organization Classification of Tumours: Tumours of haematopoietic and lymphoid tissues.* Lyon: IARC press, 2001: 225–6.

26 Schotte U, Megahed M, Jansen T *et al.* Angioimmunoblastische Lymphadenopathie mit kutanen Manifestationen bei einem 13jährigen Mädchen. *Hautarzt* 1992; **43**: 728–34.

27 Suarez-Vilela D, Izquierdo-Garcia FM. Angioimmunoblastic lymphadenopathy-like T-cell lymphoma: cutaneous clinical onset with prominent granulomatous reaction. *Am J Surg Pathol* 2003; **27**: 699–700.

28 Martel P, Laroche L, Courville P *et al.* and the French Study Group on Cutaneous Lymphoma. Cutaneous involvement in patients with angioimmunoblastic lymphadenopathy with dysproteinemia. *Arch Dermatol* 2000; **136**: 881–6.

29 Schmuth M, Ramaker J, Trautmann C *et al.* Cutaneous involvement in prelymphomatous angioimmunoblastic lymphadenopathy. *J Am Acad Dermatol* 1997; **36**: 290–5.

30 Brown HA, MacOn WR, Kurtin PJ, Gibson LE. Cutaneous involvement by angioimmunoblastic T-cell lymphoma with remarkable heterogeneous Epstein–Barr virus expression. *J Cutan Pathol* 2001; **28**: 432–8.

31 Murakami T, Ohtsuki M, Nakagawa H. Angioimmunoblastic lymphadenopathy-type peripheral T-cell lymphoma with cutaneous infiltration: report of a case and its gene expression profile. *Br J Dermatol* 2001; **144**: 878–84.

Part 2 Cutaneous B-cell lymphomas

Cutaneous B-cell lymphomas represent distinct clinical and histopathological subtypes of extranodal lymphomas. They occur far more frequently than is generally believed [1]. The widespread use of immunohistochemical and molecular genetic techniques, as well as the analysis of follow-up data, revealed that many of the cases classified in the past as cutaneous B-cell pseudolymphomas represent in fact low-grade malignant B-cell lymphomas of the skin, especially marginal zone lymphoma.

In 1997, the European Organization for Research and Treatment of Cancer (EORTC) Cutaneous Lymphoma Study Group published a classification of primary cutaneous lymphomas including three main entities of B-cell lymphoma: follicle centre cell lymphoma, marginal zone lymphoma–immunocytoma, and large B-cell lymphoma of the leg [2]. Intravascular large B-cell lymphoma and plasmacytoma were included as provisional entities. The classification of malignant lymphomas published by the World Health Organization (WHO) in 2001 does not consider cutaneous B-cell lymphomas as distinct entities, and lumps them together within different groups of nodal and extranodal lymphomas [3]. It has been demonstrated that the EORTC scheme offers some advantages in the precise diagnosis and classification of cutaneous B-cell lymphomas, especially concerning follicle centre cell lymphomas with a diffuse pattern of growth [4]. However, many problems still exist concerning the classification and nomenclature of primary cutaneous B-cell lymphomas. A suggestion that all cutaneous B-cell lymphomas should be classified as 'skin-associated lymphoid tissue (SALT)-type B-cell lymphomas' has also been put forward in the past, but it does not reflect the great variety in clinicopathological presentations of these cases, and has not gained wide acceptance [5].

A small percentage of primary cutaneous B-cell lymphomas was demonstrated to harbour *Borrelia burgdorferi* DNA sequences within specific skin lesions in studies carried out in different countries, but negative results have also been reported [6–8]. This association may be important for cutaneous immunocytomas. The presence of *B. burgdorferi* within skin lesions of cutaneous lymphoma underlines the analogies between B-cell lymphomas of the skin and those of the gastric mucosa, where, at least in some cases, infection by *Helicobacter pylori* is considered to be a causative agent. The observation of *B. burgdorferi*-specific DNA within skin lesions of cutaneous B-cell lymphoma also provided the rationale for antibiotic treatment of these patients, and indeed good results have been observed in some cases [9]. Other new treatment modalities include the use of the anti-CD20 antibody (rituximab), which has been applied intralesionally or systemically for the treatment of different types of cutaneous B-cell lymphoma. The knowledge that many patients experience a protracted course with long survival also provided the rationale for a 'watchful waiting' strategy which is now being increasingly used in low-grade cutaneous B-cell lymphomas, especially of the marginal zone type.

References

1 Kerl H, Rauch HJ, Hödl S. Cutaneous B cell lymphomas. In: Goos M, Christophers E, eds. *Lymphoproliferative Diseases of the Skin.* Berlin: Springer Verlag, 1982: 179–91.

2 Willemze R, Kerl H, Sterry W *et al.* EORTC classification for primary cutaneous lymphomas: a proposal from the Cutaneous Lymphoma Study Group of the European Organization for Research and Treatment of Cancer. *Blood* 1997; **90**: 354–71.

3 Jaffe ES, Harris NL, Stein H, Vardiman JW, eds. *World Health Organization Classification of Tumours: Tumours of Haematopoietic and Lymphoid Tissues.* Lyon: IARC Press, 2001.

4 Fink-Puches R, Zenahlik P, Bäck B *et al.* Primary cutaneous lymphomas: applicability of current classification schemes (European Organization for Research and Treatment of Cancer, World Health Organization) based on clinicopathologic features observed in a large group of patients. *Blood* 2002; **99**: 800–5.

5 Santucci M, Pimpinelli N, Arganini L. Primary cutaneous B-cell lymphoma: a unique type of low-grade lymphoma—clinicopathologic and immunologic study of 83 cases. *Cancer* 1991; **67**: 2311–26.

6 Cerroni L, Zöchling N, Pütz B, Kerl H. Infection by *Borrelia burgdorferi* and cutaneous B-cell lymphoma. *J Cutan Pathol* 1997; **24**: 457–61.

7 Goodlad JR, Davidson MM, Hollowood K *et al.* Primary cutaneous B-cell lymphoma and *Borrelia burgdorferi* infection in patients from the highlands of Scotland. *Am J Surg Pathol* 2000; **24**: 1279–85.

8 Wood GS, Kamath NV, Guitart J *et al.* Absence of *Borrelia burgdorferi* DNA in cutaneous B-cell lymphomas from the United States. *J Cutan Pathol* 2001; **28**: 502–7.

9 Zenahlik P, Fink-Puches R, Kapp KS, Kerl H, Cerroni L. Die Therapie der primären kutanen B-Zell-Lymphome. *Hautarzt* 2000; **51**: 19–24.

Chapter 9 Follicle centre cell lymphoma

Cutaneous follicle centre cell lymphoma is defined as the neoplastic proliferation of germinal centre cells confined to the skin. The pattern of growth can be either purely follicular, purely diffuse, or mixed.

Cutaneous follicle centre cell lymphoma, as it has been defined in the European Organization for Research and Treatment of Cancer (EORTC) classification, and nodal follicular lymphoma according to the World Health Organization (WHO) classification differ substantially in their definitions [1,2]. Morphologically, nodal follicular lymphoma is defined in the WHO classification as a tumour presenting with at least a partially follicular pattern, and cases with a purely diffuse pattern of growth are classified among the diffuse large B-cell lymphomas [2,3]. Phenotypically, follicular lymphomas at extracutaneous sites are characterized by the proliferation of neoplastic germinal centre cells positive for CD10 and Bcl-6 [2–5]. A background of CD21+ follicular dendritic cells is constantly found. At the genetic level, most cases exhibit the interchromosomal 14;18 translocation, usually resulting in the expression of the Bcl-2 protein by the neoplastic cells [6–9]. In contrast, in the EORTC classification, cutaneous follicle centre cell lymphoma is defined as a proliferation of centrocytes and centroblasts showing a diffuse pattern of growth in the great majority of cases and only rarely presenting a true follicular pattern [1]. CD10 and Bcl-2 are usually not expressed by the neoplastic cells and the t(14;18) is absent [10,11]. Based on the morphological, phenotypical and molecular differences, the existence of cases of true primary cutaneous follicular lymphoma has been called into question several times over the last few years [12,13]. However, previous reports and recent data clearly demonstrate that cutaneous follicle centre cell lymphoma represents an entity with distinct clinical, histopathological, immunophenotypical and molecular genetic features, and that it differs from the nodal counterpart mainly by the lack of the t(14;18) and Bcl-2 expression [14–22]. At present, a joint EORTC/WHO classification scheme is being prepared, that recognises the diffuse variant of primary cutaneous follicular lymphoma, and distinguishes it from diffuse large B-cell lymphoma.

Complete staging investigations must be performed in all patients as the clinicopathological features alone cannot distinguish with certainty between primary cutaneous follicle centre cell lymphoma and secondary involvement of extracutaneous lymphoma with a similar morphology. Primary cutaneous lymphoma is currently defined by the absence of extracutaneous manifestations after complete staging investigations have been performed (see Chapter 1) [22].

Clinical features

Patients are adults of both genders. Cutaneous follicle centre cell lymphoma presents clinically with erythematous papules, plaques and tumours, usually non-ulcerated. Lesions are located mostly on the head and neck and on the trunk (Figs 9.1–9.6). A distinct clinical presentation with plaques

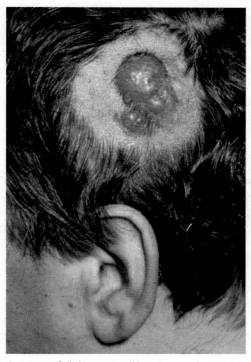

Fig. 9.1 Cutaneous follicle centre cell lymphoma. Clustered tumours on the scalp.

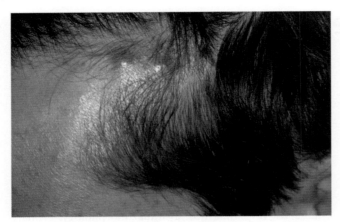

Fig. 9.2 Cutaneous follicle centre cell lymphoma (early lesions). Two papular lesions on the scalp.

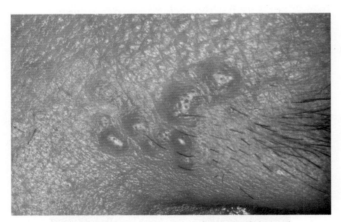

Fig. 9.3 Cutaneous follicle centre cell lymphoma (early lesions). Clustered papules on the right eyebrow.

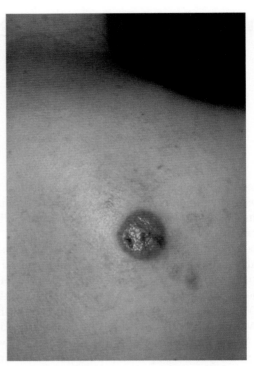

Fig. 9.4 Cutaneous follicle centre cell lymphoma. Large erythematous tumour on the shoulder. Note infiltrated erythematous patches and papules in the surroundings.

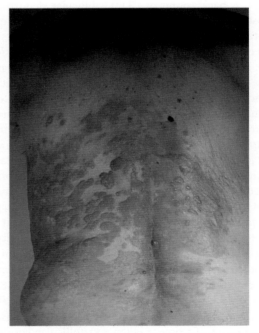

Fig. 9.5 Cutaneous follicle centre cell lymphoma. Large erythematous tumours surrounded by plaques and papules covering a large area of the back (so-called 'reticulohistiocytoma of the dorsum', 'Crosti's lymphoma').

and tumours on the back surrounded by erythematous macules and papules expanding centrifugally around the central tumours has been described in the past as 'reticulohistiocytoma of the dorsum' or 'Crosti's lymphoma' (Fig. 9.5) [24,25].

Lesions are usually clustered at a single site but may be multiple at different sites. Although there are no clear-cut differences in clinical presentation between the diffuse and follicular variants of cutaneous follicle centre cell lymphoma, cases with a follicular pattern have a predilection for the head and neck region, whereas the so-called Crosti's lymphoma corresponds in the majority of cases to a follicle centre cell lymphoma with a diffuse pattern of growth [18,24].

In some patients with the clinical presentation of Crosti's lymphoma, small erythematous papules located far from the main lesions can be observed (Fig. 9.7). These papules represent early manifestations of the disease and reveal histopathologically specific features of follicle centre cell lymphoma (Fig. 9.8). The question arises as to whether local

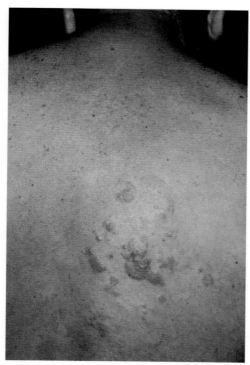

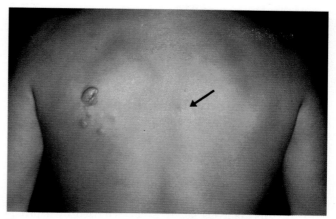

Fig. 9.7 Cutaneous follicle centre cell lymphoma. Large tumours on the left side of the back. Note small papules located at the right paravertebral area (arrow).

radiotherapy is the more appropriate treatment modality for these patients, and what the radiation field should be. The relatively high incidence of local recurrences observed in Crosti's lymphoma may be caused, at least in part, by the presence of early lesions far from the main tumour, which had not been identified clinically at the time of the planning of treatment.

Fig. 9.6 Cutaneous follicle centre cell lymphoma. Erythematous papules and plaques on the back (early lesions of 'Crosti's lymphoma').

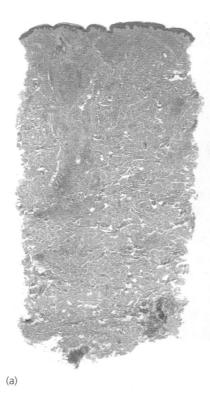

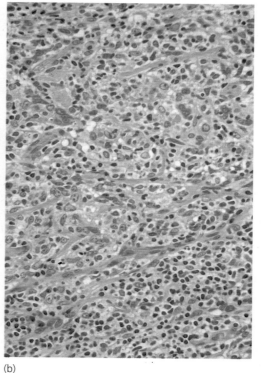

Fig. 9.8 Cutaneous follicle centre cell lymphoma, early lesion. (a) Histology reveals small nodular infiltrates throughout the dermis. (b) Cytomorphology shows small lymphocytes admixed with centrocytes and centroblasts.

(a)

(b)

Association with infections such as *Borrelia burgdorferi*, hepatitis C or human herpesvirus 8 has been described in sporadic patients but does not seem to be a major aetiological factor for cutaneous follicle centre cell lymphoma [26–29].

Histopathology, immunophenotype and molecular genetics

Histopathology

Cutaneous follicle centre cell lymphoma with a diffuse pattern of growth involves the entire dermis, often extending into the subcutaneous fat. It is characterized by a proliferation of small, medium and large cleaved cells (centrocytes) admixed with variable numbers of large cells with the morphological features of centroblasts (Figs 9.9 & 9.10) [1,30]. Centroblasts should not be arranged in 'sheets'. Small reactive T lymphocytes are almost invariably admixed with

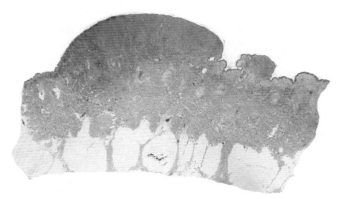

Fig. 9.9 Cutaneous follicle centre cell lymphoma, diffuse type. Dense nodular infiltrates within the dermis.

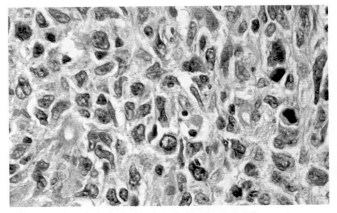

Fig. 9.10 Cutaneous follicle centre cell lymphoma, diffuse type. Centrocytes predominate, admixed with some centroblasts (detail of Fig. 9.9).

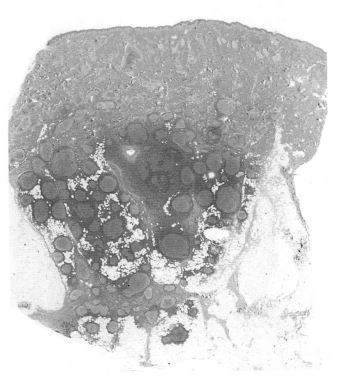

Fig. 9.11 Cutaneous follicle centre cell lymphoma, follicular type. Dense infiltrate within the deep dermis and subcutaneous fat. Note prominent lymphoid follicles.

the tumour cells. In contrast, the histopathological features of cases with a follicular pattern of growth resemble those of follicular lymphomas at extracutaneous sites [19,31]. They consist of nodular infiltrates extending into the entire dermis, usually involving the subcutaneous tissues, characterized by a prominent follicular pattern (Fig. 9.11). The epidermis is spared as a rule. Neoplastic follicles in follicular lymphoma show several morphological abnormalities, such as reduced or absent mantle zones, reduced numbers or complete lack of tingible body macrophages, and monomorphous appearance without a clear-cut distinction between dark and light areas (Fig. 9.12). These features are readily observed at low power and provide valuable clues for the diagnosis. Cytomorphologically, they consist of small and large centrocytes admixed with centroblasts, often intermingled with reactive small lymphocytes arranged within interfollicular areas.

In some cases, both patterns of growth (diffuse and follicular) can be observed in the same tumour (Fig. 9.13). In these cases, residual follicles are usually visible at the periphery of the infiltrate with a more diffuse pattern in the middle.

A morphological variant showing nodules of medium–large centrocytes admixed with some centroblasts without a

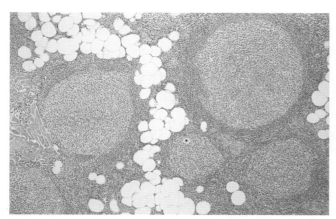

Fig. 9.12 Cutaneous follicle centre cell lymphoma, follicular type. Lymphoid follicles reveal several atypical morphological aspects: reduced mantle zone, monomorphism (lack of dark and light areas), and absence of tingible body macrophages (detail of Fig. 9.11).

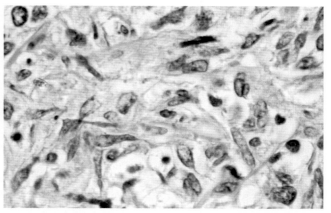

Fig. 9.14 Cutaneous follicle centre cell lymphoma, spindle cell type. Note several cells with bizarre elongated nuclei representing morphological variations of centrocytes.

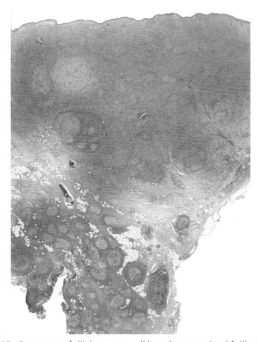

Fig. 9.13 Cutaneous follicle centre cell lymphoma, mixed follicular and diffuse type. Dense nodular infiltrates within the dermis and subcutaneous fat. Note neoplastic follicles arranged mainly at the periphery of areas with a diffuse pattern of growth.

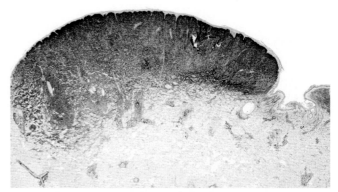

Fig. 9.15 Cutaneous follicle centre cell lymphoma, diffuse type. Positive staining for CD10 (same case as Fig. 9.9).

phoma (Fig. 9.14) [34–37]. Sclerosis and myxoid areas may also be observed in cases of cutaneous follicle centre cell lymphoma.

Immunophenotype

Neoplastic cells are positive for B-cell markers such as CD20 and CD79a in both the diffuse and follicular variants of cutaneous follicle centre cell lymphoma. Remarkably, most cases showing a diffuse pattern of growth are usually (but not always!—see Fig. 9.15) CD10⁻ and do not show a network of CD21⁺ follicular dendritic cells in the background. In contrast, cases of follicle centre cell lymphoma with a follicular pattern of growth are positive for markers of germinal centre cells such as CD10 and Bcl-6 (Figs 9.16a,b) [19,38,39]. The presence of small clusters of CD10⁺ and/or Bcl-6⁺ cells outside neoplastic follicles can be observed in a proportion of these cases [19]. This phenomenon, caused by the active

prominent interfollicular infiltrate has been termed in the past 'large cell lymphocytoma' [32,33]. It seems likely that many, if not all, of these cases represent cutaneous follicle centre cell lymphomas. Another peculiar histopathological variant is characterized by the predominance of spindle and bizarre cells, and has been termed spindle cell B-cell lym-

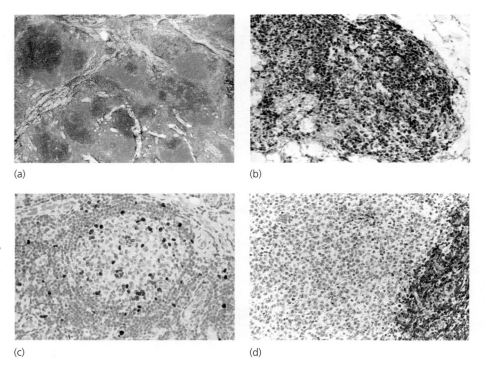

(a)

(b)

(c)

(d)

Fig. 9.16 Cutaneous follicle centre cell lymphoma, follicular type. Neoplastic follicles stain for (a) CD10 and (b) Bcl-6. (c) Reduced proliferation rate within a neoplastic follicle detected by the antibody MIB-1. (d) Negativity of neoplastic cells for Bcl-2. Note positive small lymphocytes at the edge of the neoplastic aggregate representing positive internal controls.

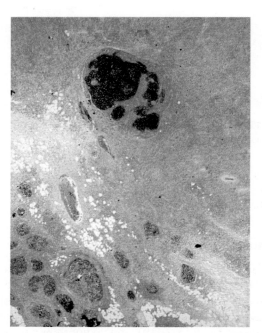

Fig. 9.17 Cutaneous follicle centre cell lymphoma, mixed follicular and diffuse type. Note large aggregates of CD21⁺ dendritic follicular cells at the margin of an area with a diffuse pattern of growth (same case as Fig. 9.13).

'migration' of follicular cells from the follicle to the interfollicular area and back, has been described in nodal follicular lymphomas as well, and is not observed as a rule in reactive lymphoid infiltrates, thus being virtually diagnostic of fol-

licular lymphoma [40]. In cases with both patterns present, CD21⁺ follicular dendritic cells are usually located at the periphery of large areas with a diffuse pattern of growth (Fig. 9.17). A good diagnostic clue for cutaneous follicle centre cell lymphoma with a follicular pattern is provided by the staining for proliferating cells (Ki67, MIB-1). Normal (reactive) germinal centres show a high degree of proliferation (more than 90% of cells), whereas neoplastic follicles often show a proliferative fraction of less than 50% of the cells (Fig. 9.16c) [19,38]. A residual network of CD21⁺ follicular dendritic cells is usually found within the neoplastic follicles. The MT2 antibody, considered by some authors as a useful marker of nodal follicular lymphoma, is only of limited value in cases of cutaneous follicle centre cell lymphoma with a diffuse or follicular pattern [41,42].

Although conflicting statements have been proposed, analysis of published reports shows that Bcl-2 expression can be found only in a minority of cases of primary cutaneous follicle centre cell lymphoma [10,19–22,30,43–45]. Bcl-2 expression is present in 10–15% of cases within a small minority of the follicular cells, and only very rarely in the whole neoplastic population (Fig. 9.16d). However, when present, Bcl-2 positivity in germinal centre cells is virtually diagnostic of follicle centre cell lymphoma and is incompatible with a reactive process.

The detection of an immunoglobulin light chain restriction is difficult in paraffin sections but can be observed more often on snap-frozen tissue sections. However, negativity for both kappa and lambda seems to be relatively common in cutaneous cases, thus hindering the diagnostic value of immunohistological staining for immunoglobulin light chains [15,19].

Molecular genetics

Cutaneous follicle centre cell lymphoma shows a monoclonal rearrangement of the J_H gene in the majority of cases, but a lack of detection of rearrangement by polymerase chain reaction (PCR) is not infrequent. This may be caused, at least in part, by the high number of somatic hypermutations that are characteristic of these tumours, thus hindering annealing of the DNA probes to neoplastic DNA.

In a recent study on cases with a follicular pattern of growth, using a laser beam-based microdissection technique, we demonstrated the presence of the same monoclonal population of B lymphocytes within different follicles from a given tumour, thus proving beyond doubt that these cases represented examples of true follicular lymphoma [19]. Remarkably, in some of the cases, a band corresponding to the same monoclonal population of follicular lymphocytes could be observed in interfollicular areas as well, confirming that neoplastic cells are actively migrating between follicles and interfollicular areas, as already suggested by the pattern of CD10 and Bcl-6 staining described above.

Analysis of data from the literature clearly shows that the interchromosomal (14;18) translocation is extremely uncommon in primary cutaneous follicle centre cell lymphoma [10,11,19–22,46,47]. At present, there are no data on specific chromosomal alterations in cases of cutaneous follicle centre cell lymphoma with either diffuse or follicular patterns. Gene expression studies using cDNA microarrays revealed that cases of cutaneous follicle centre cell lymphoma have a germinal centre cell signature [48].

A clonal evolution of neoplastic B lymphocytes has been demonstrated by single-cell PCR studies [49]. Recently, differential expression of a group of genes involved in regulation of lymphopoiesis and unalignant transformation (Polycomb-group) was found in cutaneous B-cell lymphomas arising on the head and trunk as opposed to those located on the legs, confirming that these lymphomas probably represent distinct entities [50].

Treatment

Patients are mainly treated by local radiotherapy [1,17,51–53]. Solitary tumours can be excised surgically, generally followed by local radiotherapy to the surgical field. Systemic chemotherapy is usually not necessary in these patients [1]. Interferon-α (either systemically or intralesionally) has been used for treatment of patients with cutaneous follicle centre cell lymphoma, sometimes associated with other treatment regimens [53–56]. Other modalities used sporadically include intralesional chemotherapy and antibiotic treatment [53,57].

Recently, a promising new treatment has been introduced with the use of anti-CD20 monoclonal antibodies (rituximab), which can be administered either systemically or intralesionally [58–63]. Rituximab can also be combined with systemic chemotherapy in patients with generalized skin or extracutaneous involvement [64].

Prognosis

The prognosis of patients with primary cutaneous follicle centre cell lymphoma is very good, regardless of the pattern of growth [1,17,19,65]. Although local recurrences can be frequently observed, extracutaneous involvement is uncommon. Involvement of the central nervous system has been observed rarely [66]. There is no prognostic difference between cases with a follicular pattern as compared to those with a diffuse pattern of growth [1].

RÉSUMÉ

Clinical	Adults. Solitary or grouped papules, plaques and tumours, often surrounded by erythematous patches. Preferential locations: scalp, back ('reticulohistiocytoma of the dorsum').
Morphology	Nodular or diffuse infiltrates characterized by predominance of centroblasts and centrocytes admixed with small lymphocytes. The pattern of growth can be follicular, diffuse, or mixed.
Immunology	CD20, 79a + CD10, Bcl-6 + CD5, 43 − Bcl-2 − MIB-1 reduced proliferation
Genetics	Monoclonal rearrangement of the J_H gene detected in the majority of cases. No specific genetic alterations. t(14;18) absent in most cases.
Treatment guidelines	Radiotherapy; excision of solitary lesions; interferon-α; anti-CD20 antibody. Systemic chemotherapy is reserved for generalized lesions and/or extracutaneous spread.

References

1 Willemze R, Kerl H, Sterry W *et al.* EORTC classification for primary cutaneous lymphomas: a proposal from the Cutaneous Lymphoma Study Group of the European Organization for Research and Treatment of Cancer. *Blood* 1997; **90**: 354–71.

2 Nathwani BN, Harris NL, Weisenburger D *et al.* Follicular lymphoma. In: Jaffe ES, Harris NL, Stein H, Vardiman JW, eds. *World Health Organization Classification of Tumours: Tumours of haematopoietic and lymphoid tissues.* Lyon: IARC press, 2001: 162–7.

3 Gatter KC, Warnke RA. Diffuse large B-cell lymphoma. In: Jaffe ES, Harris NL, Stein H, Vardiman JW, eds. *World Health Organization Classification of Tumours: Tumours of haematopoietic and lymphoid tissues.* Lyon: IARC press, 2001: 171–4.

4 Dogan A, Bagdi E, Munson P, Isaacson PG. CD10 and Bcl-6 expression in paraffin sections of normal lymphoid tissue and B-cell lymphomas. *Am J Surg Pathol* 2000; **24**: 846–52.

5 Isaacson PG. Malignant lymphomas with a follicular growth pattern. *Histopathology* 1996; **28**: 487–95.

6 Gaulard P, D'Agay MF, Peuchmaur M *et al.* Expression of the bcl-2 gene product in follicular lymphoma. *Am J Surg Pathol* 1992; **140**: 1089–95.

7 Tsujimoto Y, Cossman J, Jaffe E, Croce CM. Involvement of the bcl-2 gene in human follicular lymphoma. *Science* 1985; **228**: 1440–3.

8 Pezzella F, Gatter KC, Mason DY *et al.* Bcl-2 protein expression in follicular lymphomas in absence of 14;18 translocation. *Lancet* 1990; **336**: 1510–11.

9 Ngan BY, Chen-Levy Z, Weiss LM, Warnke RA, Cleary ML. Expression in non-Hodgkin's lymphoma of the bcl-2 protein associated with the t(14;18) chromosomal translocation. *N Engl J Med* 1988; **318**: 1638–44.

10 Cerroni L, Volkenandt M, Rieger E, Soyer HP, Kerl H. Bcl-2 protein expression and correlation with the interchromosomal 14;18 translocation in cutaneous lymphomas and pseudolymphomas. *J Invest Dermatol* 1994; **102**: 231–5.

11 Delia D, Borrello MG, Berti E *et al.* Clonal immunoglobulin gene rearrangements and normal T-cell receptor, bcl-2, and c-myc genes in primary cutaneous B-cell lymphomas. *Cancer Res* 1989; **49**: 4901–5.

12 Isaacson PG, Norton AJ. *Extranodal Lymphomas*, Edinburgh: Churchill Livingstone, 1994: 131–91.

13 Slater DN. Are most primary cutaneous B-cell lymphomas 'marginal cell lymphomas'?: reply. *Br J Dermatol* 1995; **133**: 953–4.

14 Berti E, Gianotti R, Alessi E, Caputo R. Primary cutaneous follicular center cell lymphoma: immunogenotypical and immunophenotypical aspects. In: van Vloten WA, Willemze R, Lange Vejlsgaard G, Thomsen K eds. *Cutaneous Lymphomas and Pseudolymphomas.* Basel: Karger, 1990: 196–202.

15 Garcia CF, Weiss LM, Warnke RA, Wood GS. Cutaneous follicular lymphoma. *Am J Surg Pathol* 1986; **10**: 454–63.

16 Kerl H, Kresbach H. Germinal center cell-derived lymphomas of the skin. *J Dermatol Surg Oncol* 1984; **10**: 291–5.

17 Pimpinelli N, Santucci M, Bosi A *et al.* Primary cutaneous follicular centre-cell lymphoma: a lymphoproliferative disease with favourable prognosis. *Clin Exp Dermatol* 1989; **14**: 12–9.

18 Pimpinelli N, Santucci M, Carli P *et al.* Primary cutaneous follicular center cell lymphoma: clinical and histological aspects. In: van Vloten WA, Willemze R, Lange Vejlsgaard G, Thomsen K eds. *Cutaneous Lymphomas and Pseudolymphomas.* Basel: Karger, 1990: 203–20.

19 Cerroni L, Arzberger E, Pütz B *et al.* Primary cutaneous follicle center cell lymphoma with follicular growth pattern. *Blood* 2000; **95**: 3922–8.

20 Goodlad JR, Krajewski AS, Batstone PJ *et al.* Primary cutaneous follicular lymphoma: a clinicopathologic and molecular study of 16 cases in support of a distinct entity. *Am J Surg Pathol* 2002; **26**: 733–41.

21 Mirza I, Macpherson N, Paproski S *et al.* Primary cutaneous follicular lymphoma: an assessment of clinical, histopathologic, immunophenotypic, and molecular features. *J Clin Oncol* 2002; **20**: 647–55.

22 Lawnicki LC, Weisenburger DD, Aoun P *et al.* The t(14;18) and bcl-2 expression are present in a subset of primary cutaneous follicular lymphoma. *Am J Clin Pathol* 2002; **118**: 765–72.

23 Fink-Puches R, Zenahlik P, Bäck B *et al.* Primary cutaneous lymphomas: applicability of current classification schemes (European Organization for Research and Treatment of Cancer, World Health Organization) based on clinicopathologic features observed in a large group of patients. *Blood* 2002; **99**: 800–5.

24 Crosti A. Micosi fungoide e reticuloistiocitomi cutanei maligni. *Min Dermatol* 1951; **26**: 3–11.

25 Berti E, Alessi E, Caputo R *et al.* Reticulohistiocytoma of the dorsum. *J Am Acad Dermatol* 1988; **19**: 259–72.

26 Cerroni L, Zöchling N, Pütz B, Kerl H. Infection by *Borrelia burgdorferi* and cutaneous B-cell lymphoma. *J Cutan Pathol* 1997; **24**: 457–61.

27 Goodlad JR, Davidson MM, Hollowood K *et al.* Primary cutaneous B-cell lymphoma and *Borrelia burgdorferi* infection in patients from the highlands of Scotland. *Am J Surg Pathol* 2000; **24**: 1279–85.

28 Zöchling N, Pütz B, Wolf P, Kerl H, Cerroni L. Human herpesvirus 8-specific DNA sequences in primary cutaneous B-cell lymphomas. *Arch Dermatol* 1998; **134**: 246–7.

29 Viguier M, River J, Agbalika F *et al.* B-cell lymphomas involving the skin associated with hepatitis C virus infection. *Int J Dermatol* 2002; **41**: 577–82.

30 Cerroni L, Kerl H. Primary cutaneous follicle center cell lymphoma. *Leuk Lymphoma* 2001; **42**: 891–900.

31 Nathwani BN, Winberg CD, Diamond LW, Bearman RM, Kim H. Morphologic criteria for the differentiation of follicular lymphoma from florid reactive follicular hyperplasia: a study of 80 cases. *Cancer* 1981; **48**: 1794–806.

32 English JSC, Smith NP, Spaull J, Wilson Jones E, Winkelmann RK. Large cell lymphocytoma: a clinicopathological study. *Clin Exp Dermatol* 1989; **14**: 181–5.

33 Winkelmann RK, Dabski K. Large cell lymphocytoma: follow-up, immunopathology studies, and comparison to cutaneous follicular and Crosti lymphoma. *Arch Dermatol Res* 1987; **279**: S81–7.

34 Cerroni L, El-Shabrawi-Caelen L, Fink-Puches R, LeBoit PE, Kerl H. Cutaneous spindle-cell B-cell lymphoma: a morphologic variant of cutaneous large B-cell lymphoma. *Am J Dermatopathol* 2000; **22**: 299–304.

35 Ferrara G, Bevilacqua M, Argenziano G. Cutaneous spindle B-cell lymphoma: a reappraisal. *Am J Dermatopathol* 2002; **24**: 526–7.

36 Cerroni L. Reply to cutaneous spindle B-cell lymphoma: a re-appraisal. *Am J Dermatopathol* 2002; **24**: 527–8.

37 Goodlad JR. Spindle-cell B-cell lymphoma presenting in the skin. *Br J Dermatol* 2001; **145**: 313–7.

38 Leinweber B, Colli C, Chott A, Kerl H, Cerroni L. Differential diagnosis of cutaneous infiltrates of B lymphocytes with follicular growth pattern. *Am J Dermatopathol*, 2004; **26**: 4–13.

39 Hoefnagel JJ, Vermeer MH, Jansen PM *et al*. Bcl-2, Bcl-6 and CD10 expression in cutaneous B-cell lymphoma: further support for a follicle centre cell origin and differential diagnostic significance. *Br J Dermatol* 2003; **149**: 1183–91.

40 Dogan AMQ, Aiello A, Diss TC *et al*. Follicular lymphomas contain a clonally linked but phenotypically distinct neoplastic B-cell population in the interfollicular zone. *Blood* 1988; **91**: 4708–14.

41 Browne G, Tobin B, Carney DN, Dervan PA. Aberrant MT2 positivity distinguishes follicular lymphoma from reactive follicular hyperplasia in B5- and formalin-fixed paraffin sections. *Am J Clin Pathol* 1991; **96**: 90–4.

42 Chimenti S, Cerroni L, Zenahlik P, Peris K, Kerl H. The role of MT2 and anti-bcl-2 protein antibodies in the differentiation of benign from malignant cutaneous infiltrates of B-lymphocytes with germinal center formation. *J Cutan Pathol* 1996; **23**: 319–22.

43 De Leval L, Harris NL, Longtine J, Ferry JA, Duncan LM. Cutaneous B-cell lymphomas of follicular and marginal zone types: use of Bcl-6, CD10, Bcl-2 and CD21 in differential diagnosis and classification. *Am J Surg Pathol* 2001; **25**: 732–41.

44 Rijlaarsdam JU, Meijer CJLM, Willemze R. Differentiation between lymphadenosis benigna cutis and primary cutaneous follicular center cell lymphomas: a comparative clinicopathologic study of 57 patients. *Cancer* 1990; **65**: 2301–6.

45 Triscott JA, Ritter JH, Swanson PE, Wick MR. Immunoreactivity for bcl-2 protein in cutaneous lymphomas and lymphoid hyperplasias. *J Cutan Pathol* 1995; **22**: 2–10.

46 Franco R, Fernandez-Vazquez A, Rodriguez-Peralto JL *et al*. Cutaneous follicular B-cell lymphoma: description of a series of 18 cases. *Am J Surg Pathol* 2001; **25**: 875–83.

47 Child FJ, Russell-Jones R, Woolford AJ *et al*. Absence of the t(14;18) chromosomal translocation in primary cutaneous B-cell lymphoma. *Br J Dermatol* 2001; **144**: 735–44.

48 Storz MN, van de Rijn M, Kim YH *et al*. Gene expression profiles of cutaneous B cell lymphoma. *J Invest Dermatol* 2003; **120**: 865–70.

49 Golembowsky S, Gellrich S, von Zimmermann M *et al*. Clonal evolution in a primary cutaneous follicle center B cell lymphoma revealed by single cell analysis in sequential biopsies. *Immunobiology* 2000; **201**: 631–44.

50 Raaphorst FM, Vermeer M, Fieret E *et al*. Site-specific expression of polycomb-group genes encoding the HPC-HPH/PRC1 complex in clinically defined primary nodal and cutaneous large B-cell lymphomas. *Am J Pathol* 2004; **164**: 533–42.

51 Rijlaarsdam JU, Toonstra J, Meijer CJLM, Noordijk EM, Willemze R. Treatment of primary cutaneous B-cell lymphomas of follicle center cell origin: a clinical follow-up study of 55 patients treated with radiotherapy or polychemotherapy. *J Clin Oncol* 1996; **14**: 549–55.

52 Piccinno R, Caccialanza M, Berti E. Dermatologic radiotherapy of primary cutaneous follicle center cell lymphoma. *Eur J Dermatol* 2003; **13**: 49–52.

53 Zenahlik P, Fink-Puches R, Kapp KS, Kerl H, Cerroni L. Die Therapie der primären kutanen B-Zell-Lymphome. *Hautarzt* 2000; **51**: 19–24.

54 Parodi A, Micalizzi C, Rebora A. Intralesional natural interferon-α in the treatment of Crosti's lymphoma (primary cutaneous B follicular centre-cell lymphoma): report of four cases. *J Dermatol Treatm* 1996; **7**: 105–7.

55 Cerroni L, Peris K, Torlone G, Chimenti S. Use of recombinant interferon-α2a in the treatment of cutaneous lymphomas of T- and B-cell lineage. In: Lambert WC, Giannotti B, van Vloten WA, eds. *Basic Mechanisms of Physiologic and Aberrant Lymphoproliferation in the Skin*. New York: Plenum Press, 1994: 545–51.

56 Trent JT, Romanelli P, Kerdel FA. Topical targretin and intralesional interferon-α for cutaneous lymphoma of the scalp. *Arch Dermatol* 2002; **138**: 1421–3.

57 Kempf W, Dummer R, Hess Schmid M *et al*. Intralesional cisplatin for the treatment of cutaneous B-cell lymphoma. *Arch Dermatol* 1998; **134**: 1343–5.

58 Heinzerling LM, Urbanek M, Funk JO *et al*. Reduction of tumor burden and stabilization of disease by systemic therapy with anti-CD20 antibody (rituximab) in patients with primary cutaneous B-cell lymphoma. *Cancer* 2000; **89**: 1835–44.

59 Schmook T, Stockfleth E, Lischner S *et al*. Remarkable remission of a follicular lymphoma treated with rituximab and polychemotherapy (CHOP). *Clin Exp Dermatol* 2003; **28**: 31–3.

60 Paul T, Radny P, Kröber SM *et al*. Intralesional rituximab for cutaneous B-cell lymphoma. *Br J Dermatol* 2001; **144**: 1239–43.

61 Gellrich S, Muche JM, Pelzer K, Audring H, Sterry W. Der Anti-CD20-Antikörper bei primär kutanen B-Zell-Lymphomen. *Hautarzt* 2001; **52**: 205–10.

62 Heinzerling L, Dummer R, Kempf W, Hess Schmid M, Burg G. Intralesional therapy with anti-CD20 monoclonal antibody rituximab in primary cutaneous B-cell lymphoma. *Arch Dermatol* 2000; **136**: 374–8.

63 Kennedy GA, Blum R, McCormack C, Prince HM. Treatment of primary cutaneous follicular centre lymphoma with rituximab: a report of two cases. *Australas J Dermatol* 2004; **45**: 54–7.

64 Fierro MT, Savoia P, Quaglino P *et al*. Systemic therapy with cyclophosphamide and anti-CD20 antibody (rituximab) in relapsed primary cutaneous B-cell lymphoma: a report of 7 cases. *J Am Acad Dermatol* 2003; **49**: 281–7.

65 Willemze R, Meijer CJLM, Sentis HJ *et al*. Primary cutaneous large cell lymphomas of follicular center cell origin: a clinical follow-up study of 19 patients. *J Am Acad Dermatol* 1987; **16**: 518–26.

66 Bekkenk MW, Postma TJ, Meijer CJLM, Willemze R. Frequency of central nervous system involvement in primary cutaneous B-cell lymphoma. *Cancer* 2000; **89**: 913–9.

Chapter 10 Marginal zone lymphoma and cutaneous immunocytoma

In the first edition of this book, we discussed cutaneous marginal zone lymphoma and immunocytoma in two separate chapters [1]. In recent years, most authors have agreed that these two entities represent subtypes of a single entity of low-grade malignant cutaneous B-cell lymphoma, and the term 'marginal zone lymphoma' has been widely used to refer to both [2–9]. There is no doubt that cutaneous marginal zone lymphoma and immunocytoma are closely related. However, we believe that some differences do exist and that for the moment we should still try to characterize each separately, in order to check whether the differences are substantial or not. In our view, the main differences between cutaneous marginal zone lymphoma and immunocytoma are the following:

1 Cutaneous marginal zone lymphoma is a tumour of younger adults and adults, whereas cutaneous immunocytoma is seen more often in the elderly.

2 The preferential location differs (trunk and upper extremities for cutaneous marginal zone lymphoma, lower extremities for immunocytoma).

3 Association with *Borrelia burgdorferi* infection is more common in cutaneous immunocytoma [10]. We have observed cases of immunocytoma, but not of marginal zone lymphoma, arising on the background of acrodermatitis chronica atrophicans.

4 The histopathological pattern differs (see below); intranuclear inclusions (Dutcher bodies) are seen only in cutaneous immunocytoma.

However, we fully acknowledge that the differences may be just variations on the theme of a single entity of low-grade cutaneous B-cell lymphoma and have therefore decided to include both of them in a single chapter in this edition of the book. The terminology, notwithstanding the term adopted, is still not correct. Marginal zone lymphoma of the skin is different from extranodal marginal zone lymphoma (which in turn is different from nodal marginal zone lymphoma and from splenic marginal zone lymphoma); in addition, immunocytoma of the skin has probably no relationship with lymphoplasmacytic lymphoma (formerly immunocytoma) of the lymph nodes, as features of Waldenström macroglobulinaemia are constantly absent in cutaneous cases. In short, a confusing terminology is being used and better terms for these entities will have to be found in due course. The original proposal of Santucci *et al.* [11] to term all cutaneous B-cell lymphomas 'skin-associated lymphoid tissue—SALT-type B-cell lymphomas' seems impractical in the light of the different clinical, histopathological, phenotypical and molecular features of the various B-cell lymphomas of the skin.

MARGINAL ZONE LYMPHOMA

Primary cutaneous marginal zone lymphoma is one of the major subtypes of the low-grade malignant cutaneous B-cell lymphomas. In the European Organization for Research and Treatment of Cancer (EORTC) classification it is grouped together with immunocytomas, whereas in the World Health Organization (WHO) classification it is listed among the extranodal marginal zone lymphomas of mucosa-associated lymphoid tissue (MALT) lymphoma [12,13]. Cases reported in the past as 'cutaneous follicular lymphoid hyperplasia with monotypic plasma cells' probably represent examples of marginal zone lymphoma of the skin [14].

Association with *B. burgdorferi* has been detected in some cases in areas both with and without endemic infection [10,15,16]. However, this association may be regional, as two other studies on cutaneous marginal zone lymphoma did not show evidence of infection by *B. burgdorferi* [17,18]. A link with *Helicobacter pylori* infection has been ruled out [19], and association with hepatitis C virus infection seems unlikely [20,21]. In spite of rare positive cases, there seems to be no involvement of human herpesviruses 7 and 8 in the pathogenesis of cutaneous marginal zone lymphoma [22,23].

In two patients, the onset of cutaneous marginal zone lymphoma followed successful treatment of nodal Hodgkin lymphoma [24].

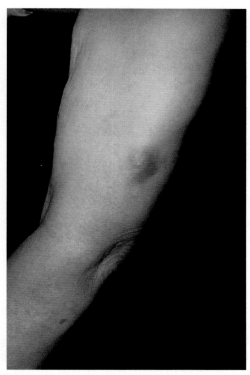

Fig. 10.1 Marginal zone lymphoma. Solitary erythematous nodule on the arm.

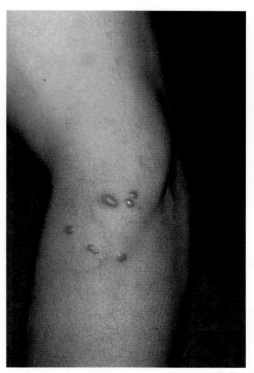

Fig. 10.3 Marginal zone lymphoma. Cluster of small erythematous nodules on the arm.

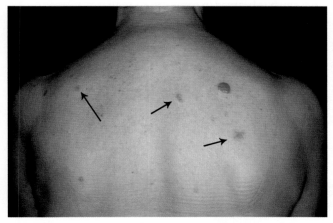

Fig. 10.2 Marginal zone lymphoma. Large erythematous nodule on the right shoulder. Note an earlier lesion on the left shoulder (long arrow) and two scars from previous excisions of similar lesions on the back (short arrows).

Clinical features

Patients are typically younger adults, with a male predominance [3]. An onset in childhood has been observed [25,26]. They present with red to reddish brown papules, plaques and nodules localized particularly to the upper extremities or the trunk. Lesions are commonly solitary but may be multiple, characterized either by localized clusters of papules and small nodules or by several lesions scattered on the trunk and upper extremities (Figs 10.1–10.3). Cutaneous recurrences are frequent and may be distant from the primary site of involvement. The clinical picture of 'Crosti's lymphoma' (see Chapter 9) is never seen in patients with cutaneous marginal zone lymphoma.

The onset of anetoderma in some lesions of cutaneous marginal zone lymphoma has been reported [27,28].

Histopathology, immunophenotype and molecular genetics

Histopathology

Histology shows patchy, nodular or diffuse infiltrates involving the dermis and sometimes the superficial part of the subcutaneous fat. The epidermis is not involved. A characteristic pattern can be observed at scanning magnification: nodular infiltrates with follicles, sometimes containing reactive

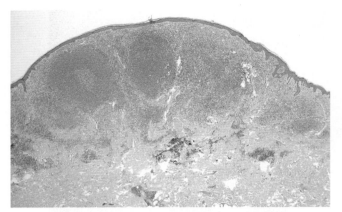

Fig. 10.4 Marginal zone lymphoma. Dense nodular infiltrates within the dermis. Note characteristic arrangement of the cells with central nodules of reactive lymphocytes, one with a germinal centre, surrounded by small amounts of neoplastic cells (see text).

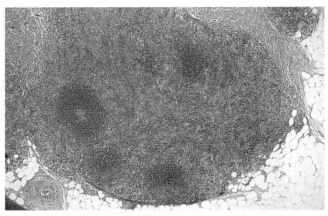

Fig. 10.5 Marginal zone lymphoma. Dense nodule within the deep dermis and superficial subcutaneous fat. Note small nodules of reactive lymphocytes (dark), one with a germinal centre, surrounded by large numbers of neoplastic cells (pale) (see text).

germinal centres, are surrounded by a pale-staining peri- and interfollicular population of small- to medium-sized cells with indented nuclei, inconspicuous nucleoli and abundant pale cytoplasm (marginal zone cells, centrocyte-like cells) (Figs 10.4 & 10.5) [3]. In addition, plasma cells (at the margins of the infiltrate), lymphoplasmacytoid cells, small lymphocytes and occasional large blasts are observed. The number of neoplastic cells within the infiltrate is variable and can be very low.

In typical cases, the neoplastic population is composed of marginal zone cells, a few lymphoplasmacytoid lymphocytes and several plasma cells. Usually marginal zone cells represent only a proportion of the neoplastic population (Fig. 10.6a) but in rare cases they predominate, forming sheets without plasma cell differentiation (Fig. 10.6b). In other lesions, neoplastic plasma cells predominate admixed with a few marginal zone cells, resembling the picture of

cutaneous plasmacytoma (Fig. 10.6c) [29]. Cases with predominance of blasts are rare (Fig. 10.7) and should be distinguished from examples of follicle centre cell lymphoma by accurate immunophenotyping (see below). Even in cases with predominance of blasts, reactive cells are a prominent component of the infiltrate and neoplastic cells are usually a minority of it. Eosinophils, as well as a granulomatous reaction, can be observed in some cases [3,30].

It should be emphasized that reactive cells (T and B lymphocytes, histiocytes, eosinophils) represent often the majority of the infiltrating cells in lesions of cutaneous marginal zone lymphoma, thus creating diagnostic problems.

Immunophenotype

The marginal zone cells reveal a CD20$^+$, CD79a$^+$, CD5$^-$, CD10$^-$ and Bcl-6$^-$ phenotype. Bcl-6 and CD10 antibodies are

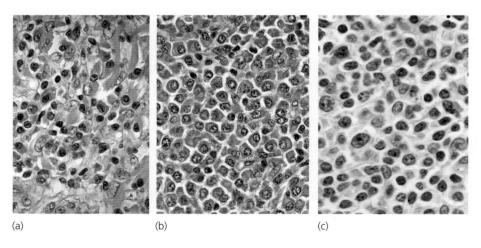

(a) (b) (c)

Fig. 10.6 Marginal zone lymphoma. (a) Marginal zone cells ('centrocyte-like') with abundant cytoplasm admixed with plasma cells, small lymphocytes and eosinophils. (b) Marginal zone cells, some with blastic morphology, predominate. (c) Lymphoplasmacytoid cells and plasma cells predominate, admixed with some blastic cells.

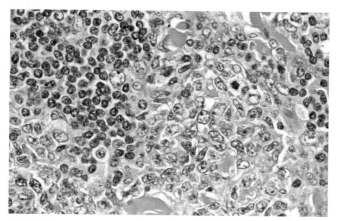

Fig. 10.7 Marginal zone lymphoma. Note several blastic cells admixed with small reactive lymphocytes.

particularly useful for differentiation of cutaneous marginal zone lymphoma with blastic differentiation from follicle centre cell lymphoma [31–33]. Coexpression of CD20 and CD43 is usually not found [34]. In approximately 75–85% of cases, intracytoplasmic monotypic expression of immuno-globulin light chains can be observed (Fig. 10.8). Staining for Ki67 (MIB-1) shows that the proliferating monoclonal population of B lymphocytes is characteristically disposed at the periphery of the cellular aggregates.

Nuclear Bcl-10 expression has been observed in a small number of cases in the absence of Bcl-10 gene mutations [17].

Molecular genetics

A monoclonal rearrangement of the J_H gene can be observed in approximately 50–60% of cases. The t(11;18) and the t(1;14) are not present in cutaneous cases [17,35]. Recently, a specific interchromosomal 14;18 translocation involving *IgH* and *MALT1* has been described in a subset of cutaneous marginal zone lymphomas as well as of marginal zone lymphomas of other organs including the liver, ocular adnexa and salivary glands, indicating the relationship of cutaneous cases to those arising at extracutaneous sites [35]. Gene expression studies using cDNA microarrays revealed that cases of cutaneous marginal zone lymphoma have a plasma cell signature [36].

Hypermethylation of *p15* and/or *p16* and expression of p15 and/or p16 protein have been observed in some patients with cutaneous marginal zone lymphoma [37].

Treatment

Solitary lesions may be excised. Complete responses have also been achieved after administration of systemic steroids. Many patients can be managed with a so-called 'watchful waiting' strategy. Patients with multiple lesions can be treated with interferon-α or with anti-CD20 antibodies (rituximab) [38–41]. Complete responses after systemic antibiotics have been reported, and this should probably be the primary treatment for patients with evidence of *B. burgdorferi* infection

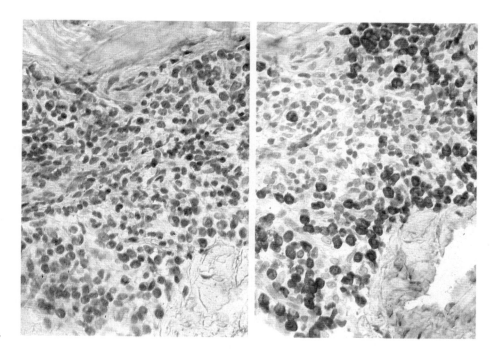

Fig. 10.8 Marginal zone lymphoma. Monoclonal lambda expression of plasma cells at the periphery of nodular infiltrates.

[39,42,43]. Systemic chemotherapy should be reserved for those rare cases with extracutaneous dissemination.

Prognosis

The prognosis is excellent, and the estimated 5-year survival is 98% [44]. Recurrences can be observed in 40–50% of patients after successful treatment but retain the low-grade features of the primary tumour. At present, the prognostic significance of different histopathological subtypes (mixed cell, predominance of marginal zone cells, predominance of plasma cells), if any, is unclear. Blastic transformation in recurrent lesions has been associated with a worse prognosis [45]. It has been suggested that cases with Bcl-10 nuclear expression have a locally more aggressive behaviour [17].

RÉSUMÉ

Marginal zone lymphoma

Clinical	Young adults and adults; cases in children reported. Solitary or grouped papules or small nodules. Preferential locations: upper extremities, trunk.
Morphology	Patchy, nodular or diffuse infiltrates. Characteristic pattern with central nodular dark area composed of small reactive lymphocytes with or without formation of germinal centres, surrounded by a pale area where neoplastic marginal zone cells and plasma cells predominate.
Immunology	CD20, 79a + CD5, 10, 43, Bcl-6 – cIg + (monoclonal)
Genetics	Monoclonal rearrangement of the J_H gene detected in 50–60% of cases. t(14;18)(q32;q21) in a minority of cases.
Treatment guidelines	Excision of solitary lesions; systemic steroids; radiotherapy; 'watchful waiting'. Interferon-α and anti-CD20 antibody (rituximab) are effective. Antibiotic treatment may be effective. Systemic chemotherapy reserved for patients with extracutaneous spread.

IMMUNOCYTOMA

Immunocytoma is defined as a proliferation of small lymphocytes, lymphoplasmacytoid cells and plasma cells showing monotypic intracytoplasmic immunoglobulins. Primary cutaneous immunocytoma differs from nodal immunocytoma: patients do not show the features of Waldenström macroglobulinaemia and have an excellent prognosis and response to treatment. Rare reports on skin lesions of lymphoplasmacytic lymphoma in patients with Waldenström macroglobulinaemia probably represent secondary cutaneous involvement rather than primary cutaneous immunocytomas [46]. In the WHO classification, cutaneous immunocytoma probably would not be classified among the lymphoplasmacytic lymphomas, but rather within the category of extranodal marginal zone B-cell lymphoma of mucosa-associated lymphoid tissue (MALT lymphoma) [13]. However, we have encountered some cases that fit into the definition of lymphoplasmacytic lymphoma as proposed by the WHO (a neoplasm of small B lymphocytes, plasmacytoid monocytes and plasma cells, without features of other lymphomas such as pseudofollicles, neoplastic follicles and marginal zone or monocytoid B cells). In the EORTC classification, cutaneous immunocytoma is listed in a category together with marginal zone lymphoma [12]. At least some of the cases reported in the recent past as cutaneous immunocytomas would probably be classified today as marginal zone lymphoma [47,48].

There may be a link between primary cutaneous immunocytoma and infection by *B. burgdorferi*. In the past, cases of cutaneous immunocytoma have been observed arising within skin lesions of acrodermatitis chronica atrophicans [49]. In a study using the highly sensitive polymerase chain reaction (PCR) technique, 75% of cases classified as cutaneous immunocytoma were positive compared to 10% of cases of marginal zone lymphoma [10].

Clinical features

Patients are typically elderly, of both sexes. Clinical examination reveals erythematous reddish brown plaques or dome-shaped tumours located especially on the lower extremities (Fig. 10.9). Ulceration is uncommon. Generalized tumours are never encountered; rarely, patients present with miliary lesions restricted to an anatomical area (Fig. 10.10) [50].

Anetoderma may develop within skin lesions of cutaneous immunocytoma (Fig. 10.11) [51].

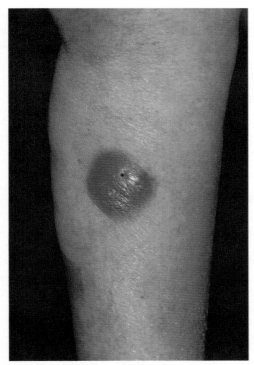

Fig. 10.9 Immunocytoma. Large dome-shaped tumour on the lower leg.

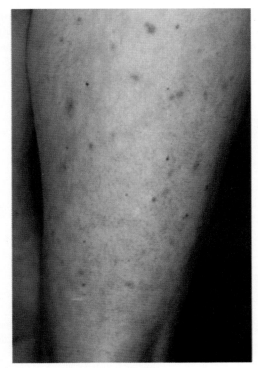

Fig. 10.10 Immunocytoma. Miliary lesions on the upper leg.

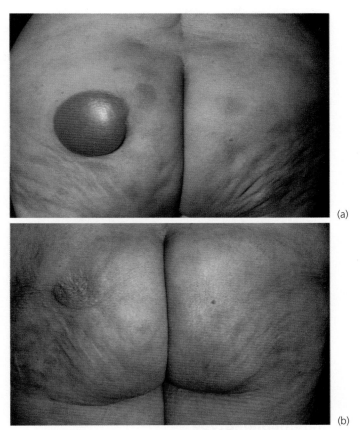

(a)

(b)

Fig. 10.11 Immunocytoma. (a) Large dome-shaped tumour on the buttock. (b) Note resolution with anetoderma after radiotherapy.

Histopathology, immunophenotype and molecular genetics

Histopathology

The architectural pattern is characterized by dense, monomorphous, nodular or diffuse infiltrates with involvement of the dermis and subcutis (Fig. 10.12). The epidermis is usually spared. At scanning power, the typical 'peripheral' pattern of cutaneous marginal zone lymphoma is not seen because the infiltrate is monomorphous. In addition, the neoplastic cells do not possess the abundant clear cytoplasm of marginal zone cells, giving the tumour a 'darker' appearance compared to marginal zone lymphoma.

The predominating cell types are lymphoplasmacytoid cells and small lymphocytes (Fig. 10.13a). In addition, plasma cells are usually present, often located at the periphery of the infiltrates. Periodic acid–Schiff (PAS)-positive intranuclear inclusions (Dutcher bodies) are observed as a rule

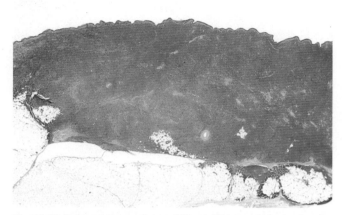

Fig. 10.12 Immunocytoma. Dense diffuse infiltrates within the dermis and the subcutaneous fat.

and represent a valuable diagnostic clue (Fig. 10.13b). React-ive follicles and germinal centres are rare.

In contrast to cutaneous marginal zone lymphoma, neo-plastic cells in cutaneous immunocytoma represent the great majority of the infiltrate, and reactive T and B lymphocytes and histiocytes only a minority. Eosinophils are absent.

Immunophenotype

The neoplastic cells express monoclonal cytoplasmic immu-noglobulins. Unlike nodal lymphoplasmacytic lymphoma, which is characterized by intracytoplasmic IgM, cutaneous

cases more often show IgG positivity. B-cell-associated markers are positive and CD5, CD10 and Bcl-6 are negative. Staining for CD43 reveals positivity in the neoplastic cells in some cases.

Molecular genetics

Molecular analysis reveals monoclonal rearrangement of the J_H gene in most cases. There are no specific genetic abnorm-alities associated with cutaneous immunocytoma.

Treatment

Small solitary nodules can be surgically excised. Larger lesions can be treated by local radiotherapy. As for other types of low-grade lymphoma, a 'watchful waiting' strategy may be appropriate in some patients. Cases with proven asso-ciation with *B. burgdorferi* infection should be managed with systemic antibiotics first. Systemic chemotherapy usually is not used for primary cutaneous immunocytoma.

Prognosis

The prognosis of cutaneous immunocytoma is excellent, with only a few patients experiencing a more aggressive course [52]. Recurrences can be observed after treatment, usually at the same site. Cutaneous recurrences (without extracutaneous disease) have also been observed after sys-temic chemotherapy [53].

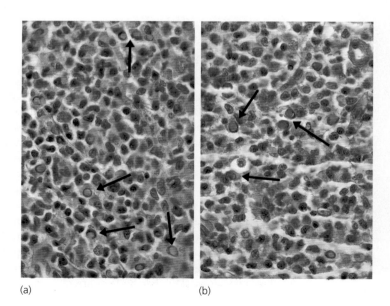

(a)   (b)

Fig. 10.13 Immunocytoma. (a) Lymphoplasmacytoid lymphocytes predominate. Note several eosinophilic intranuclear inclusions ('Dutcher bodies') (arrows). (b) Intranuclear inclusions ('Dutcher bodies') stain bright purple–red with periodic acid–Schiff (PAS) (arrows).

RÉSUMÉ

Immunocytoma

Clinical	Adults and elderly. Solitary or grouped plaques or dome-shaped tumours. Preferential location: lower extremities.
Morphology	Monomorphous, nodular or diffuse infiltrates characterized by predominance of lymphoplasmacytoid lymphocytes, small lymphocytes and plasma cells. Often Dutcher bodies.
Immunology	CD20, 79a + CD5, 10, Bcl-6 − CD43 +/− cIg + (monoclonal)
Genetics	Monoclonal rearrangement of the J_H gene detected in the majority of cases.
Treatment guidelines	Radiotherapy; surgical excision of small solitary lesions; 'watchful waiting'. Antibiotic treatment may be effective.

References

1 Cerroni L, Kerl H, Gatter K. *An Illustrated Guide to Skin Lymphoma.* Oxford: Blackwell Science, 1998.

2 Bailey EM, Ferry JA, Harris NL *et al.* Marginal zone lymphoma (low-grade B-cell lymphoma of mucosa-associated lymphoid tissue type) of skin and subcutaneous tissue: a study of 15 patients. *Am J Surg Pathol* 1996; **20**: 1011–23.

3 Cerroni L, Signoretti S, Höfler G *et al.* Primary cutaneous marginal zone B-cell lymphoma: a recently described entity of low-grade malignant cutaneous B-cell lymphoma. *Am J Surg Pathol* 1997; **21**: 1307–15.

4 de la Fouchardiére A, Balme B, Chouvet B *et al.* Primary cutaneous marginal zone B-cell lymphoma: a report of 9 cases. *J Am Acad Dermatol* 1999; **41**: 181–8.

5 Duncan LN, LeBoit PE. Are primary cutaneous immunocytoma and marginal zone lymphoma the same disease? *Am J Surg Pathol* 1997; **21**: 1368–72.

6 Sander CA, Kaudewitz P, Schirren CG, Jaffe ES, Kind P. Immunocytoma and marginal zone B-cell lymphoma (MALT lymphoma), presenting in skin: different entities or a spectrum of disease? *J Cutan Pathol* 1996; **23**: 59.

7 Servitje O, Gallardo F, Estrach T *et al.* Primary cutaneous marginal zone B-cell lymphoma: a clinical, histopathological, immunophe-notypic and molecular genetic study of 22 cases. *Br J Dermatol* 2002; **147**: 1147–58.

8 Tomaszewski MM, Abbondanzo SL, Lupton GP. Extranodal marginal zone B-cell lymphoma of the skin: a morphologic and immunophenotypic study of 11 cases. *Am J Dermatopathol* 2000; **22**: 205–11.

9 Yang B, Tubbs RR, Finn W *et al.* Clinicopathologic reassessment of primary cutaneous B-cell lymphomas with immunophenotypic and molecular genetic characterization. *Am J Surg Pathol* 2000; **24**: 694–702.

10 Cerroni L, Zöchling N, Pütz B, Kerl H. Infection by *Borrelia burgdorferi* and cutaneous B-cell lymphoma. *J Cutan Pathol* 1997; **24**: 457–61.

11 Santucci M, Pimpinelli N, Arganini L. Primary cutaneous B-cell lymphoma: a unique type of low-grade lymphoma—clinicopathologic and immunologic study of 83 cases. *Cancer* 1991; **67**: 2311–26.

12 Willemze R, Kerl H, Sterry W *et al.* EORTC classification for primary cutaneous lymphomas: a proposal from the Cutaneous Lymphoma Study Group of the European Organization for Research and Treatment of Cancer. *Blood* 1997; **90**: 354–71.

13 Isaacson PG, Müller-Hermelink HK, Piris MA *et al.* Extranodal marginal zone B-cell lymphoma of mucosa-associated lymphoid tissue (MALT lymphoma). In: Jaffe ES, Harris NL, Stein H, Vardiman JW, eds. *World Health Organization Classification of Tumours: Tumours of Haematopoietic and Lymphoid Tissues.* Lyon: IARC Press, 2001: 157–60.

14 Schmid U, Eckert F, Griesser H *et al.* Cutaneous follicular lymphoid hyperplasia with monotypic plasma cells: a clinicopathologic study of 18 patients. *Am J Surg Pathol* 1995; **19**: 12–20.

15 Goodlad JR, Davidson MM, Hollowood K *et al.* Primary cutaneous B-cell lymphoma and *Borrelia burgdorferi* infection in patients from the highlands of Scotland. *Am J Surg Pathol* 2000; **24**: 1279–85.

16 de la Fouchardiére A, Vandenesch F, Berger F. *Borrelia*-associated primary cutaneous MALT lymphoma in a non-endemic region. *Am J Surg Pathol* 2003; **27**: 702–3.

17 Li C, Inagaki H, Kuo TT *et al.* Primary cutaneous marginal zone B-cell lymphoma: a molecular and clinicopathologic study of 24 Asian cases. *Am J Surg Pathol* 2003; **27**: 1061–9.

18 Wood GS, Kamath NV, Guitart J *et al.* Absence of *Borrelia burgdorferi* DNA in cutaneous B-cell lymphomas from the United States. *J Cutan Pathol* 2001; **28**: 502–7.

19 Yazdi AS, Puchta U, Flaig MJ, Sander CA. *Helicobacter pylori* not detected in cutaneous mucosa-associated lymphoid tissue (MALT) lymphomas. *Arch Dermatol Res* 2003; **294**: 447–8.

20 Viguier M, River J, Agbalika F *et al.* B-cell lymphomas involving the skin associated with hepatitis C virus infection. *Int J Dermatol* 2002; **41**: 577–82.

21 Prati D, Zanella A, De Mattei C *et al.* Chronic hepatitis C virus infection and primary cutaneous B-cell lymphoma. *Br J Haematol* 1999; **105**: 841.

22 Zöchling N, Pütz B, Wolf P, Kerl H, Cerroni L. Human herpesvirus 8-specific DNA sequences in primary cutaneous B-cell lymphomas. *Arch Dermatol* 1998; **134**: 246–7.

23 Nagore E, Ledesma E, Collado C *et al.* Detection of Epstein–Barr virus and human herpesvirus 7 and 8 genomes in primary cutaneous T- and B-cell lymphomas. *Br J Dermatol* 2000; **143**: 320–3.

24 Servitje O, Marti RM, Estrach T *et al.* Occurrence of Hodgkin's disease and cutaneous B cell lymphoma in the same patient: a report of two cases. *Eur J Dermatol* 2000; **10**: 43–6.

25 Fink-Puches R, Chott A, Ardigo M *et al.* The spectrum of cutaneous lymphomas in patients under 20 years of age. *Pediatr Dermatol,* in press.

26 Taddesse-Heath L, Pittaluga S, Sorbara L *et al.* Marginal zone B-cell lymphoma in children and young adults. *Am J Surg Pathol* 2003; **27**: 522–31.

27 Kasper RC, Wood GS, Nihal M, LeBoit PE. Anetoderma arising in cutaneous B-cell lymphoproliferative disease. *Am J Dermatopathol* 2001; **23**: 124–32.

28 Child FJ, Woollons A, Price ML, Calonje E, Russell-Jones R. Multiple cutaneous immunocytoma with secondary anetoderma: a report of two cases. *Br J Dermatol* 2000; **143**: 165–70.

29 Kiyohara T, Kumakiri M, Kobayashi H, Nakamura H, Ohkawara A. Cutaneous marginal zone B-cell lymphoma: a case accompanied by massive plasmacytoid cells. *J Am Acad Dermatol* 2003; **48**: s82–s85.

30 Cerroni L. Cutaneous granulomas and malignant lymphomas. *Dermatology* 2003; **206**: 78–80.

31 Leinweber B, Colli C, Chott A, Kerl H, Cerroni L. Differential diagnosis of cutaneous infiltrates of B lymphocytes with follicular growth pattern. *Am J Dermatopathol,* 2004; **26**: 4–13.

32 de Leval L, Harris NL, Longtine J, Ferry JA, Duncan LM. Cutaneous B-cell lymphomas of follicular and marginal zone types: use of Bcl-6, CD10, Bcl-2, and CD21 in differential diagnosis and classification. *Am J Surg Pathol* 2001; **25**: 732–41.

33 Cerroni L, Kerl H. Diagnostic immunohistology: cutaneous lymphomas and pseudolymphomas. *Semin Cutan Med Surg* 1999; **18**: 64–70.

34 Baldassano MF, Bailey EM, Ferry JA, Harris NL, Duncan LM. Cutaneous lymphoid hyperplasia and cutaneous marginal zone lymphoma: comparison of morphologic and immunophenotypic features. *Am J Surg Pathol* 1999; **23**: 88–96.

35 Streubel B, Lamprecht A, Dierlamm J *et al.* T(14;18)(q32;q21) involving *IGH* and *MALT1* is a frequent chromosomal aberration in MALT lymphoma. *Blood* 2003; **101**: 2335–9.

36 Storz MN, van de Rijn M, Kim YH *et al.* Gene expression profiles of cutaneous B cell lymphoma. *J Invest Dermatol* 2003; **120**: 865–70.

37 Child FJ, Scarisbrick JJ, Calonje E *et al.* Inactivation of tumor suppressor genes p15^{INK4b} and p16^{INK4a} in primary cutaneous B cell lymphoma. *J Invest Dermatol* 2002; **118**: 941–8.

38 Soda R, Costanzo A, Cantonetti M *et al.* Systemic therapy of primary cutaneous B-cell lymphoma, marginal zone type, with rituximab, a chimeric anti-CD20 monoclonal antibody. *Acta Derm Venereol (Stockh)* 2001; **81**: 207–8.

39 Zenahlik P, Fink-Puches R, Kapp KS, Kerl H, Cerroni L. Die Therapie der primären kutanen B-Zell-Lymphome. *Hautarzt* 2000; **51**: 19–24.

40 Wollina U, Hahnfeld S, Kosmehl H. Primary cutaneous marginal center lymphoma: complete remission induced by interferon-α2a. *J Cancer Res Clin Oncol* 1999; **125**: 305–8.

41 Massengale WT, McBurney E, Gurtler J. CD20-negative relapse of cutaneous B-cell lymphoma after anti-CD20 monoclonal antibody therapy. *J Am Acad Dermatol* 2002; **46**: 441–3.

42 Roggero E, Zucca E, Mainetti C *et al.* Eradication of *Borrelia burgdorferi* infection in primary marginal zone B-cell lymphoma of the skin. *Hum Pathol* 2000; **31**: 263–8.

43 Kütting B, Bonsmann G, Metze D, Luger TA, Cerroni L. *Borrelia burgdorferi*-associated primary cutaneous B cell lymphoma: complete clearing of skin lesions after antibiotic pulse therapy or intralesional injection of interferon-α2a. *J Am Acad Dermatol* 1997; **36**: 311–4.

44 Fink-Puches R, Zenahlik P, Bäck B *et al.* Primary cutaneous lymphomas: applicability of current classification schemes (European Organization for Research and Treatment of Cancer, World Health Organization) based on clinicopathologic features observed in a large group of patients. *Blood* 2002; **99**: 800–5.

45 Gronbaeck K, Moller PH, Nedergaard T *et al.* Primary cutaneous B-cell lymphoma: a clinical, histological, phenotypic and genotypic study of 21 cases. *Br J Dermatol* 2000; **142**: 913–23.

46 Lin P, Bueso-Ramos C, Wilson CS, Mansoor A, Medeiros LJ. Waldenström macroglobulinemia involving extramedullary sites: morphologic and immunophenotypic findings in 44 patients. *Am J Surg Pathol* 2003; **27**: 1104–13.

47 LeBoit PE, McNutt NS, Reed JA, Jacobson M, Weiss LM. Primary cutaneous immunocytoma: a B-cell lymphoma that can easily be mistaken for cutaneous lymphoid hyperplasia. *Am J Surg Pathol* 1994; **18**: 969–78.

48 Rijlaarsdam JU, van der Putte SCJ, Berti E *et al.* Cutaneous immunocytomas: a clinicopathologic study of 26 cases. *Histopathology* 1993; **23**: 117–25.

49 Goos N. Acrodermatitis chronica atrophicans and malignant lymphoma. *Acta Derm Venereol (Stockh)* 1971; **51**: 457–9.

50 Aberer E, Cerroni L, Kerl H. Cutaneous immunocytoma presenting with multiple infiltrated macules and papules. *J Am Acad Dermatol* 2001; **44**: 324–9.

51 Machet MC, Machet L, Vaillant L *et al.* Acquired localized cutis laxa due to cutaneous lymphoplasmacytoid lymphoma. *Arch Dermatol* 1995; **131**: 110–1.

52 Sangueza OP, Burket JM, Sacks Y. Primary cutaneous immunocytoma: report of an unusual case with secondary spreading to the gastrointestinal tract. *J Cutan Pathol* 1997; **24**: 43–6.

53 Allbritton JI, Horn TD. Cutaneous lymphoplasmacytic lymphoma. *J Am Acad Dermatol* 1998; **38**: 820–4.

Chapter 11 Plasmacytoma

Cutaneous plasmacytoma is a B-cell lymphoma characterized by the clonal proliferation of plasma cells primarily affecting the skin, in the absence of bone marrow involvement (extramedullary plasmacytoma) [1–8]. This type of cutaneous B-cell lymphoma is exceedingly rare and in most instances skin lesions represent secondary involvement from multiple myeloma [9]. It is possible that most cases of primary cutaneous plasmacytoma are in fact examples of marginal zone lymphoma with a prominent plasma cell differentiation (see Chapter 10). In fact, we have observed patients with cutaneous 'plasmacytoma' who, after successful treatment, relapsed with skin lesions showing histopathological and phenotypical features of marginal zone lymphoma. In addition, in a workshop on cutaneous plasmacytoma organized by the European Organization for Research and Treatment of Cancer (EORTC)—Cutaneous Lymphomas Task Force in Bilbao in 2001, no clean-cut cases of primary cutaneous plasmacytoma could be identified.

Clinical features

Patients present clinically with solitary, clustered or, in exceptional cases, generalized [10,11] erythematous, reddish brown or violaceous cutaneous or subcutaneous plaques or tumours. There is a predilection for the head and trunk (Fig. 11.1). Cutaneous plasmacytoma occurs mostly in elderly male patients. Associated symptoms (serum paraproteinaemia, Bence Jones proteins in the urine) are usually absent.

Primary cutaneous plasmacytoma has been described as a secondary lymphoma in a patient with B-cell chronic lymphocytic leukaemia [12].

Histopathology, immunophenotype and molecular genetics

Histopathology

Cutaneous tumours of plasmacytoma consist of dense

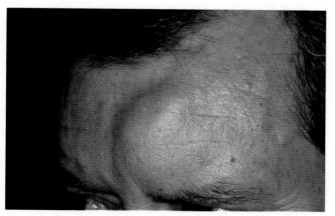

Fig. 11.1 Cutaneous plasmacytoma. Large subcutaneous tumour on the forehead.

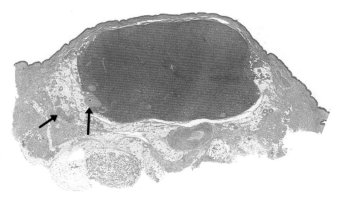

Fig. 11.2 Cutaneous plasmacytoma. Dense diffuse infiltrate of plasma cells within the entire dermis. Note amyloid deposits around blood vessels (arrows).

nodules and/or sheets of cells within the entire dermis and subcutis (Fig. 11.2). Mature and immature plasma cells with varying degrees of atypia predominate (Fig. 11.3). Dutcher bodies and Russell bodies are found occasionally. Small reactive lymphocytes are few or absent.

In rare cases, amyloid deposits are present within and/ or surrounding the neoplastic infiltrates (amyloid deposits

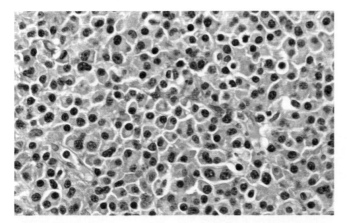

Fig. 11.3 Cutaneous plasmacytoma. The nodule is composed mainly of typical and atypical plasma cells.

are more common in secondary cutaneous involvement by plasmacytoma). Crystalloid intracytoplasmic inclusions within histiocytes and macrophages may also occur [13,14].

Immunophenotype

Neoplastic plasma cells contain cytoplasmic immunoglobulin (usually IgA) and show monoclonal expression of one immunoglobulin light chain. Leucocyte common antigen (CD45) and most B-cell-associated markers are negative, but cells can be stained by antibodies specific for CD38 or CD138 in most cases, and for CD79a in some cases. Immunohistochemical expression of cytokeratins, HMB45 and CD30 can be observed within neoplastic plasma cells, representing a source of diagnostic error.

Molecular genetics

Molecular analysis usually reveals a monoclonal rearrangement of the J_H gene. No specific genetic alterations associated with primary cutaneous plasmacytoma have been detected.

Treatment and prognosis

The treatment of choice is radiotherapy or surgical excision. Systemic treatment (usually melphalan and corticosteroids) should be given only to patients who have generalized skin lesions. A case of primary multiple cutaneous plasmacytoma has been treated with intralesional tumour necrosis factor-α with a marked reduction in tumour size [10].

The prognosis of primary cutaneous plasmacytoma is much more favourable than that of patients with secondary skin involvement associated with multiple myeloma, and seems to be related to the tumour burden [4]. Analysis of

data published in the literature is hindered by possible overlap of cutaneous plasmacytoma with cases of marginal zone lymphoma of the skin with prominent plasma cell differentiation. An overlap between these two entities has also been suggested for lesions arising at extramedullary sites other than the skin [15].

RÉSUMÉ

Clinical	Elderly; more males than females. Solitary, grouped or, rarely, generalized (sub)cutaneous plaques and tumours. Preferential locations: head, trunk.
Morphology	Nodular or diffuse infiltrates characterized by predominance of mature and immature plasma cells.
Immunology	CD45(LCA), CD20 – CD38, 138 + CD79a +/– CIg + (monoclonal)
Genetics	Monoclonal rearrangement of the J_H gene detected in the majority of cases. No specific genetic alterations.
Treatment guidelines	Radiotherapy; excision of solitary lesions. Systemic treatment only in cases with generalized lesions.

References

1 Torne R, Su WPD, Winkelmann RK, Smolle J, Kerl H. Clinicopathologic study of cutaneous plasmacytoma. *Int J Dermatol* 1990; **29**: 562–6.

2 Wong KF, Chan JKC, Li LPK, Yau TK, Lee AWM. Primary cutaneous plasmacytoma: report of two cases and review of the literature. *Am J Dermatopathol* 1994; **16**: 392–7.

3 Tüting T, Bork K. Primary plasmacytoma of the skin. *J Am Acad Dermatol* 1996; **34**: 386–90.

4 Muscardin LM, Pulsoni A, Cerroni L. Primary cutaneous plasmacytoma: report of a case with review of the literature. *J Am Acad Dermatol* 2000; **43**: 962–5.

5 Chang YT, Wong CK. Primary cutaneous plasmacytomas. *Clin Exp Dermatol* 1994; **19**: 177–80.

6 Llamas-Martin R, Postigo-Iorente C, Vanaclocha-Sebastian F, Gil-Martin R, Iglesias-Diez L. Primary cutaneous extramedullary plasmacytoma secreting lambda IgG. *Clin Exp Dermatol* 1993; **18**: 351–5.

7 Miyamoto T, Kobayashi T, Hagari Y, Mihara M. The value of genotypic analysis in the assessment of cutaneous plasmacytomas. *Br J Dermatol* 1997; **137**: 418–21.

8 Müller RPA, Krausse S, Rahlf G. Primär kutanes Plasmozytom: Fallbericht und Literaturübersicht. *Hautarzt* 1990; **41**: 232–5.

9 Requena L, Kutzner H, Palmedo G *et al*. Cutaneous involvement in multiple myeloma: a clinicopathologic, immunohistochemical, and cytogenetic study of 8 cases. *Arch Dermatol* 2003; **139**: 475–86.

10 Tsuboi R, Morioka R, Yaguchi H *et al*. Primary cutaneous plasmacytoma: treatment with intralesional tumor necrosis factor-α. *Br J Dermatol* 1992; **126**: 395–7.

11 Green T, Grant J, Pye R, Marcus R. Multiple primary cutaneous plasmacytomas. *Arch Dermatol* 1992; **128**: 962–5.

12 Belinchon I, Ramos JM, Onrubia J, Mayol MJ. Primary cutaneous plasmacytoma in a patient with chronic lymphatic leukemia. *J Am Acad Dermatol* 1996; **35**: 777–8.

13 Jenkins RE, Calonje E, Fawcett H, Greaves MW, Wilson-Jones E. Cutaneous crystalline deposits in myeloma. *Arch Dermatol* 1994; **130**: 484–8.

14 El-Shabrawi-Caelen L, Cerroni L, Kerl H. Crystal storing histiocytosis. *Dermatopathol Pract Concept* 2001; **7**: 305–6.

15 Hussong JW, Perkins SL, Schnitzer B, Hargreaves H, Frizzera G. Extramedullary plasmacytoma: a form of marginal zone cell lymphoma? *Am J Clin Pathol* 1999; **111**: 111–6.

Chapter 12 Large B-cell lymphoma, leg type

Large B-cell lymphoma, leg type, is a malignant lymphoma of intermediate behaviour, occurring mostly on the leg(s) in elderly patients [1,2]. The terminology of this entity is controversial and is not widely accepted. However, one could compare conceptually the leg-type large B-cell lymphoma to the nasal-type NK/T-cell lymphoma that can arise either in the nasal mucosa or at other sites of the body but has been named after the most typical site of involvement. Large B-cell lymphomas, leg type, are included as 'large B-cell lymphoma of the leg' in the European Organization for the Research and Treatment of Cancer (EORTC) classification [3], whereas in the World Health Organization (WHO) classification they would be classified as diffuse large B-cell lymphomas [4].

It is important to distinguish cutaneous leg-type large B-cell lymphoma from follicle centre cell lymphoma with a predominance of centroblasts and large centrocytes. The latter has similar clinical and prognostic features to other types of cutaneous follicle centre cell lymphomas. Cleaved cells predominate in the large cell variant of follicle centre cell lymphoma, whereas round cells are in the majority in leg-type large B-cell lymphoma. Differentiation between the two may be difficult or even impossible in given cases. In fact, it is well documented that leg-type large B-cell lymphoma is a tumour of postgerminal centre B lymphocytes so that overlapping features with follicle centre cell lymphoma are to be expected (see Immunophenotype, Molecular genetics; see also Chapter 9).

Large B-cell lymphoma, leg type, can be seen in immunocompromised patients and has been observed in association with Kaposi sarcoma, but does not seem to be specifically linked to infection by human herpesvirus 8 [5–8]. The presence of specific sequences of *Borrelia burgdorferi* DNA has been demonstrated in rare cases [9,10].

Clinical features

The disease predominantly affects elderly patients (over 70 years of age), especially females. Patients present with solitary

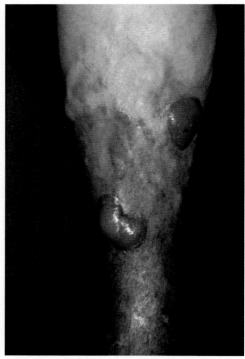

Fig. 12.1 Large B-cell lymphoma, leg type. Large tumours on the lower extremity. Note features of chronic venous insufficiency.

or clustered erythematous or reddish brown tumours, mostly located on the distal extremity of one leg (Fig. 12.1). Sometimes both legs are involved. Early lesions may be difficult to diagnose clinically (Fig. 12.2). Ulceration is common. Small erythematous papules can be seen adjacent to larger nodules in some cases. Large ulcers may lead to the misdiagnosis of chronic venous ulceration (Fig. 12.3) [11]. Large B-cell lymphoma, leg type, has been observed on the background of chronic lymphoedema [12].

It is important to stress that lesions with similar histopathological and phenotypical features can arise at cutaneous sites other than the legs (large B-cell lymphoma, leg type, occurs in approximately 60% of cases on the leg(s) only).

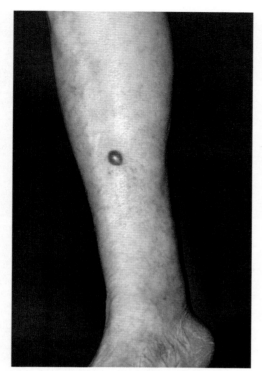

Fig. 12.2 Large B-cell lymphoma, leg type. Small solitary tumour on the right lower extremity.

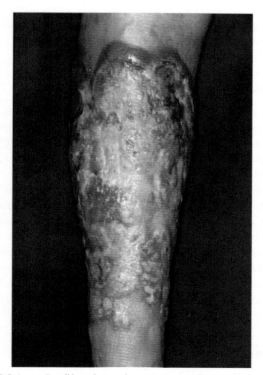

Fig. 12.3 Large B-cell lymphoma, leg type. Large ulcerated lesion with infiltrated margins involving the entire lower leg.

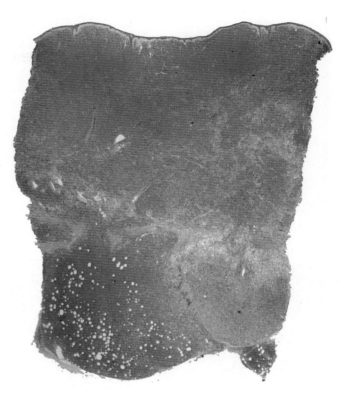

Fig. 12.4 Large B-cell lymphoma, leg type. Dense diffuse infiltrate involving the entire dermis and subcutaneous fat.

Rarely, patients present with typical tumours on the legs and concomitant lesions at other body sites.

Histopathology, immunophenotype and molecular genetics

Histopathology

There is a dense diffuse infiltrate within the entire dermis and subcutis (Fig. 12.4). Involvement of the epidermis by large neoplastic cells, simulating a T-cell lymphoma, is not uncommon (Fig. 12.5). Rare cases may even show band-like infiltrates in the superficial and mid-dermis, simulating the architectonic features of mycosis fungoides [13]. The neoplastic infiltrate consists predominantly of immunoblasts and centroblasts (Fig. 12.6). Other cell types include large cleaved cells, anaplastic large cells and multilobated cells. Cases with predominance of large cleaved cells (large centrocytes) should probably be better classified as cutaneous follicle centre cell lymphoma, diffuse type (see Chapter 9). Reactive small lymphocytes are few or absent. Mitoses are frequent.

A rare histopathological variant of leg-type large B-cell lymphoma shows a starry sky and/or mosaic stone-like

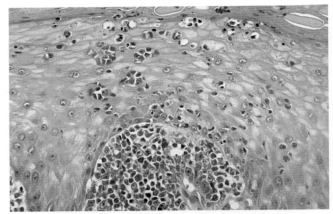

Fig. 12.5 Large B-cell lymphoma, leg type. Epidermotropism of neoplastic B lymphocytes.

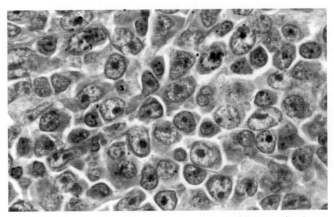

Fig. 12.6 Large B-cell lymphoma, leg type. Immunoblasts predominate in this case.

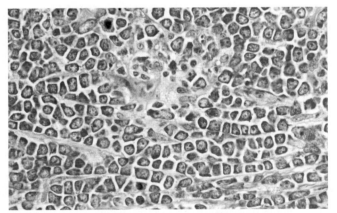

Fig. 12.7 Large B-cell lymphoma, leg type. 'Mosaic stone'-like arrangement of neoplastic cells resembling features of Burkitt lymphoma or of lymphoblastic lymphoma.

pattern similar to that of Burkitt-like lymphoma (Fig. 12.7). In rare instances, large B-cell lymphoma, leg type, may relapse with the clinicopathological features of intravascular large B-cell lymphoma [14].

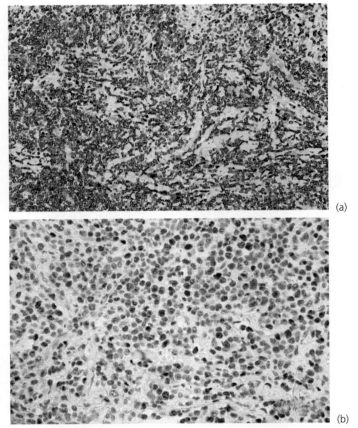

Fig. 12.8 Large B-cell lymphoma, leg type. (a) Positive staining for Bcl-2. (b) Positive nuclear staining for Bcl-6.

Immunophenotype

Neoplastic cells express B-cell markers (CD20, CD79a), but there can be (partial) loss of antigen expression. Bcl-2 protein is positive in the great majority of cases (Fig. 12.8a) [15,16]. The proliferation markers usually stain a large proportion of the cells.

In the majority of cases, neoplastic cells express Bcl-6 or CD10, or both, demonstrating a derivation from germinal centre cells (Fig. 12.8b) [17–20]. Markers of plasma cell differentiation (CD138) are only rarely positive.

A rare variant of leg-type large B-cell lymphoma is positive for CD30 and should not be misinterpreted as anaplastic large cell lymphoma [21]. Expression of CD30 does not have any particular diagnostic or prognostic meaning in large B-cell lymphoma, leg type.

Molecular genetics

The tumours reveal monoclonal rearrangement of the J_H gene. The t(14;18) is not present. Analysis of single cells by micromanipulation and polymerase chain reaction (PCR) revealed that leg-type large B-cell lymphomas are characterized by a proliferation of postgerminal centre cells [22,23]. Hypermethylation of *p15* and/or *p16* and expression of p15 and/or p16 protein have been observed in some patients [24].

In nodal diffuse large B-cell lymphomas, analysis of gene expression profiles by DNA microarray revealed the presence of distinct subgroups with prognostic differences [25]. In the skin, gene expression studies using cDNA microarray revealed that cases of large B-cell lymphoma have a germinal centre cell signature [26].

A t(14;18)(q32;q21) has been detected in one case of cutaneous large B-cell lymphoma, leg type, but the case may have represented in truth secondary cutaneous spread from an extracutaneous B-cell lymphoma [27]. Recently, differences in expression of polycomb-group genes, that are involved in regulation of lymphopoiesis and malignant transformation, have been detected between cutaneous and extracutaneous diffuse large B-cell lymphomas, supporting the concept that skin cases represent a distinct entity [28]. In addition, a site-specific expression pattern observed in skin cases arising on the head, neck and trunk, as opposed to those located on the leg, confirmed that these tumours represent probably distinct subtypes of cutaneous B-cell lymphoma (see also Chapter 9) [28].

Treatment

The treatment of choice of solitary lesions is radiotherapy, eventually followed by surgical excision of smaller nodules [29]. Systemic chemotherapy is preferable for multiple lesions but can be difficult to administer because of the advanced age of most patients (often over 80 years). Intralesional administration of interferon-α has been used with a complete response reported in one patient [30]. Short-term response to antibiotic treatment has also been observed [31]. Recently, a promising new treatment has been made available using the anti-CD20 antibody (rituximab), either alone or in combination with systemic chemotherapy [11,32–38].

Prognosis

Large B-cell lymphoma, leg type, has an intermediate behaviour and the estimated 5-year survival is 58% [39]. Relapse after treatment is common and extracutaneous spread often occurs a few years after the onset of the disease. Involvement of the central nervous system can be observed in some cases [40]. In multivariate analyses, the main prognostic factors were the morphology of the cells (cases with a predominance of round cells have a worse prognosis than those with predominance of cleaved cells), the number of lesions at presentation and a location on the leg (worse prognosis) [19,41].

The prognostic value of Bcl-2 expression in cutaneous cases is unclear (in the lymph nodes, Bcl-2$^+$ cases have a worse prognosis). Histopathological evaluation of the sentinel lymph node has been proposed for the assessment of extracutaneous spread of leg-type large B-cell lymphoma [42].

RÉSUMÉ

Clinical	Elderly; female to male ratio 3 : 1. Solitary or clustered tumours, often ulcerated. Preferential locations: distal portion of one leg.
Morphology	Dense diffuse infiltrates characterized by predominance of large cells (centroblasts, immunoblasts). Occasionally shows epidermotropism.
Immunology	CD20, 79a + sIg (cIg) + (monoclonal) Bcl-2 + Bcl-6 +
Genetics	Monoclonal rearrangement of the J$_H$ gene detected in the majority of cases. No specific genetic alterations.
Treatment guidelines	*Solitary lesions*: radiotherapy; surgical excision. *Multiple lesions*: systemic chemotherapy; rituximab.

References

1 Vermeer MH, Geelen FAMJ, van Haselen CW *et al*. Primary cutaneous large B-cell lymphomas of the legs: a distinct type of cutaneous B-cell lymphoma with an intermediate prognosis. *Arch Dermatol* 1996; **132**: 1304–8.

2 Paulli M, Viglio A, Vivenza D *et al*. Primary cutaneous large B-cell lymphoma of the leg: histogenetic analysis of a controversial entity. *Hum Pathol* 2002; **33**: 937–43.

3 Willemze R, Kerl H, Sterry W *et al*. EORTC classification for primary cutaneous lymphomas: a proposal from the Cutaneous Lymphoma Study Group of the European Organization for Research and Treatment of Cancer. *Blood* 1997; **90**: 354–71.

4 Gatter KC, Warnke RA. Diffuse large B-cell lymphoma. In: Jaffe ES, Harris NL, Stein H, Vardiman JW, eds. *World Health Organization Classification of Tumours: Tumours of Haematopoietic and Lymphoid Tissues.* Lyon: IARC Press, 2001: 171–4.

5 Berti E, Marzano AV, Decleva I *et al*. Simultaneous onset of primary cutaneous B-cell lymphoma and human herpesvirus 8-associated Kaposi's sarcoma. *Br J Dermatol* 1997; **136**: 924–9.

6 Beylot-Barry M, Vergier B, Masquelier B *et al*. The spectrum of

cutaneous lymphomas in HIV infection: a study of 21 cases. *Am J Surg Pathol* 1999; **23**: 1208–16.

7 Engels EA, Pittaluga S, Whitby D *et al.* Immunoblastic lymphoma in persons with AIDS-associated Kaposi's sarcoma: a role for Kaposi's sarcoma-associated herpesvirus. *Mod Pathol* 2003; **16**: 424–9.

8 Zöchling N, Pütz B, Wolf P, Kerl H, Cerroni L. Human herpesvirus 8-specific DNA sequences in primary cutaneous B-cell lymphomas. *Arch Dermatol* 1998; **134**: 246–7.

9 Cerroni L, Zöchling N, Pütz B, Kerl H. Infection by *Borrelia burgdorferi* and cutaneous B-cell lymphoma. *J Cutan Pathol* 1997; **24**: 457–61.

10 Goodlad JR, Davidson MM, Hollowood K *et al.* Primary cutaneous B-cell lymphoma and *Borrelia burgdorferi* infection in patients from the highlands of Scotland. *Am J Surg Pathol* 2000; **24**: 1279–85.

11 Garbea A, Dippel E, Hildenbrand R *et al.* Cutaneous large B-cell lymphoma of the leg masquerading as a chronic venous ulcer. *Br J Dermatol* 2002; **146**: 144–7.

12 Torres-Paoli D, Sanchez JL. Primary cutaneous B-cell lymphoma of the leg in a chronic lymphoedematous extremity. *Am J Dermatopathol* 2000; **22**: 257–60.

13 Cerroni L, Peris K, Amantea A *et al.* Primary cutaneous B-cell lymphoma with histopathologic features of mycosis fungoides. *Am J Dermatopathol* 1992; **14**: 82.

14 Kamath NV, Gilliam AC, Nihal M, Spiro TP, Wood GS. Primary cutaneous large B-cell lymphoma of the leg relapsing as cutaneous intravascular large B-cell lymphoma. *Arch Dermatol* 2001; **137**: 1637–8.

15 Geelen FAMJ, Vermeer MH, Meijer CJLM *et al.* Bcl-2 protein expression in primary cutaneous large B-cell lymphoma is site-related. *J Clin Oncol* 1998; **16**: 2080–5.

16 Gronbaeck K, Moller PH, Nedergaard T *et al.* Primary cutaneous B-cell lymphoma: a clinical, histological, phenotypic and genotypic study of 21 cases. *Br J Dermatol* 2000; **142**: 913–23.

17 Kim BK, Surti U, Pandya A, Swerdlow SH. Primary and secondary cutaneous diffuse large B-cell lymphomas: a multiparameter analysis of 25 cases including fluorescence *in situ* hybridization for t(14;18) translocation. *Am J Surg Pathol* 2003; **27**: 356–64.

18 Fernandez-Vazquez A, Rodriguez-Peralto JL, Martinez MA *et al.* Primary cutaneous large B-cell lymphoma: the relation between morphology, clinical presentation, immunohistochemical markers, and survival. *Am J Surg Pathol* 2001; **25**: 307–15.

19 Goodlad JR, Krajewski AS, Batstone PJ *et al.* Primary cutaneous diffuse large B-cell lymphoma: Prognostic significance of clinicopathological subtypes. *Am J Surg Pathol* 2003; **27**: 1538–45.

20 Hoefnagel JJ, Vermeer MH, Jansen PM *et al.* Bcl-2, Bcl-6 and CD10 expression in cutaneous B-cell lymphoma: further support for a follicle centre cell origin and differential diagnostic significance. *Br J Dermatol* 2003; **149**: 1183–91.

21 Herrera E, Gallardo M, Bosch R *et al.* Primary cutaneous CD30 (Ki-1)-positive non-anaplastic B-cell lymphoma. *J Cutan Pathol* 2002; **29**: 181–4.

22 Gellrich S, Golembowski S, Audring H, Jahn S, Sterry W. Molecular analysis of the immunoglobulin VH gene rearrangement in a primary cutaneous immunoblastic B-cell lymphoma by micromanipulation and single-cell PCR. *J Invest Dermatol* 1997; **109**: 541–5.

23 Gellrich S, Rutz S, Golembowski S *et al.* Primary cutaneous follicle center cell lymphomas and large B cell lymphomas of the leg descend from germinal center cells: a single cell polymerase chain reaction analysis. *J Invest Dermatol* 2001; **117**: 1512–20.

24 Child FJ, Scarisbrick JJ, Calonje E *et al.* Inactivation of tumor suppressor genes p15^{INK4b} and p16^{INK4a} in primary cutaneous B cell lymphoma. *J Invest Dermatol* 2002; **118**: 941–8.

25 Alizadeh AA, Eisen MB, Davis RE *et al.* Distinct types of diffuse large B-cell lymphoma identified by gene expression profiling. *Nature* 2000; **403**: 503–11.

26 Storz MN, van de Rijn M, Kim YH *et al.* Gene expression profiles of cutaneous B cell lymphoma. *J Invest Dermatol* 2003; **120**: 865–70.

27 Cook JR, Sherer M, Craig FE, Shekhter-Levin S, Swerdlow SH. t(14;18)(q32;q21) involving *MALT1* and *IGH* genes in an extranodal diffuse large B-cell lymphoma. *Hum Pathol* 2003; **34**: 1212–5.

28 Raaphorst FM, Vermeer M, Fieret E *et al.* Site-specific expression of polycomb-group genes encoding the HPC-HPH/PRC1 complex in clinically defined primary nodal and cutaneous large B-cell lymphomas. *Am J Pathol* 2004; **164**: 533–42.

29 Zenahlik P, Fink-Puches R, Kapp KS, Kerl H, Cerroni L. Die Therapie der primären kutanen B-Zell-Lymphome. *Hautarzt* 2000; **51**: 19–24.

30 Wollina U, Mentzel T, Graefe T. Large B-cell lymphoma of the leg: complete remission with perilesional interferon-α. *Dermatology* 2001; **203**: 165–7.

31 Hofbauer GFL, Kessler B, Kempf W *et al.* Multilesional primary cutaneous diffuse large B-cell lymphoma responsive to antibiotic treatment. *Dermatology* 2001; **203**: 168–70.

32 Aboulafia DM. Primary cutaneous large B-cell lymphoma of the legs: a distinct clinical pathologic entity treated with CD20 monoclonal antibody (rituximab). *Am J Clin Oncol* 2001; **24**: 237–40.

33 Bonnekoh B, Schulz M, Franke I, Gollnick H. Complete remission of a primary cutaneous B-cell lymphoma of the lower leg by first-line monotherapy with the CD20-antibody rituximab. *J Cancer Res Clin Oncol* 2002; **128**: 161–6.

34 Heinzerling LM, Urbanek M, Funk JO *et al.* Reduction of tumor burden and stabilization of disease by systemic therapy with anti-CD20 antibody (rituximab) in patients with primary cutaneous B-cell lymphoma. *Cancer* 2000; **89**: 1835–44.

35 Sabroe RA, Child FJ, Woolford AJ, Spittle MF, Russell-Jones R. Rituximab in cutaneous B-cell lymphoma: a report of two cases. *Br J Dermatol* 2000; **143**: 157–61.

36 Viguier M, Bachelez H, Brice P, Rivet J, Dubertret L. Lymphomes cutanes B traites par rituximab: deux cas. *Ann Dermatol Vénéréol* 2002; **129**: 1152–5.

37 Fierro MT, Savoia P, Quaglino P *et al.* Systemic therapy with cyclophosphamide and anti-CD20 antibody (rituximab) in relapsed primary cutaneous B-cell lymphoma: a report of 7 cases. *J Am Acad Dermatol* 2003; **49**: 281–7.

38 Brogan BL, Zic JA, Kinney MC *et al.* Large B-cell lymphoma of the leg: clinical and pathologic characteristics in a North American series. *J Am Acad Dermatol* 2003; **49**: 223–8.

39 Fink-Puches R, Zenahlik P, Bäck B *et al.* Primary cutaneous lymphomas: applicability of current classification schemes (European Organization for Research and Treatment of Cancer, World Health Organization) based on clinicopathologic features observed in a large group of patients. *Blood* 2002; **99**: 800–5.

40 Bekkenk MW, Postma TJ, Meijer CJLM, Willemze R. Frequency of central nervous system involvement in primary cutaneous B-cell lymphoma. *Cancer* 2000; **89**: 913–9.

41 Grange F, Bekkenk MW, Wechsler J *et al.* Prognostic factors in primary cutaneous large B-cell lymphomas: a European multicenter study. *J Clin Oncol* 2001; **19**: 3602–10.

42 Starz H, Balda BR, Bachter D, Büchels H, Vogt H. Secondary lymph node involvement from primary cutaneous large B-cell lymphoma of the leg: sentinel lymph nodectomy as a new strategy for staging circumscribed cutaneous lymphoma. *Cancer* 1999; **85**: 199–207.

Chapter 13 B-lymphoblastic lymphoma

B-lymphoblastic lymphomas are malignant proliferations of precursor B lymphocytes [1]. Cutaneous involvement is not rare but exact data are not available. Although patients usually have secondary skin manifestations of acute lymphoblastic leukaemia with bone marrow and peripheral blood involvement, primary skin involvement has been observed occasionally [2–8].

It must be stressed that histological features alone do not allow one to differentiate lymphoblastic lymphomas of B phenotype from those of T-cell lineage (see Chapter 8). Rarely, lymphoblastic lymphomas do not express B- or T-cell markers having a so-called null phenotype.

Clinical features

Children and young adults are usually affected [2,3]. Cases in neonates have been observed [5–13]. Clinically, patients present with large erythematous tumours, usually solitary, commonly located on the head and neck (Fig. 13.1). In patients with precursor B-lymphoblastic leukaemia, cutaneous involvement may be the first sign of recurrence after successful first-line treatment. In these cases, skin manifestations may be characterized by solitary or localized papules and tumours that may be difficult to recognize (Fig. 13.2).

Histopathology, immunophenotype and molecular genetics

Histopathology

Dense diffuse monomorphous infiltrates are found within the dermis and the subcutaneous fat. Cytomorphologically, the lymphoblasts are medium-sized cells with round, oval or convoluted nuclei, fine chromatin, inconspicuous nucleoli and scant cytoplasm (Fig. 13.3). Mitoses and necrotic ('apoptotic') cells are frequent, and 'starry sky' or 'mosaic stone'-like patterns may be seen (Figs 13.4 & 13.5). In secondary skin involvement from B-lymphoblastic leukaemia, the

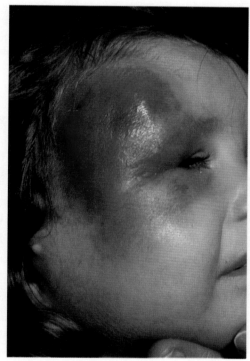

Fig. 13.1 Cutaneous B-lymphoblastic lymphoma. Large tumour on the face of an 18-month-old child.

pattern at low power may mimic that of an inflammatory skin condition, emphasizing the need for careful histological and immunohistochemical examination to make a confident diagnosis (Fig. 13.6).

Immunophenotype

The cutaneous lymphoblastic lymphomas express usually CD79a, CD20, TdT, CD10 (CALLA) and cytoplasmic μ heavy-chains without surface immunoglobulins (Figs 13.6c,d & 13.7). A proportion of the cases are also positive for CD99 and CD34. Expression of the various markers is related to the stage of differentiation of the cells and B-cell markers may be negative in some cases.

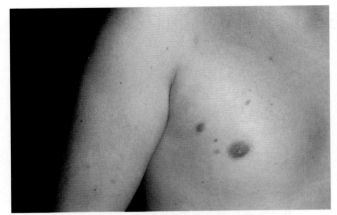

Fig. 13.2 Cutaneous B-lymphoblastic lymphoma. Small erythematous papule on the chest as first sign of recurrence of acute lymphoblastic leukaemia in a 28-year-old man (histopathological and immunophenotypical features are depicted in Fig. 13.6).

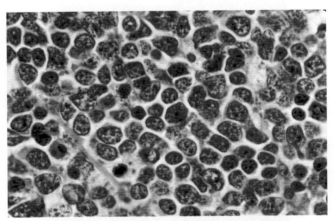

Fig. 13.3 Cutaneous B-lymphoblastic lymphoma. B lymphoblasts with round nuclei and finely dispersed chromatin.

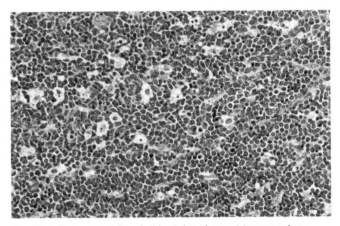

Fig. 13.4 Cutaneous B-lymphoblastic lymphoma. Monomorphous proliferation of medium-sized cells. Note 'starry sky' pattern.

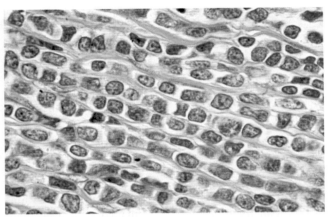

Fig. 13.5 Cutaneous B-lymphoblastic lymphoma. Note 'mosaic stone'-like arrangement of neoplastic cells.

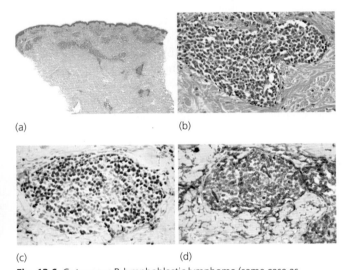

(a) (b)

(c) (d)

Fig. 13.6 Cutaneous B-lymphoblastic lymphoma (same case as Fig. 13.2). (a) Dense perivascular infiltrates in the superficial and mid-dermis. (b) Monomorphous medium-sized cells predominate. Most neoplastic cells show nuclear positivity for (c) TdT and (d) CD34.

Molecular genetics

Molecular genetics usually shows a monoclonal rearrangement of the J_H gene and a polyclonal pattern of the T-cell receptor (TCR) gene. In rare instances, a concomitant monoclonal rearrangement of the TCR gene can be observed, giving rise to potential pitfalls in the molecular diagnosis of the tumour.

The differential diagnosis of B-lymphoblastic lymphoma includes several entities that may show similar morphological features. Mantle cell lymphoma contains cells with more cleaved or irregularly shaped nuclei and a characteristic immunophenotype (CD5+, cyclin-D1+, CD10−, TdT−) (see Chapter 15). Myelomonocytic leukaemia shows a prolifera-

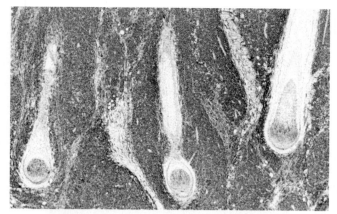

Fig. 13.7 Cutaneous B-lymphoblastic lymphoma. Most neoplastic cells show positivity for CD10.

tion of immature myeloid cells with figurate or 'Indian-line' patterns that stain positive for myeloid markers (naphthol-ASD-chloracetate-esterase, myeloperoxidase) and do not reveal a monoclonal rearrangement of the J_H gene (see Chapter 18). Blastic NK-cell lymphoma is characterized by a strong positivity for CD4 and CD56 in addition to a variable positivity for TdT, as well as by a lack of rearrangement of the J_H gene (see Chapter 16). The differential diagnosis may also include cutaneous Merkel cell tumours and metastatic neuroendocrine carcinomas, which are characterized by the coexpression of cytokeratin filaments, neurofilament proteins and various other markers (chromogranin A) in addition to the lack of expression of lymphoid markers and presence of J_H gene rearrangement.

RÉSUMÉ

Clinical	Childen, young adults. Solitary tumours. Preferential location: head and neck.
Morphology	Nodular or diffuse infiltrates characterized by monomorphous proliferations of lymphoblasts.
Immunology	CD20, 79a + CD10 + CD34 +/− TdT +
Genetics	Monoclonal rearrangement of the J_H gene detected in the majority of cases.
Treatment guidelines	Systemic chemotherapy; bone marrow transplantation.

Treatment and prognosis

These patients should be managed in a haematological setting. The treatment of choice is systemic chemotherapy, often with bone marrow transplantation. Patients with localized skin disease appear to have a relatively good prognosis, but treatment strategies should be the same as those for systemic variants of the disease.

References

1 Brunning RD, Borowitz M, Matutes E *et al.* Precursor B lymphoblastic leukaemia/lymphoblastic lymphoma (precursor B-cell acute lymphoblastic leukaemia). In: Jaffe ES, Harris NL, Stein H, Vardiman JW, eds. *World Health Organization Classification of Tumours: Tumours of Haematopoietic and Lymphoid Tissues.* Lyon: IARC Press, 2001: 111–4.

2 Sander CA, Medeiros LJ, Abruzzo LV, Horak ID, Jaffe ES. Lymphoblastic lymphoma presenting in cutaneous sites: a clinicopathologic analysis of six cases. *J Am Acad Dermatol* 1991; **25**: 1023–31.

3 Chimenti S, Fink-Puches R, Peris K *et al.* Cutaneous involvement in lymphoblastic lymphoma. *J Cutan Pathol* 1999; **26**: 379–85.

4 Schmitt IM, Manente L, Di Matteo A *et al.* Lymphoblastic lymphoma of the pre-B phenotype with cutaneous presentation. *Dermatology* 1997; **195**: 289–92.

5 Trupiano JK, Bringelsen K, Hsi E. Primary cutaneous lymphoblastic lymphoma presenting in an 8-week-old infant. *J Cutan Pathol* 2002; **29**: 107–12.

6 Grümayer ER, Ladenstein RL, Slavc I *et al.* B-cell differentiation pattern of cutaneous lymphomas in infancy and childhood. *Cancer* 1988; **61**: 303–8.

7 Kamps WA, Poppema S. Pre-B-cell non-Hodgkin's lymphoma in childhood. *Am J Clin Pathol* 1988; **90**: 103–7.

8 Knowles DM. Lymphoblastic lymphoma. In: Knowles DM, ed. *Neoplastic Hematopathology.* Philadelphia: Lippincott, 2001: 915–51.

9 Kahwash SB, Qualman SJ. Cutaneous lymphoblastic lymphoma in children: report of six cases with precursor B-cell lineage. *Pediatr Dev Pathol* 2002; **5**: 45–53.

10 Momoi A, Toba K, Kawai K *et al.* Cutaneous lymphoblastic lymphoma of putative plasmacytoid dendritic cell-precursor origin: two cases. *Leuk Res* 2002; **26**: 693–8.

11 Maitra A, McKenna RW, Weinberg AG, Schneider NR, Kroft SH. Precursor B-cell lymphoblastic lymphoma: a study of nine cases lacking blood and bone marrow involvement and review of the literature. *Am J Clin Pathol* 2001; **115**: 868–75.

12 Lin P, Jones D, Dorfman DM, Medeiros LJ. Precursor B-cell lymphoblastic lymphoma: a predominantly extranodal tumor with low propensity for leukemic involvement. *Am J Surg Pathol* 2000; **24**: 1480–90.

13 Yen A, Sanchez R, Oblender M, Raimer S. Leukemia cutis: Darier's sign in a neonate with acute lymphoblastic leukemia. *J Am Acad Dermatol* 1996; **34**: 375–8.

Chapter 14 B-cell chronic lymphocytic leukaemia

B-cell chronic lymphocytic leukaemia (B-CLL) represents the most frequent type of chronic lymphocytic leukaemia. Cutaneous lesions in patients affected by B-CLL are common. In most instances they represent non-specific manifestations related to the impaired immune competence of these patients or to the ingestion of drugs. In some cases, neoplastic B lymphocytes are found within the skin [1]. Such lesions are referred to as specific cutaneous manifestations of the disease or 'leukaemia cutis'.

Clinical features

Clinically, patients present with localized or generalized erythematous papules, plaques or tumours [1–3]. Peculiar clinical presentations include the so-called 'facies leonina' and the onset of specific skin lesions at sites of previous herpes simplex or herpes zoster eruptions (Figs 14.1 & 14.2) [4]. These latter were often classified in the past as pseudolymphoma [5,6], but are in fact specific cutaneous manifestations of the disease [4,7]. It has been recently demonstrated that lesions arising at typical sites of *Borrelia burgdorferi* infection (nipple, scrotum, earlobe) represent specific manifestations of B-CLL triggered by infection with *B. burgdorferi* (Fig. 14.3) [8]. Lesions arising on the nipple were well known in the past and were termed 'leukaemia lymphatica mamillae' in old textbooks.

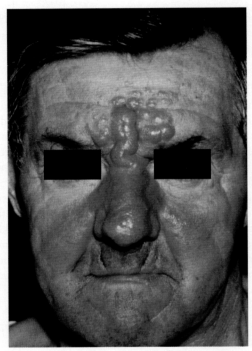

Fig. 14.1 Cutaneous B-cell chronic lymphocytic leukaemia (B-CLL). Nodules on the face conferring the aspect of the so-called 'facies leonina'.

Histopathology, immunophenotype and molecular genetics

Histopathology

Histology may show either a patchy perivascular and periadnexal pattern, or the presence of dense, monomorphous, diffuse or nodular infiltrates of lymphocytes (Fig. 14.4) [4]. The subcutaneous fat is involved as a rule. The tumour is composed predominantly of small lymphocytes without atypical features (Fig. 14.5). Small nodular areas with larger cells showing features of prolymphocytes or paraimmunoblasts (so-called 'proliferation centres') can be observed occasionally [4]. In some cases, other cells such as eosinophils and epithelioid histiocytes can be found.

In patients with B-CLL, infiltrates of neoplastic lymphocytes may be observed in biopsy specimens of different cutaneous conditions, representing specific manifestations of the disease at sites of skin inflammation caused by different aetiological factors [4,8,9]. A case of cutaneous 'composite' lymphoma with features of both mycosis fungoides and B-CLL has been observed [10], probably representing a further example of the phenomenon just described.

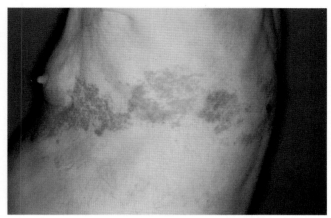

Fig. 14.2 Cutaneous B-CLL. Specific skin manifestations at the site of a previous herpes zoster eruption.

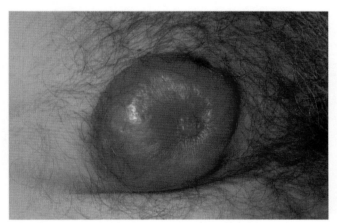

Fig. 14.3 Cutaneous B-CLL. Specific skin manifestation at the site of a *Borrelia burgdorferi* infection (so-called 'leukaemia lymphatica mamillae').

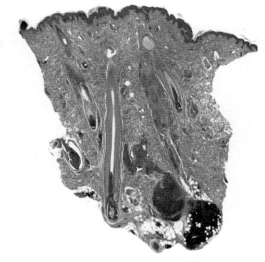

Fig. 14.4 Cutaneous B-CLL. Dense lymphoid infiltrates within the dermis and subcutaneous fat.

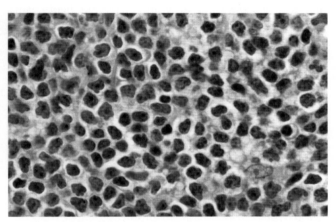

Fig. 14.5 Cutaneous B-CLL. Monomorphous infiltrate of small lymphocytes.

Immunophenotype and molecular genetics

Immunohistology reveals the presence of B lymphocytes characterized by an aberrant immunophenotype (CD20+, CD5+, CD43+) and monoclonal expression of immunoglobulin light-chains (Fig. 14.6) [4]. CD5 may be negative in some cases. A variable population of reactive T lymphocytes is usually present. Molecular genetics shows in most cases a monoclonal rearrangement of the J_H gene.

Treatment and prognosis

The prognosis seems not to be affected by skin involvement [4]. The treatment must be planned according to the haematological findings. Small solitary or clustered skin lesions may be removed surgically or by carbon dioxide laser vaporization [2]. Larger lesions may be treated by radiotherapy. Positive responses to UVB therapy have been reported [11]. Rarely, skin manifestations may regress slowly without any specific treatment [12].

Richter syndrome

Large cell transformation of B-CLL (Richter syndrome) has been reported occasionally in the skin [4,13,14]. Patients present clinically with solitary large cutaneous tumours. Histology reveals features of a large B-cell lymphoma with many centroblasts and immunoblasts. Immunohistology shows positivity for B-cell markers, often with an aberrant profile

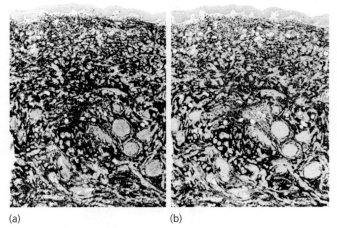

(a)   (b)

Fig. 14.6 Cutaneous B-CLL. The neoplastic cells are positive for both (a) CD20 and (b) CD5.

similar to that described above (CD20$^+$, CD5$^+$, CD43$^+$), and monoclonal expression of immunoglobulin light-chains. Molecular genetics reveals the presence of a monoclonal rearrangement of the J_H gene. The clone may or may not be

the same as that observed in the lymphocytes of the preceding B-CLL, meaning that in some cases Richter syndrome represents the occurrence of a high-grade lymphoma unrelated to the previous B-CLL (a so-called 'second lymphoma'). The prognosis of patients with cutaneous Richter syndrome is very poor and treatment is usually ineffective.

True skin lesions of Richter syndrome should be distinguished from the rare onset of primary cutaneous B-cell lymphoma in patients with B-CLL, as the prognosis and management are different [14].

RÉSUMÉ

Clinical	Elderly. Solitary, grouped or generalized cutaneous papules, plaques and tumours. Possible onset at sites of previous inflammation (e.g. herpes simplex or herpes zoster infection, infection by *Borrelia burgdorferi*).
Morphology	Patchy or nodular infiltrates characterized by predominance of small lymphocytes. Predominance of large cells in Richter syndrome.
Immunology	CD20 + CD5 + (−) CD43 + sIg + (monoclonal)
Genetics	Monoclonal rearrangement of the J_H gene detected in the majority of cases.
Treatment guidelines	Radiotherapy; excision of solitary lesions.

References

1 Cerroni L, Zenahlik P, Höfler G *et al.* Specific cutaneous infiltrates of B-cell chronic lymphocytic leukemia: a clinicopathologic and prognostic study of 42 patients. *Am J Surg Pathol* 1996; **20**: 1000–10.

2 Paydas S, Zorludemir S. Leukaemia cutis and leukaemic vasculitis. *Br J Dermatol* 2000; **143**: 773–9.

3 Schmid-Wendtner MH, Sander C, Volkenandt M, Wendtner CM. Chronic lymphocytic leukemia presenting with cutaneous lesions. *J Clin Oncol* 1999; **17**: 1083–5.

4 Cerroni L, Zenahlik P, Kerl H. Specific infiltrates of B-cell chronic lymphocytic leukemia (B-CLL) arising at sites of herpes simplex and herpes zoster scars. *Cancer* 1995; **76**: 26–31.

5 Winkelmann RK, Connolly SM, Yiannias JA, Muenter MD, Harmon CB. Postzoster eruptions: granuloma annulare, granulomatous vasculitis and pseudolymphoma. *Eur J Dermatol* 1995; **5**: 470–6.

6 Roo E, Villegas C, Lopez-Bran E *et al.* Postzoster cutaneous pseudolymphoma. *Arch Dermatol* 1994; **130**: 661–3.

7 Cerroni L. Pseudolymphoma? *Arch Dermatol* 1995; **131**: 226.

8 Cerroni L, Höfler G, Bäck B *et al.* Specific cutaneous infiltrates of B-cell chronic lymphocytic leukemia (B-CLL) at sites typical for *Borrelia burgdorferi* infection. *J Cutan Pathol* 2002; **29**: 142–7.

9 Smoller BR, Warnke RA. Cutaneous infiltrate of chronic lymphocytic leukemia and relationship to primary cutaneous epithelial neoplasms. *J Cutan Pathol* 1998; **25**: 160–4.

10 Hull PR, Saxena A. Mycosis fungoides and chronic lymphocytic leukaemia: composite T-cell and B-cell lymphomas presenting in the skin. *Br J Dermatol* 2000; **143**: 439–44.

11 Porter WM, Sidwell RU, Catovsky D, Bunker CB. Cutaneous presentation of chronic lymphatic leukaemia and response to ultraviolet B phototherapy. *Br J Dermatol* 2001; **144**: 1092–4.

12 Kazakov DV, Belousova IE, Michaelis S *et al.* Unusual manifestation of specific cutaneous involvement by B-cell chronic lymphocytic leukemia: spontaneous regression with scar formation. *Dermatology* 2003; **207**: 111–5.

13 Robertson LE, Pugh W, O'Brien S *et al.* Richter's syndrome: a report on 39 patients. *J Clin Oncol* 1993; **11**: 1985–9.

14 Ratnavel RC, Dunn-Walters DK, Boursier L *et al.* B-cell lymphoma associated with chronic lymphatic leukaemia: two cases with contrasting aggressive and indolent behaviour. *Br J Dermatol* 1999; **140**: 708–14.

Chapter 15 Other cutaneous B-cell lymphomas

There are a few reports on other entities of B-cell lymphoma arising primarily in the skin. In addition, most malignant B-cell lymphomas observed at extracutaneous sites may secondarily involve the skin, especially in their later stages. The text below summarizes the clinicopathological aspects of skin manifestations in the most important of these cases.

INTRAVASCULAR LARGE B-CELL LYMPHOMA

Intravascular large B-cell lymphoma (also termed angiotropic lymphoma) is a malignant proliferation of large B lymphocytes within blood vessels. This disease was formerly classified as a vascular neoplasm (malignant angioendotheliomatosis) [1]. In rare cases, the skin may be the only affected site, although more often it is disseminated, with involvement of the central nervous system being common. Most cases of cutaneous intravascular lymphoma show a B-cell phenotype but a T-cell variant of the disease has been reported (see Chapter 8). Intravascular large B-cell lymphoma is included as a provisional entity in the European Organization for Research and Treatment of Cancer (EORTC) classification and as a distinct entity in the World Health Organization (WHO) classification [2,3].

The reason(s) why neoplastic cells in intravascular large B-cell lymphoma are confined within the vessels is unclear. The absence of molecules crucial for adhesion of lymphocytes to endothelial cells and migration out of the vessels (CD29, CD54) has been observed in some cases, leading to the hypothesis that neoplastic lymphocytes in intravascular large B-cell lymphoma are unable to escape outside of the vessel walls [4].

Intravascular large B-cell lymphoma may arise in patients with pre-existing cutaneous or, more often, nodal large B-cell lymphoma, probably representing in these cases recurrence of the original disease [5,6].

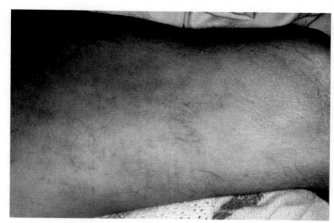

Fig. 15.1 Erythematous, infiltrated lesions of intravascular large B-cell lymphoma on the thigh. (Courtesy of Professor Alain Townsend, Oxford.)

Clinical features

Patients present with indurated, erythematous or violaceous patches and plaques, preferentially located on the trunk and thighs (Fig. 15.1). The clinical appearance is not typical of lymphoma and may sometimes suggest a diagnosis of panniculitis or of purpura [7–11]. Generalized telangiectasia has been observed in one patient [12]. Neurological symptoms as a sign of involvement of the central nervous system are commonly present [13]. Other organs that are frequently involved are the liver and kidneys.

Histopathology, immunophenotype and molecular genetics

Histology reveals a proliferation of large lymphocytes filling dilated blood vessels within the dermis and subcutaneous tissues (Fig. 15.2). A perivascular infiltrate of large atypical

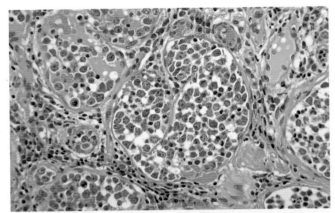

Fig. 15.2 Cutaneous intravascular large B-cell lymphoma. Angiotropic infiltrate of medium- and large-sized neoplastic cells.

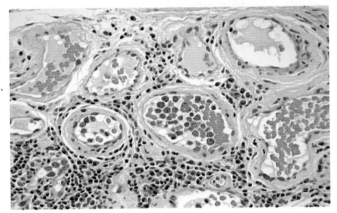

Fig. 15.3 Cutaneous intravascular large B-cell lymphoma within capillaries of a pre-existent haemangioma.

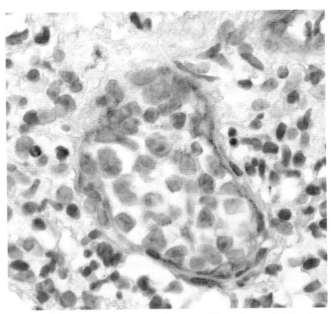

Fig. 15.4 Cutaneous intravascular large B-cell lymphoma. Staining for factor VIII highlights the intravascular arrangement of neoplastic large lymphocytes.

cells is present in some cases. The malignant cells are large with scanty cytoplasm, often with prominent nucleoli (immunoblasts). In rare cases, colonization of capillaries of cutaneous haemangiomas by large B cells (intravascular large B-cell lymphoma within haemangioma) has been observed (Fig. 15.3) [14–18]. In two patients, the diagnosis of intravascular large B-cell lymphoma could be achieved by biopsy of senile ('cherry') haemangiomas in the absence of other specific skin manifestations [16,17].

Neoplastic cells are positive for B-cell-associated markers and in a subset of cases show aberrant CD5 expression [19]. Staining with endothelial cell-related antibodies (CD31, CD34) highlights the characteristic intravascular location of the cells (Fig. 15.4). Molecular analysis shows monoclonal rearrangement of the J_H gene. Fluorescence *in situ* hybridization (FISH) studies revealed karyotype abnormalities in cases of intravascular large B-cell lymphoma, but observations were limited to small numbers of cases [20].

Intravascular large B-cell lymphoma should be distinguished from reactive angioendotheliomatosis, which is a benign skin condition characterized by an intravascular proliferation of either endothelial or histiocytic cells (see Chapter 19) [21].

Treatment and prognosis

The treatment of choice of intravascular large B-cell lymphoma is systemic chemotherapy. Autologous peripheral blood stem cell transplantation has been used in one patient achieving a complete remission with a 15-month disease-free survival [22], but data on large numbers of patients are lacking. The prognosis of cases limited to the skin may be better than that of the generalized (multisystem) disease but only a very limited number of patients have been followed up to date.

T-CELL-RICH B-CELL LYMPHOMA

T-cell-rich B-cell lymphoma is characterized by the malignant proliferation of B lymphocytes admixed with a predominant population of reactive T lymphocytes. For a diagnosis of T-cell-rich B-cell lymphoma, neoplastic large B cells should not exceed 10% of the infiltrate. T-cell-rich B-cell lymphoma

RÉSUMÉ

Intravascular large B-cell lymphoma

Clinical	Adults. Solitary or multiple indurated patches and plaques, sometimes resembling panniculitis. Preferential locations: trunk, thighs.
Morphology	Intravascular proliferation of large atypical lymphoid cells.
Immunology	CD20, 79a + (a few cases CD3, 5+) sIg + (monoclonal)
Genetics	Monoclonal rearrangement of the J_H gene. No specific genetic alterations.
Treatment guidelines	Systemic chemotherapy. Role of peripheral blood stem cell transplantation should be evaluated.

is considered to be a variant of the diffuse large B-cell lymphomas and is included as 'T-cell/histiocyte-rich B-cell lymphoma' in the WHO classification [23]. Cutaneous involvement seems to be extremely uncommon but rare cases arising primarily in the skin have been reported [24–28].

Clinical features

Patients with T-cell-rich B-cell lymphoma are adults of both genders. Clinically, they present with erythematous papules, plaques or nodules usually on the face and trunk. The occurrence of cutaneous T-cell-rich B-cell lymphoma followed by nodal Hodgkin lymphoma has been observed in a patient with Gardner syndrome [29].

Histopathology, immunophenotype and molecular genetics

Histology shows large blasts admixed with a predominant population of small lymphocytes (Fig. 15.5a). In a few patients, a biphasic pattern has been observed suggesting that, at least in some cases, cutaneous T-cell-rich B-cell lymphoma represents progression from a pre-existing low-grade B-cell lymphoma of the skin. Angiocentricity may be observed rarely [30].

Immunohistology reveals the B-cell phenotype of the large cells (CD20+, CD30−), often with positivity for markers of germinal centre derivation (Bcl-6) (Fig. 15.5b). The small lymphocytes express a T-helper phenotype (CD3+, CD4+, CD8−). Molecular genetics shows a polyclonal pattern of T-cell receptor (TCR) genes, and in most cases a monoclonal rearrangement of the J_H gene. In cases showing no evidence of monoclonal rearrangement of the J_H gene, the negativity is probably brought about by the small number of neoplastic

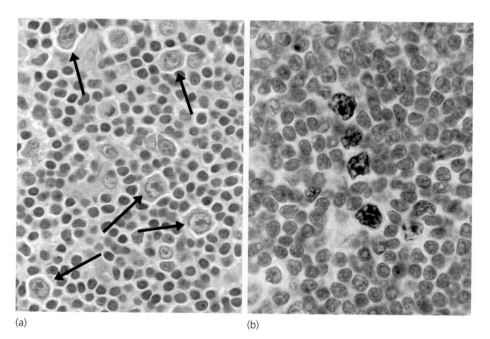

Fig. 15.5 Cutaneous 'T-cell-rich' large B-cell lymphoma. (a) Large blasts scattered among a predominant population of small T lymphocytes and histiocytes (arrows). (b) Nuclear positivity of the large cells for Bcl-6.

(a)

(b)

RÉSUMÉ

T-cell-rich B-cell lymphoma

Clinical	Adults. Erythematous papules, plaques and nodules. Preferential locations: face, trunk. Variant of the diffuse large B-cell lymphoma.
Morphology	< 10% of large B cells in the background of a predominant T-cell population.
Immunology	CD20, 79a + Bcl-6 +
Genetics	Monoclonal rearrangement of the J_H gene.
Treatment guidelines	Radiotherapy; role of systemic chemotherapy unclear.

cells admixed with a high number of reactive lymphocytes. Polymerase chain reaction (PCR) analysis after microdissection of large cells may be a useful tool for confirmation of monoclonality in such cases.

Treatment and prognosis

As in the other primary cutaneous B-cell lymphomas, therapy of those cases confined to the skin should probably not be aggressive (surgical excision and/or local radiotherapy), at least as first-line treatment strategy. An indolent behaviour has been described in a small number of cases arising primarily in the skin.

MANTLE CELL LYMPHOMA

Mantle cell lymphoma is a rare B-cell lymphoma deriving from the inner mantle zone of lymphoid follicles. Cutaneous involvement is uncommon but in rare cases specific skin lesions may be the first manifestation of the disease [31–34]. A few cases of mantle cell lymphoma arising primarily in the skin have been reported but the uniform good prognosis observed in these patients casts doubt on the classification of these cases [35].

Clinical features

Patients are middle-aged or older individuals, with a pre-

dominance of males. Clinically, the lesions are characterized by multiple reddish tumours.

Histopathology, immunophenotype and molecular genetics

Histology shows diffuse monomorphous infiltrates throughout the entire dermis and subcutis composed of small- to medium-sized lymphocytes with irregular nuclei (Fig. 15.6). It has been reported that the blastoid variant, with either lymphoblast-like or large cleaved cells, is frequently found in cutaneous infiltrates.

Immunohistology is characterized by positivity for CD20 and CD5, and negativity for other T-cell markers. Nuclear staining for cyclin-D1 is a helpful tool for the differentiation

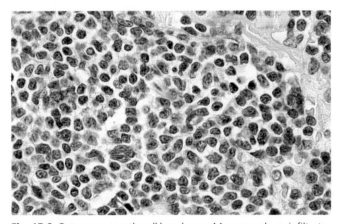

Fig. 15.6 Cutaneous mantle cell lymphoma. Monomorphous infiltrate of medium-sized cells with irregular nuclei.

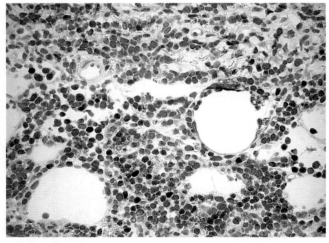

Fig. 15.7 Cutaneous mantle cell lymphoma. Positive nuclear staining for cyclin-D1.

RÉSUMÉ

Mantle cell lymphoma

Clinical	Adults. Usually multiple tumours. Existence of true primary cases questionable.
Morphology	Monomorphous proliferation of small- to medium-sized lymphocytes with irregular nuclei.
Immunology	CD20 +
	CD5 +
	Cyclin-D1 +
Genetics	Monoclonal rearrangement of the J_H gene. t(11;14)(q13;q32).
Treatment guidelines	Systemic chemotherapy; bone marrow transplantation.

of cutaneous mantle cell lymphoma from other malignant B-cell lymphomas, especially B-cell chronic lymphocytic leukaemia (B-CLL) and B-lymphoblastic lymphoma (Fig. 15.7) [36]. Molecular analyses reveal a monoclonal rearrangement of the J_H gene in the majority of cases. The typical t(11;14)(q13;q32) can be demonstrated by conventional cytogenetics, FISH or PCR.

Treatment and prognosis

The treatment of choice is systemic chemotherapy, often associated with bone marrow transplantation. The prognosis is poor and the median survival is less than 5 years.

LYMPHOMATOID GRANULOMATOSIS

Lymphomatoid granulomatosis is a B-cell lymphoproliferative disorder associated with Epstein–Barr virus (EBV) infection. The disease may progress to an overt diffuse large B-cell lymphoma. Lymphomatoid granulomatosis was described first by Liebow *et al.* [37] in 1972 as an angiocentric and angiodestructive lymphoproliferative process in the lungs. It is currently divided into three grades according to the proportion of EBV+ B cells in relation to the reactive infiltrate [38]. Grade 3 lesions are considered as a variant of diffuse large B-cell lymphoma [38].

Clinical features

The skin is often involved although the most common site affected is the lungs [39–43]. Patients are usually adults but skin lesions have been observed in children [44]. The clinical presentation usually is characterized by multiple erythematous papules, plaques or tumours, commonly ulcerated. Sites of predilection are the trunk and extremities. Pulmonary and/or constitutional symptoms are almost invariably present. Cutaneous lesions may precede the onset of pulmonary symptoms although true primary cases have not been observed.

Histopathology, immunophenotype and molecular genetics

The histopathological features of cutaneous manifestations of lymphomatoid granulomatosis depend on the grade of disease and type of lesion. In some cases, only a non-specific perivascular and periadnexal infiltrate of small- to medium-sized cells can be seen. Cutaneous tumours of lymphomatoid granulomatosis are characterized usually by the presence of an angiocentric/angiodestructive infiltrate with variable numbers of large B lymphocytes (Figs 15.8a,b). Granulomatous features are often present.

Immunohistology shows that the larger cells have a B-cell phenotype (Fig. 15.8c). It is important to remember that reactive small- to medium-sized lymphocytes with a T-helper phenotype are the predominant cells within the infiltrates.

RÉSUMÉ

Lymphomatoid granulomatosis

Clinical	Adults. Usually multiple tumours. Lungs usually involved.
Morphology	Grade 3 lesions show angiocentric/angiodestructive infiltrates with presence of variable numbers of large B lymphocytes. Reactive T lymphocytes predominate.
Immunology	CD20 + (large B lymphocytes)
	CD3, 4 + (reactive small lymphocytes)
	EBV + (large B lymphocytes)
Genetics	Monoclonal rearrangement of the J_H gene.
Treatment guidelines	Systemic chemotherapy; interferon-α.

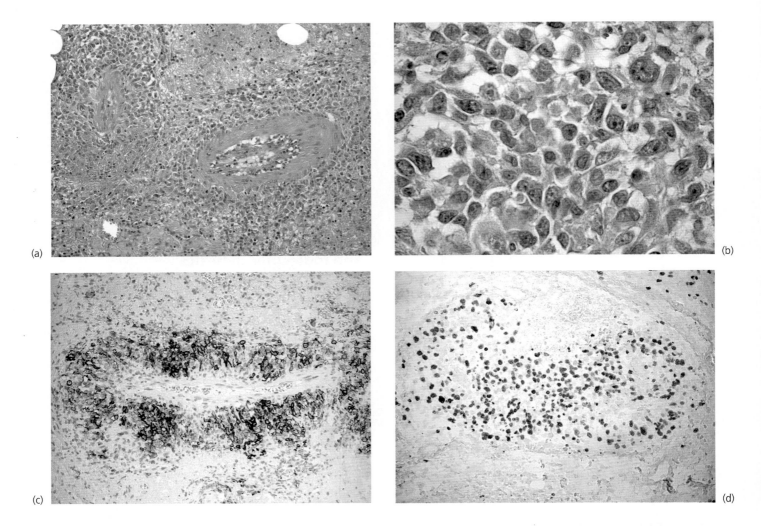

Fig. 15.8 Cutaneous lymphomatoid granulomatosis. (a) Angiocentric infiltrate with large perivascular lymphocytes and areas of necrosis. (b) Detail of large atypical cells. (c) Expression of CD20 by perivascular large lymphocytes. (d) The large B lymphocytes reveal a positive signal after *in situ* hybridization for Epstein–Barr virus (EBER-1).

The neoplastic B lymphocytes show a positive hybridization signal for EBV (Fig. 15.8d). Molecular analyses reveal in some cases a monoclonal rearrangement of the J_H gene.

In the absence of a previous or concomitant diagnosis of typical lymphomatoid granulomatosis in the respiratory tract, a diagnosis of cutaneous lymphomatoid granulomatosis should be made only when all of the features described above are present.

Treatment and prognosis

Different treatment modalities have been used for patients with cutaneous lesions of lymphomatoid granulomatosis (interferon-α, systemic chemotherapy) determined by the grade of lesions at extracutaneous sites. The prognosis depends on the grade and extent of extracutaneous involvement.

References

1 Sheibani K, Battifora H, Winberg CD *et al.* Further evidence that 'malignant angioendotheliomatosis' is an angiotropic large-cell lymphoma. *N Engl J Med* 1986; **314**: 943–8.
2 Willemze R, Kerl H, Sterry W *et al.* EORTC classification for primary cutaneous lymphomas: a proposal from the Cutaneous Lymphoma Study Group of the European Organization for Research and Treatment of Cancer. *Blood* 1997; **90**: 354–71.
3 Gatter KC, Warnke RA. Intravascular large B-cell lymphoma. In: Jaffe ES, Harris NL, Stein H, Vardiman JW, eds. *World Health Organization Classification of Tumours: Tumours of Haematopoietic and Lymphoid Tissues.* Lyon: IARC Press, 2001: 177–8.

4 Ponzoni M, Arrigoni G, Gould VE et al. Lack of CD29 (beta1 integrin) and CD54 (ICAM-1) adhesion molecules in intravascular lymphomatosis. *Hum Pathol* 2000; **31**: 220–6.

5 Asagoe K, Fujimoto W, Yoshino T et al. Intravascular lymphomatosis of the skin as a manifestation of recurrent B-cell lymphoma. *J Am Acad Dermatol* 2003; **48**: S1–4.

6 Kamath NV, Gilliam AC, Nihal M, Spiro TP, Wood GS. Primary cutaneous large B-cell lymphoma of the leg relapsing as cutaneous intravascular large B-cell lymphoma. *Arch Dermatol* 2001; **137**: 1637–8.

7 Chang A, Zic JA, Boyd AS. Intravascular large cell lymphoma: a patient with asymptomatic purpuric patches and a chronic clinical course. *J Am Acad Dermatol* 1998; **39**: 318–21.

8 Di Giuseppe JA, Nelson WG, Seifter EJ, Boitnott JK, Mann RB. Intravascular lymphomatosis: a clinicopathologic study of 10 cases and assessment of response to chemotherapy. *J Clin Oncol* 1994; **12**: 2573–9.

9 Kiyohara T, Kumakiri M, Kobayashi H et al. A case of intravascular large B-cell lymphoma mimicking erythema nodosum: the importance of multiple skin biopsies. *J Cutan Pathol* 2000; **27**: 413–8.

10 Stroup RM, Sheibani K, Moncada A, Purdy LJ, Battifora H. Angiotropic (intravascular) lymphoma: a clinicopathologic study of seven cases with unique clinical presentations. *Cancer* 1990; **66**: 1781–8.

11 Yegappan S, Coupland R, Arber DA et al. Angiotropic lymphoma: an immunophenotypically and clinically heterogeneous lymphoma. *Mod Pathol* 2001; **14**: 1147–56.

12 Özgüroglu E, Büyülbabani N, Ögzüroglu M, Baykal C. Generalized telangiectasia as the major manifestation of angiotropic (intravascular) lymphoma. *Br J Dermatol* 1997; **137**: 422–5.

13 Glass J, Hochberg FH, Miller DC. Intravascular lymphomatosis: a systemic disease with neurologic manifestations. *Cancer* 1993; **71**: 3156–64.

14 Kobayashi T, Munakata S, Sugiura H et al. Angiotropic lymphoma: proliferation of B cells in the capillaries of cutaneous angiomas. *Br J Dermatol* 2000; **143**: 162–4.

15 Rubin MA, Cossman J, Freter CE, Azumi N. Intravascular large cell lymphoma coexisting within hemangiomas of the skin. *Am J Surg Pathol* 1997; **21**: 860–4.

16 Satoh S, Yamazaki M, Yahikozawa H et al. Intravascular large B-cell lymphoma diagnosed by senile angioma biopsy. *Intern Med* 2003; **42**: 117–20.

17 Cerroni L, Zalaudek I, Kerl H. Intravascular large B-cell lymphoma colonizing cutaneous hemangiomas. *Dermatology*, in press.

18 Cerroni L. Hemangiomas with (bad) surprise. *Dermatology*, in press.

19 Khalidi HS, Brynes RK, Browne P et al. Intravascular large B-cell lymphoma: the CD5 antigen is expressed by a subset of cases. *Mod Pathol* 1998; **11**: 983–8.

20 Khoury H, Lestou VS, Gascoyne RD et al. Multicolor karyotyping and clinicopathologic analysis of three intravascular lymphoma cases. *Mod Pathol* 2003; **16**: 716–24.

21 Wick MR, Rocamora A. Reactive and malignant 'angioendotheliomatosis': a discriminant clinicopathological study. *J Cutan Pathol* 1988; **15**: 260–71.

22 Koizumi M, Nishimura M, Yokota A et al. Successful treatment of intravascular malignant lymphomatosis with high-dose chemotherapy and autologous peripheral blood stem cell transplantation. *Bone Marrow Transplant* 2001; **27**: 1101–3.

23 Gatter KC, Warnke RA. Diffuse large B-cell lymphoma. In: Jaffe ES, Harris NL, Stein H, Vardiman JW, eds. *World Health Organization Classification of Tumours: Tumours of haematopoietic and lymphoid tissues.* Lyon: IARC press, 2001: 171–4.

24 Arai E, Sakurai M, Nakayama H, Morinaga S, Katayama I. Primary cutaneous T-cell-rich B-cell lymphoma. *Br J Dermatol* 1993; **129**: 196–200.

25 Dommann SN, Dommann-Scherrer CC, Zimmerman D et al. Primary cutaneous T-cell-rich B-cell lymphoma: a case report with a 13-year follow-up. *Am J Dermatopathol* 1995; **17**: 618–24.

26 Dunphy CH, Nahass GT. Primary cutaneous T-cell-rich B-cell lymphomas with flow cytometric immunophenotypic findings: report of 3 cases and review of the literature. *Arch Pathol Lab Med* 1999; **123**: 1236–40.

27 Li S, Griffin CA, Mann RB, Borowitz MJ. Primary cutaneous T-cell-rich B-cell lymphoma: clinically distinct from its nodal counterpart? *Mod Pathol* 2001; **14**: 10–3.

28 Sander CA, Kaudewitz P, Kutzner H et al. T-cell-rich B-cell lymphoma presenting in skin: a clinicopathologic analysis of six cases. *J Cutan Pathol* 1996; **23**: 101–8.

29 Kamarashev J, Dummer R, Hess Schmid M et al. Primary cutaneous T-cell-rich B-cell lymphoma and Hodgkin's disease in a patient with Gardner's syndrome. *Dermatology* 2000; **201**: 362–5.

30 Gogstetter D, Brown M, Seab J, Scott G. Angiocentric primary cutaneous T-cell-rich B-cell lymphoma: a case report and review of the literature. *J Cutan Pathol* 2000; **27**: 516–25.

31 Sen F, Medeiros LJ, Lu D et al. Mantle cell lymphoma involving skin: cutaneous lesions may be the first manifestation of disease and tumors often have blastoid cytologic features. *Am J Surg Pathol* 2002; **26**: 1312–8.

32 Dubus P, Young P, Beylot-Barry M et al. Value of interphase FISH for the diagnosis of t(11;14)(q13;q32) on skin lesions of mantle cell lymphoma. *Am J Clin Pathol* 2002; **118**: 832–41.

33 Marti RM, Campo E, Bosch F, Palou J, Estrach T. Cutaneous lymphocyte-associated antigen (CLA) expression in a lymphoblastoid mantle cell lymphoma presenting with skin lesions: comparison with other clinicopathologic presentations of mantle cell lymphoma. *J Cutan Pathol* 2001; **28**: 256–64.

34 Geerts ML, Busschots AM. Mantle-cell lymphomas of the skin. *Dermatol Clin* 1994; **12**: 409–17.

35 Bertero M, Novelli M, Fierro MT, Bernengo MG. Mantle zone lymphoma: an immunohistologic study of skin lesions. *J Am Acad Dermatol* 1994; **30**: 23–30.

36 Moody BR, Bartlett NL, George DW et al. Cyclin D1 as an aid in the diagnosis of mantle cell lymphoma in skin biopsies: a case report. *Am J Dermatopathol* 2001; **23**: 470–6.

37 Liebow AA, Carrington CR, Friedman PJ. Lymphomatoid granulomatosis. *Hum Pathol* 1972; **3**: 457–558.

38 Jaffe ES, Wilson WH. Lymphomatoid granulomatosis. In: Jaffe ES, Harris NL, Stein H, Vardiman JW, eds. *World Health Organization Classification of Tumours: Tumours of haematopoietic and lymphoid tissues.* Lyon: IARC press, 2001: 185–7.

39 Beaty MW, Toro J, Sorbara L et al. Cutaneous lymphomatoid granulomatosis: correlation of clinical and biologic features. *Am J Surg Pathol* 2001; **25**: 1111–20.

40 Carlson KC, Gibson LE. Cutaneous signs of lymphomatoid granulomatosis. *Arch Dermatol* 1991; **127**: 1693–8.

41 Katzenstein ALA, Carrington CB, Liebow AA. Lymphomatoid granulomatosis: a clinicopathologic study of 152 cases. *Cancer* 1979; **43**: 360–73.

42 McNiff JM, Cooper D, Howe G *et al.* Lymphomatoid granulomatosis of the skin and lung: an angiocentric T-cell-rich B-cell lymphoproliferative disorder. *Arch Dermatol* 1996; **132**: 1464–70.

43 Tong MM, Cooke B, Barnetson RSC. Lymphomatoid granulomatosis. *J Am Acad Dermatol* 1992; **27**: 872–6.

44 LeSueur BW, Ellsworth L, Bangert JL, Hansen RC. Lymphomatoid granulomatosis in a 4-year-old boy. *Pediatr Dermatol* 2000; **17**: 369–72.

Part 3 Blastic NK-cell lymphoma

Chapter 16 Blastic NK-cell lymphoma

Blastic NK-cell lymphoma is an aggressive systemic neoplasm commonly involving the skin. Although the term 'blastic NK-cell lymphoma' implies a derivation from natural killer cells, there is a considerable body of evidence pointing to a derivation from a common myeloid and lymphoid cell precursor, identified recently as the plasmacytoid type-2 dendritic cell (DC2, 'plasmacytoid monocyte') [1–4]. Malignant transformation would occur at a very early stage of differentiation. Recently, there has been a proposal to rename this entity as 'early plasmacytoid dendritic cell leukaemia–lymphoma' [5].

Blastic NK-cell lymphoma is not included in the European Organization for Research and Treatment of Cancer (EORTC) classification but is included within the precursor T-cell lymphomas as a neoplasm of uncertain lineage and stage of differentiation in the World Health Organization (WHO) classification [6,7]. Cases with histopathological and phenotypical features similar to those of blastic NK-cell lymphoma have also been termed 'agranular CD4+ CD56+ haematodermic neoplasms' [2,4,8–10].

Although a relationship between blastic NK-cell lymphoma and myelogenous leukaemia has been postulated [11–15], with evolution into myelogenous leukaemia being documented in a few patients [12], typical cases of acute myeloid leukaemia involving the skin usually have a different phenotype, being almost always negative for CD56 (see Chapter 18) [16]. However, overlapping myeloid and lymphoid features are known also in other neoplasms such as chronic myelogenous leukaemia, in which blast crisis in 10% of the cases reveals a B- or, more rarely, a T-cell phenotype.

In most cases, at presentation, blastic NK-cell lymphoma is confined to the skin or skin lesions are the first manifestation of the disease [17–22]. Leukaemic spread after variable periods of time is the rule [18], indicating that primary cutaneous cases most likely represent examples of so-called 'aleukaemic leukaemia cutis' [23]. The recent identification of plasmacytoid monocytes resident within the skin provides a theoretical background to the frequent occurrence of these lymphomas with lesions confined to the skin [24].

In contrast to true NK-cell neoplasms, which are more frequently reported in Asians, blastic NK-cell lymphoma has been observed in all races. Another different feature from lymphomas of true NK-cell origin is the constant absence of Epstein–Barr virus (EBV) in blastic NK-cell lymphoma.

Clinical features

Patients are mostly elderly adults although cases in younger individuals, including small children, have been reported [8,18–21,25]. There is a predominance of males. Clinically, they present with solitary (rarely), localized or, more commonly, generalized plaques and tumours with a characteristic 'bruise-like' violaceous aspect (Figs 16.1 & 16.2). Ulceration is uncommon. Mucosal regions may be involved (Fig. 16.3). The morphology of cutaneous lesions is similar to that of the skin manifestations of myelogenous leukaemia. In a distinct proportion of patients (approximately 30–40%), skin lesions are accompanied by general symptoms and extracutaneous manifestations in the blood, bone marrow and/or other organs. Lymph nodes are involved in approximately half of cases at presentation. Thrombocytopenia, anaemia and neutropenia are commonly found [2].

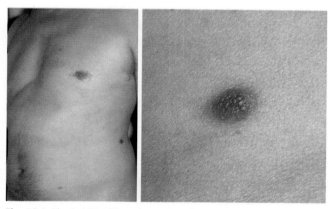

Fig. 16.1 Blastic NK-cell lymphoma. Small solitary tumour on the flank. Note deep red colour.

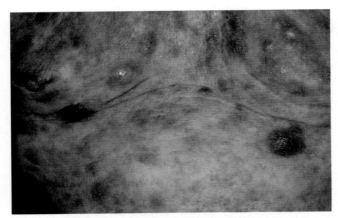

Fig. 16.2 Blastic NK-cell lymphoma. Multiple plaques and tumours on the chest. Note 'bruise-like' violaceous aspect. (Reprinted with permission from *The American Journal of Surgical Pathology*, in press.)

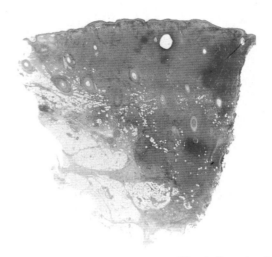

Fig. 16.4 Blastic NK-cell lymphoma. Dense diffuse infiltrate involving the entire dermis and the superficial part of the subcutaneous fat.

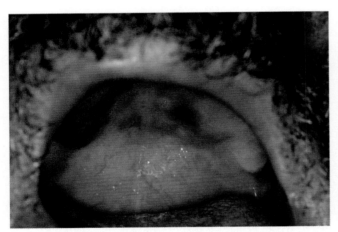

Fig. 16.3 Blastic NK-cell lymphoma. Involvement of the oral mucosa.

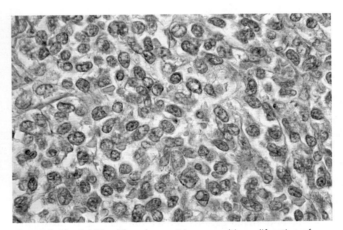

Fig. 16.5 Blastic NK-cell lymphoma. Monomorphic proliferation of medium-sized cells.

Skin lesions are the first manifestation of the disease in over 90% of patients. In patients with primary cutaneous disease, the time interval between the onset of skin lesions and leukaemic spread is variable, usually between a few weeks and several months. In one exceptional case there was a 15-year history of multiple cutaneous nodules [26].

Histopathology, immunophenotype and molecular genetics

Histopathology

Histologically, blastic NK-cell lymphoma is characterized by a diffuse monomorphous infiltrate of medium-sized neoplastic cells with a blastoid morphology (Figs 16.4 & 16.5). The epidermis is not involved as a rule, whereas involvement of the subcutaneous tissues is common. Angiocentricity and/

or angiodestruction, necrosis and granulomatous reactions are uncommon. The morphological features are similar to those of skin involvement in myelogenous leukaemia or myeloid sarcoma.

Immunophenotype

Immunophenotypically, the neoplastic cells are positive for CD4 and CD56 (Fig. 16.6), and negative for TIA-1 (Fig. 16.7d) [4,18,19,27]. CD56 was negative in one exceptional case [28]. Other markers that may be positive in a proportion of cases are CD2, CD7, CD43, CD45Ra and HLA-DR, whereas other T- and B-cell antigens, as well as myeloid and NK-cell antigens, are negative (Fig. 16.7b). Cases positive for TdT and CD68 have been reported, but in our experience

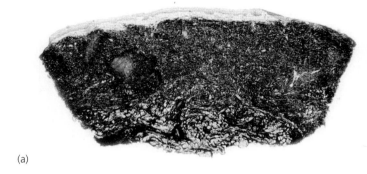

(a)

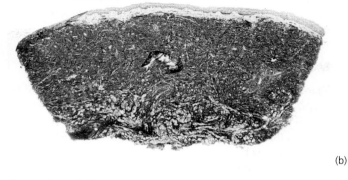

(b)

Fig. 16.6 Blastic NK-cell lymphoma. Positive reaction for (a) CD56 and (b) CD4. (Reprinted with permission from *The American Journal of Surgical Pathology*, in press.)

Fig. 16.7 Blastic NK-cell lymphoma. Positivity for (a) TdT and negativity for (b) myeloperoxidase, (c) CD68 and (d) TIA-1.

CD68 is usually negative (Figs 16.7a,c) [4,10,19,29,30]. Petrella *et al.* described positivity for CD123 in all of their cases in one series, a finding confirmed in subsequent studies [4,31]. The positivity for CD123 could underline the relationship with DC2s, while the positivity for TdT confirms the origin from a precursor cell.

Recently, expression of the lymphoid proto-oncogene *TCL1* was demonstrated in the majority of blastic NK-cell

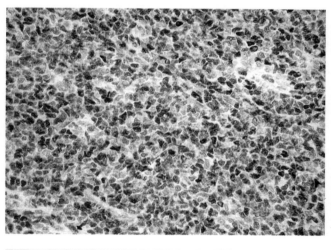

(a)

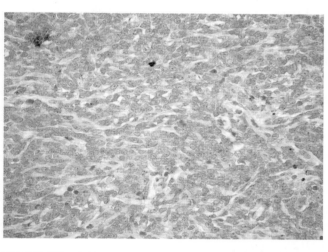

(b)

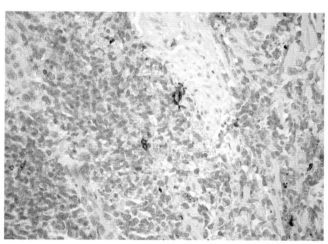

(c)

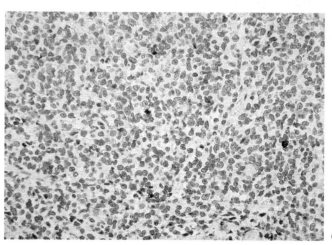

(d)

lymphomas in one series, as well as in lymph node plasmacytoid DC2s, again emphasizing the likely derivation of this unusual neoplasm from these cells [31].

Molecular genetics

There is no association with EBV. Molecular genetic studies reveal that the T-cell receptor (TCR) and J_H genes are in germline configuration. A monoclonal rearrangement of the TCR and/or J_H genes rules out the diagnosis of blastic NK-cell lymphoma by definition.

Complex karyotypes and chromosomal abnormalities involving chromosomes 5q, 6q, 12p, 13q, 15q and 9 have been observed in blastic NK-cell lymphoma [3].

Treatment

Treatment of patients with blastic NK-cell lymphoma should be carried out in a haematological setting. The neoplasm should be considered as a form of aleukaemic leukaemia cutis and treated accordingly. The therapy of choice is systemic chemotherapy, eventually with bone marrow transplantation. Solitary lesions may be treated with radiotherapy but systemic chemotherapy should be administered as well. Although different treatment schemes (for myelogenous leukaemia as well as for precursor lymphomas) have been applied, often with good primary responses, remissions are short and recurrences are the rule [32]. It seems that, at present, there is no advantage to any conventional chemotherapeutic scheme for lymphoid or myeloid malignancies. Allogeneic stem cell transplantation revealed more promising results, possibly with complete cure in a few patients [2,5].

Future strategies may also include the use of immunotherapy against surface markers of neoplastic cells such as CD123.

Prognosis

Blastic NK-cell lymphoma is a very aggressive neoplasm, and the prognosis is very poor. The estimated 5-year survival is 0% [33]. Patients usually succumb to their lymphoma within 1 year, and only in exceptional cases have longer survivals been reported [2,5,8,26]. Although presentation with solitary or localized skin lesions may be associated with a longer survival, at present there is no evidence that long-term survival can be achieved with conventional treatments even for these patients. It has been suggested that allogeneic stem cell transplantation may yield better results, and should be offered as the first therapeutic option whenever possible [2,5].

RÉSUMÉ

Clinical — Adults, elderly. Localized or generalized 'bruise-like' violaceous plaques and tumours. Ulceration uncommon. No preferential location reported.

Morphology — Monomorphous infiltrate of medium-sized cells within the entire dermis and subcutis. The epidermis is spared. Cytomorphology: blastoid cells.

Immunology

CD4	+
CD56	+
CD123 (frozen)	+
TIA-1	−
CD3, 5, 20, 57	−
CD68, TdT	+/−

Genetics — Germline configuration of the TCR and J_H genes. No evidence of Epstein–Barr virus infection.

Treatment guidelines — Systemic chemotherapy.

References

1 Chaperot L, Bendriss N, Manches O et al. Identification of a leukemic counterpart of the plasmacytoid dendritic cells. *Blood* 2001; **97**: 3210–7.
2 Feuillard J, Jacob MC, Valensi F et al. Clinical and biologic features of CD4+ CD56+ malignancies. *Blood* 2002; **99**: 1556–63.
3 Leroux D, Mugneret F, Callanan M et al. CD4+, CD56+ DC2 acute leukemia is characterized by recurrent clonal chromosomal changes affecting 6 major targets: a study of 21 cases by the Groupe Français de Cytogenetique Hematologique. *Blood* 2002; **99**: 4154–9.
4 Petrella T, Comeau MR, Maynadié M et al. Agranular CD4+ CD56+ hematodermic neoplasm (blastic NK-cell lymphoma) originates from a population of CD56+ precursor cells related to plasmacytoid monocytes. *Am J Surg Pathol* 2002; **26**: 852–62.
5 Jacob MC, Chaperot L, Mossuz P et al. CD4+ CD56+ lineage negative malignancies: a new entity developed from malignant early plasmacytoid dendritic cells. *Haematologica* 2003; **88**: 941–55.
6 Chan JKC, Jaffe ES, Ralfkiaer E. Blastic NK-cell lymphoma. In: Jaffe ES, Harris NL, Stein H, Vardiman JW, eds. *World Health Organization Classification of Tumours: Tumours of haematopoietic and lymphoid tissues.* Lyon: IARC press, 2001: 214–5.
7 Willemze R, Kerl H, Sterry W et al. EORTC classification for primary cutaneous lymphomas: a proposal from the Cutaneous Lymphoma Study Group of the European Organization for Research and Treatment of Cancer. *Blood* 1997; **90**: 354–71.

8 Dummer R, Potoczna N, Haffner AC *et al*. A primary cutaneous non-T, non-B CD4⁺, CD56⁺ lymphoma. *Arch Dermatol* 1996; **132**: 550–3.

9 Kato N, Yasukawa K, Kimura K *et al*. CD2⁻ CD4⁺ CD56⁺ hematodermic/hematolymphoid malignancy. *J Am Acad Dermatol* 2001; **44**: 231–8.

10 Petrella T, Dalac S, Maynadie M *et al*. CD4⁺ CD56⁺ cutaneous neoplasms: a distinct hematological entity? Groupe Français d'Etude des Lymphomes Cutanés (GFELC). *Am J Surg Pathol* 1999; **23**: 137–46.

11 Bagot M, Bouloc A, Charue D *et al*. Do primary cutaneous non-T non-B CD4⁺ CD56⁺ lymphomas belong to the myelo-monocytic lineage? *J Invest Dermatol* 1998; **111**: 1242–4.

12 Khoury JD, Medeiros LJ, Manning JT *et al*. CD56⁺ TdT⁺ blastic natural killer cell tumor of the skin: primitive systemic malignancy related to myelomonocytic leukemia. *Cancer* 2002; **94**: 2401–8.

13 Scott AA, Head DR, Kopecky KJ *et al*. HLA-DR⁻, CD33⁺, CD56⁺, CD16⁻ myeloid/natural killer cell acute leukemia: a previously unrecognized form of acute leukemia potentially misdiagnosed as French–American–British acute myeloid leukemia-M3. *Blood* 1994; **84**: 244–55.

14 Suzuki R, Nakamura S. Malignancies of natural killer (NK) cell precursor: myeloid/NK cell precursor acute leukemia and blastic NK cell lymphoma/leukemia. *Leuk Res* 1999; **23**: 615–24.

15 Kazakov DV, Mentzel T, Burg G, Dummer R, Kempf W. Blastic natural killer-cell lymphoma of the skin associated with myelodysplastic syndrome of myelogenous leukaemia: a coincidence or more? *Br J Dermatol* 2003; **149**: 869–76.

16 Kaddu S, Zenahlik P, Beham-Schmid C, Kerl H, Cerroni L. Specific cutaneous infiltrates in patients with myelogenous leukemia: a clinicopathologic study of 26 patients with assessment of diagnostic criteria. *J Am Acad Dermatol* 1999; **40**: 966–78.

17 Bower CP, Standen GR, Pawade J, Knechtli CJ, Kennedy CTC. Cutaneous presentation of steroid responsive blastoid natural killer cell lymphoma. *Br J Dermatol* 2000; **142**: 1017–20.

18 Chan JKC, Jaffe ES, Ralfkiaer E. Blastic NK-cell lymphoma. In: Jaffe ES, Harris NL, Stein H *et al*. eds. *World Health Organization Classification of Tumours: Tumours of Haematopoietic and Lymphoid Tissues*. Lyon: IARC Press, 2001: 214–5.

19 Massone C, Chott A, Metze D *et al*. Subcutaneous, blastic natural killer (NK) NK/T-cell and other cytotoxic lymphomas of the skin: a morphologic, immunophenotypic and molecular study of 50 patients. *Am J Surg Pathol* in press.

20 Nagatani T, Okazawa H, Kambara T *et al*. Cutaneous monomorphous CD4- and CD56-positive large-cell lymphoma. *Dermatology* 2000; **200**: 202–8.

21 Radonich MA, Lazova R, Bolognia J. Cutaneous natural killer/T-cell lymphoma. *J Am Acad Dermatol* 2002; **46**: 451–6.

22 Child FJ, Mitchell TJ, Whittaker SJ *et al*. Blastic natural killer cell and extranodal natural killer cell-like T-cell lymphoma presenting in the skin: report of six cases from the UK. *Br J Dermatol* 2003; **148**: 507–15.

23 Husak R, Blume-Peytaki U, Orfanos CE. Aleukemic leukemia cutis in an adolescent boy. *N Engl J Med* 1999; **340**: 893–4.

24 Wollenberg A, Wagner M, Gunther S *et al*. Plasmacytoid dendritic cells: a new cutaneous dendritic cell subset with distinct role in inflammatory skin diseases. *J Invest Dermatol* 2002; **119**: 1096–102.

25 Chang SE, Choi HJ, Huh J *et al*. A case of primary cutaneous CD56⁺, TdT⁺, CD4⁺, blastic NK-cell lymphoma in a 19-year-old woman. *Am J Dermatopathol* 2002; **24**: 72–5.

26 Brody J, Allen S, Schulman P *et al*. Acute agranular CD4-positive natural killer cell leukemia: comprehensive clinicopathologic studies including virologic and *in vitro* culture with inducing agents. *Cancer* 1995; **75**: 2474–83.

27 Santucci M, Pimpinelli N, Massi D *et al*. Cytotoxic/natural killer cell cutaneous lymphomas: report of the EORTC cutaneous lymphoma task force workshop. *Cancer* 2003; **97**: 610–27.

28 Petrella T, Teitell MA, Spiekermann C *et al*. A CD56-negative case of blastic natural killer-cell lymphoma (agranular CD4⁺/CD56⁺ haematodermic neoplasm). *Br J Dermatol* 2004; **150**: 174–6.

29 Ko YH, Kim SH, Ree HJ. Blastic NK-cell lymphoma expressing terminal deoxynucleotidyl transferase with Homer–Wright type pseudorosettes formation. *Histopathology* 1998; **33**: 547–53.

30 Nakamura S, Koshikawa T, Yatabe Y, Suchi T. Lymphoblastic lymphoma expressing CD56 and TdT. *Am J Surg Pathol* 1998; **22**: 135–7.

31 Herling M, Teitell MA, Shen RR, Medeiros LJ, Jones D. TCL1 expression in plasmacytoid dendritic cells (DC2s) and the related CD4⁺ CD56⁺ blastic tumors of skin. *Blood* 2003; **101**: 5007–9.

32 DiGiuseppe JA, Louie DC, Williams JE *et al*. Blastic natural killer cell leukemia–lymphoma: a clinicopathologic study. *Am J Surg Pathol* 1997; **21**: 1223–30.

33 Fink-Puches R, Zenahlik P, Bäck B *et al*. Primary cutaneous lymphomas: applicability of current classification schemes (European Organization for Research and Treatment of Cancer, World Health Organization) based on clinicopathologic features observed in a large group of patients. *Blood* 2002; **99**: 800–5.

Part 4 Cutaneous Hodgkin lymphoma

Chapter 17 Cutaneous Hodgkin lymphoma

Hodgkin lymphoma is regarded as a distinct malignant lymphoma characterized by the presence of neoplastic Reed–Sternberg cells in association with different patterns of reactive cells. Recent studies of the Reed–Sternberg cell have shown in most examples an origin from a germinal centre B lymphocyte suggesting that more than 90% of cases of Hodgkin lymphoma represent variants of B-cell lymphomas. A viral aetiology is possible because the Epstein–Barr virus genome has been detected frequently. Skin manifestations of nodal Hodgkin lymphoma were not uncommon in the past [1–8]. Modern treatment modalities have resulted in a dramatic decrease in cutaneous involvement although occasional cases are still reported [9–12]. Rare cases of Hodgkin lymphoma presenting as primary disease in the skin have also been described [13–15]. It should be noted that some authors consider these to be examples of cutaneous anaplastic large cell lymphoma or lymphomatoid papulosis rather than true cases of primary cutaneous Hodgkin lymphoma.

Nodal Hodgkin lymphoma may be preceded by, concomitant with or followed by other cutaneous lymphoproliferative disorders including mycosis fungoides, lymphomatoid papulosis and anaplastic large cell lymphoma (see also Chapters 2 and 4) [16–23]. Cases of Hodgkin lymphoma associated with granulomatous slack skin have also been described [24,25]. These may represent examples of mycosis fungoides-associated granulomatous slack skin in patients with Hodgkin lymphoma rather than true specific cutaneous manifestations of the Hodgkin lymphoma. Similarly, the patient reported as having 'follicular mucinosis' in association with Hodgkin lymphoma [26] may perhaps have had coexistent mycosis fungoides-associated follicular mucinosis.

The onset of cutaneous manifestations of Hodgkin lymphoma has been observed in a HIV-infected patient [27].

Clinical features

Clinically, skin lesions in Hodgkin lymphoma are usually confined to the drainage area of affected lymph nodes

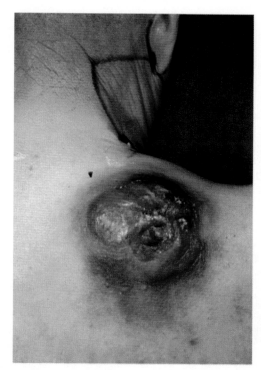

Fig. 17.1 Cutaneous Hodgkin lymphoma. Large ulcerated tumour on the right shoulder.

(retrograde lymphatic spread) [8,28]. Papules, plaques and tumours may all be observed (Figs 17.1 & 17.2) [28,29]. Ulceration is not uncommon. In some cases lesions are generalized.

Histopathology, immunophenotype and molecular genetics

Histology shows the typical features of Hodgkin lymphoma with Reed–Sternberg and Hodgkin cells on the background of small lymphocytes, histiocytes, eosinophils and plasma

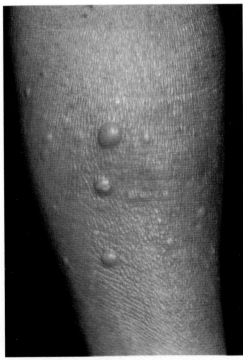

Fig. 17.2 Cutaneous Hodgkin lymphoma. Papules and small nodules on the arm.

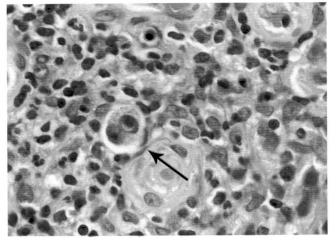

Fig. 17.3 Cutaneous Hodgkin lymphoma. Reed–Sternberg cell (arrow) on the background of small lymphocytes, histiocytes and eosinophils.

cells (Figs 17.3 & 17.4) [28]. Reed–Sternberg cells may be absent in some cutaneous lesions. It is not possible to classify skin lesions according to the histopathological subtypes seen in lymph nodes and recognized in the World Health

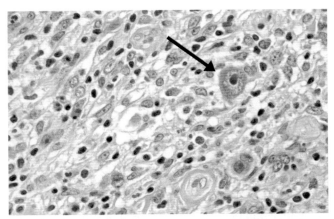

Fig. 17.4 Cutaneous Hodgkin lymphoma. Large Hodgkin cell with eosinophilic nucleolus (arrow) admixed with small lymphocytes, histiocytes and eosinophils.

Organization (WHO) classification of lymphoid tumours (nodular lymphocyte-predominant Hodgkin lymphoma, classical Hodgkin lymphoma, nodular sclerosis classical Hodgkin lymphoma, mixed cellularity classical Hodgkin lymphoma, lymphocyte-depleted classical Hodgkin lymphoma) [30].

It should be noted that Hodgkin and Reed–Sternberg-like cells may be found in a variety of other conditions including mainly lymphomatoid papulosis and anaplastic large cell lymphoma.

Immunohistology reveals in most cases a CD30[+], CD15[+] phenotype of Reed–Sternberg and Hodgkin cells although CD15 may be negative in some cases [28,31]. The small lymphocytes are of both B- and T-cell lineages.

There are no molecular data on cutaneous cases of Hodgkin lymphoma.

Treatment and prognosis

Patients with specific cutaneous manifestations of Hodgkin lymphoma should be treated in a haematological setting according to schemes tailored for the underlying disease.

In the past, the prognosis for patients with skin manifestations of nodal Hodgkin lymphoma was poor in spite of aggressive treatment. Modern treatment modalities have resulted in a decline in the onset of specific skin manifestations. Because only occasional patients present with cutaneous involvement, there is little information on which to base prognosis and therapeutic options. However, cutaneous Hodgkin lymphoma usually represents advanced (stage IV) disease and carries a bad prognosis.

RÉSUMÉ

Clinical Adults. Solitary, grouped or, rarely, generalized cutaneous papules, plaques and tumours.
Lesions are commonly located at the drainage area of affected lymph nodes.

Morphology Nodular or diffuse infiltrates characterized by presence of Reed–Sternberg and Hodgkin cells on a background of small lymphocytes, histiocytes and eosinophils.

Immunology CD30 +
CD15 +(–)

Genetics Data on genetic features of specific skin manifestations are not available.

Treatment guidelines Treatment planned on the basis of the underlying disease.
Radiotherapy of isolated skin tumours.

References

1 Gordon RA, Lookingbill DP, Abt AB. Skin infiltration in Hodgkin's disease. *Arch Dermatol* 1980; **116**: 1038–40.
2 Heyd J, Weissberg N, Gottschalk S. Hodgkin's disease of the skin: a case report. *Cancer* 1989; **63**: 924–9.
3 O'Bryan-Tear CG, Burke M, Coulson IH, Marsden RA. Hodgkin's disease presenting in the skin. *Clin Exp Dermatol* 1987; **12**: 69–71.
4 Silverman CL, Strayer DS, Wasserman TH. Cutaneous Hodgkin's disease. *Arch Dermatol* 1982; **118**: 918–21.
5 Smith JL, Butler JJ. Skin involvement in Hodgkin's disease. *Cancer* 1980; **45**: 354–61.
6 Torne R, Umbert P. Hodgkin's disease presenting with superficial lymph nodes and tumors of the scalp. *Dermatologica* 1986; **172**: 225–8.
7 White RM, Patterson JW. Cutaneous involvement in Hodgkin's disease. *Cancer* 1985; **55**: 1136–45.
8 Benninghoff DL, Medina A, Alexander LL, Camiel MR. The mode of spread of Hodgkin's disease to the skin. *Cancer* 1970; **26**: 1135–40.
9 Derrick EK, Deutsch GP, Price ML. Cutaneous extension of Hodgkin's disease. *J R Soc Med* 1991; **84**: 684–5.
10 Nelson MC, Petrik JH, Lack EE *et al.* Lymphocyte-predominant Hodgkin disease manifested as a subcutaneous arm mass. *Am J Radiol* 1990; **155**: 658–9.
11 Tassies D, Sierra J, Montserrat E *et al.* Specific cutaneous involvement in Hodgkin's disease. *Hematol Oncol* 1992; **10**: 75–9.
12 Takagawa S, Maruyama R, Yokozeki H *et al.* Skin invasion of Hodgkin's disease mimicking scrofuloderma. *Dermatology* 1999; **199**: 268–70.
13 Sioutos N, Kerl H, Murphy SB, Kadin ME. Primary cutaneous Hodgkin disease: unique clinical, morphologic and immunophenotypic findings. *Am J Dermatopathol* 1994; **16**: 2–8.
14 Kumar S, Kingma DW, Weiss WB, Raffeld M, Jaffe ES. Primary cutaneous Hodgkin's disease with evolution to systemic disease: association with Epstein–Barr virus. *Am J Surg Pathol* 1996; **20**: 754–9.
15 Guitart J, Fretzin D. Skin as the primary site of Hodgkin's disease: a case report of primary cutaneous Hodgkin's disease and review of its relationship with non-Hodgkin's lymphoma. *Am J Dermatopathol* 1998; **20**: 218–22.
16 Caya JG, Choi H, Tieu TM, Wollenberg NJ, Almagro UA. Hodgkin's disease followed by mycosis fungoides in the same patient: case report and review of the literature. *Cancer* 1984; **53**: 463–7.
17 Clement M, Bhakri H, Monk B *et al.* Mycosis fungoides and Hodgkin's disease. *J R Soc Med* 1984; **77**: 1037–8.
18 Davis TH, Morton CC, Miller-Cassman R, Balk SP, Kadin ME. Hodgkin's disease, lymphomatoid papulosis, and cutaneous T-cell lymphoma derived from a common T-cell clone. *N Engl J Med* 1992; **326**: 1115–22.
19 Hawkins KA, Schinella R, Schwartz M *et al.* Simultaneous occurrence of mycosis fungoides and Hodgkin disease. *Am J Hematol* 1983; **14**: 355–62.
20 Kadin ME. Lymphomatoid papulosis and associated lymphomas: how are they related? *Arch Dermatol* 1993; **129**: 351–3.
21 Kamarashev J, Dummer R, Hess Schmid M *et al.* Primary cutaneous T-cell-rich B-cell lymphoma and Hodgkin's disease in a patient with Gardner's syndrome. *Dermatology* 2000; **201**: 362–5.
22 Simrell CR, Boccia RV, Longo DL, Jaffe ES. Coexisting Hodgkin's disease and mycosis fungoides. *Arch Pathol Lab Med* 1986; **110**: 1029–34.
23 Weinman VF, Ackerman AB. Lymphomatoid papulosis: a critical review and new findings. *Am J Dermatopathol* 1981; **3**: 129–62.
24 DeGregorio R, Fenske NA, Glass LF. Granulomatous slack skin: a possible precursor of Hodgkin's disease. *J Am Acad Dermatol* 1995; **33**: 1044–7.
25 Noto G, Pravatà G, Miceli S, Aricò M. Granulomatous slack skin: report of a case associated with Hodgkin's disease and a review of the literature. *Br J Dermatol* 1994; **131**: 275–9.
26 Stewart M, Smoller BR. Follicular mucinosis in Hodgkin's disease: a poor prognostic sign? *J Am Acad Dermatol* 1991; **24**: 784–5.
27 Shaw MT, Jacobs SR. Cutaneous Hodgkin's disease in a patient with human immunodeficiency virus infection. *Cancer* 1989; **64**: 2585–7.
28 Cerroni L, Beham-Schmid C, Kerl H. Cutaneous Hodgkin's disease: an immunohistochemical analysis. *J Cutan Pathol* 1995; **22**: 229–35.
29 Hayes TG, Rabin VR, Rosen T, Zubler MA. Hodgkin's disease presenting in the skin: case report and review of the literature. *J Am Acad Dermatol* 1990; **22**: 944–7.
30 Stein H, Delsol G, Pileri S *et al.* Hodgkin lymphoma. In: Jaffe ES, Harris NL, Stein H, Vardiman JW, eds. *World Health Organization Classification of Tumours: Tumours of Haematopoietic and Lymphoid Tissues.* Lyon: IARC Press, 2001: 237–53.
31 Moretti S, Pimpinelli N, Di Lollo S, Vallecchi C, Bosi A. *In situ* immunologic characterization of cutaneous involvement in Hodgkin's disease. *Cancer* 1989; **63**: 661–6.

Part 5 Other cutaneous lymphomas/leukaemias

Chapter 18 Cutaneous myelogenous leukaemia

Myelogenous leukaemias are a spectrum of diseases encompassing chronic myeloproliferative diseases, myelodysplastic disorders and acute myeloid leukaemias. Skin manifestations are more common in patients with acute myelogenous leukaemia of the French–American–British (FAB) classification subtypes M4 and M5 (acute myelomonocytic leukaemia, acute monoblastic leukaemia, acute monocytic leukaemia), but can be observed rarely in other subtypes of acute myeloid leukaemia, in a small percentage of patients with chronic myelogenous leukaemia and also in patients with myelodysplastic syndromes [1–11].

Cases showing isolated extramedullary tumours with myeloid differentiation have been referred to as chloroma or granulocytic sarcoma in the past but are currently referred to as myeloid sarcomas [12–14]. Myeloid sarcoma may precede or be concomitant with myelogenous leukaemia.

There may be a relationship between myelogenous leukaemia and blastic NK-cell lymphomas (see Chapter 16).

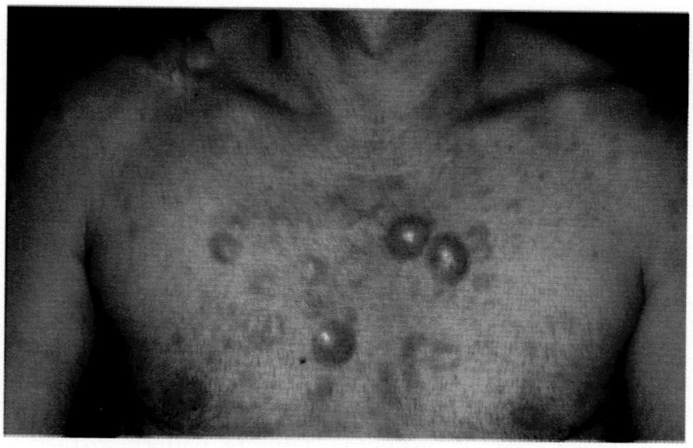

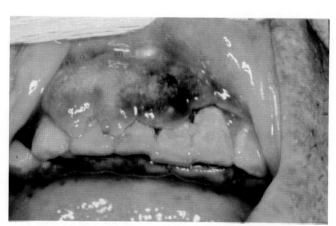

Fig. 18.1 Cutaneous manifestations of myelogenous leukaemia. Large tumours on the chest in a 40-year-old patient without a leukaemic picture who developed overt leukaemia 2 months after the onset of skin lesions ('aleukaemic leukaemia cutis').

Clinical features

The majority of cases present in adult patients as multiple, localized or generalized papules, plaques and nodules with a characteristic reddish brown or violaceous colour in the context of a known leukaemia (Fig. 18.1) [1]. Cases in children and even neonates have been reported [15,16]. Involvement of the mucosal regions is common (Fig. 18.2). Diagnosis of specific cutaneous infiltrates may be difficult in cases presenting with unusual clinical features such as solitary skin nodules, maculopapular eruptions clinically resembling drug or viral eruptions or other uncommon presentations [1,17,18].

Specific skin infiltrates of acute myelogenous leukaemia have been observed in the skin lesions of Sweet syndrome, psoriasis and basal cell carcinoma, suggesting that there may be a selective predilection for pre-existing cutaneous lesions in some cases [19–22].

Fig. 18.2 Cutaneous manifestations of myelogenous leukaemia. Involvement of the gingiva with characteristic violaceous plaques.

In a distinct proportion of patients, specific skin infiltrates represent the first clinical manifestation of the disease, preceding blood and/or bone marrow changes by weeks or even months ('aleukaemic leukaemia cutis') [23,24].

Histopathology and immunophenotype

Histopathology

There are no differences in the histopathological features of skin involvement by acute or chronic myelogenous leukaemia [1]. Specific cutaneous lesions show mild, moderate or dense, diffuse or nodular dermal infiltrates often with perivascular and periadnexal accentuation and sparing of the upper papillary dermis. Involvement of the subcutis is common. The infiltrate is composed of medium-sized round to oval cells with a slightly eosinophilic cytoplasm and distinct, sometimes indented, bilobular or kidney-shaped basophilic nuclei (atypical monocytoid cells) (Fig. 18.3). Large cells may also be seen. Variable numbers of mitotic figures (including atypical mitoses) and apoptotic cells can be found. Reactive cells (e.g. lymphocytes, mast cells) are present in some cases. A granulomatous reaction may also be observed [1,25,26].

Prominent single files of neoplastic cells between collagen bundles can be observed in the majority of cases ('Indian filing') (Fig. 18.4). A distinctive 'figurate' pattern characterized by concentric layering of neoplastic cells around blood vessels and adnexal structures is typical of the skin lesions in acute myelomonocytic leukaemia, acute monoblastic leukaemia and acute monocytic leukaemia (Fig. 18.5).

Cutaneous lesions of myeloid sarcoma present with large cutaneous or subcutaneous tumours composed of myeloblasts or monoblasts.

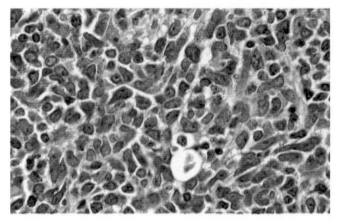

Fig. 18.3 Cutaneous manifestations of myelogenous leukaemia. Monomorphous infiltrate of atypical monocytoid cells.

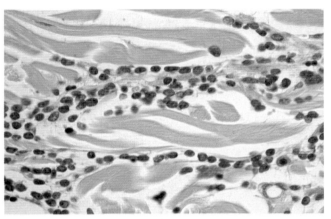

Fig. 18.4 Cutaneous manifestations of myelogenous leukaemia. Linear arrangement of neoplastic cells ('Indian filing').

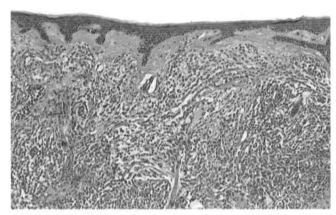

Fig. 18.5 Cutaneous manifestations of myelogenous leukaemia. Typical disposition of neoplastic cells with 'layering' around vessels and adnexal structures ('figurate' pattern).

Immunophenotype

Cutaneous lesions of myelogenous leukaemia show the simultaneous expression of lysozyme, myeloperoxidase, CD45, CD43 and CD74 (Fig. 18.6). Other myeloid markers useful for the classification of these tumours (e.g. CD13, CD14, CD33, CD116, CD117) do not work in routinely fixed, paraffin-embedded sections of tissue. Staining for naphthol-ASD-chloracetate-esterase (NASDCl, Leder stain) is positive, mainly in cases with a more mature phenotype, but tends to be negative in more immature cells. Staining for CD56 is positive only in a minority of cases, usually allowing a differentiation to be made from the lesions of blastic NK-cell lymphoma [1,5,27]. There seems to be no correlation between features seen in specific skin infiltrates and the subtype of the underlying myelogenous leukaemia.

A diagnostic pitfall is the finding of little or no reactivity for lysozyme and myeloperoxidase in association with

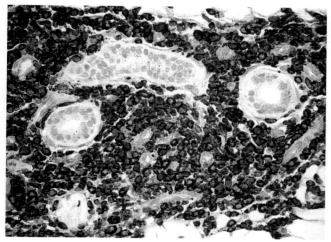

Fig. 18.6 Cutaneous manifestations of myelogenous leukaemia. Positive staining of neoplastic cells for myeloperoxidase.

CD43 positivity, suggesting an erroneous diagnosis of a T-cell lymphoma. A full immunophenotype of T and myeloid markers usually reveals the true diagnosis.

Treatment and prognosis

The skin manifestations are managed by treating the underlying myelogenous leukaemia. Patients with 'aleukaemic leukaemia cutis' should be managed in the same way as patients with blood and/or medullary involvement, as the disease inevitably progresses over short periods of time [28].

There seems to be no differences in survival between patients with specific skin manifestations of acute or chronic myelogenous leukaemia. The course is aggressive, and survival is usually a few months only.

RÉSUMÉ

Clinical	Adults. Generalized cutaneous papules, plaques and tumours. Common involvement of mucosal regions.
Morphology	Nodular or diffuse infiltrates characterized by predominance of atypical myeloid cells. 'Indian filing', 'figurate' pattern.
Immunology	Myeloperoxidase + NASDCI + CD43, 74 + Lysozyme +
Treatment guidelines	Systemic chemotherapy.

References

1 Kaddu S, Zenahlik P, Beham-Schmid C, Kerl H, Cerroni L. Specific cutaneous infiltrates in patients with myelogenous leukemia: a clinicopathologic study of 26 patients with assessment of diagnostic criteria. *J Am Acad Dermatol* 1999; **40**: 966–78.

2 Desch JK, Smoller BR. The spectrum of cutaneous disease in leukemias. *J Cutan Pathol* 1993; **20**: 407–10.

3 Janier M, Raynaud E, Blanche P, Daniel F, Herreman G. Leukaemia cutis and erythroleukaemia. *Br J Dermatol* 1999; **141**: 372–3.

4 Kaiserling E, Horny HP, Geerts ML, Schmid U. Skin involvement in myelogenous leukemia: morphologic and immunophenotypic heterogeneity of skin infiltrates. *Mod Pathol* 1994; **7**: 771–9.

5 Kuwabara H, Nagai M, Yamaoka G, Ohnishi H, Kawakami K. Specific skin manifestations in CD56 positive acute myeloid leukemia. *J Cutan Pathol* 1999; **26**: 1–5.

6 Nagao K, Kikuchi A, Kawai Y *et al.* Skin infiltration in acute promyelocytic leukemia. *Dermatology* 1997; **194**: 168–71.

7 Namba Y, Koizumi H, Nakamura H *et al.* Specific cutaneous lesions of the scalp in myelodysplastic syndrome with deletion of 20q. *J Dermatol* 1999; **26**: 220–4.

8 Sepp N, Radaszkiewicz T, Meijer CJLM *et al.* Specific skin manifestations in acute leukemia with monocytic differentiation: a morphologic and immunohistochemical study of 11 cases. *Cancer* 1993; **71**: 124–32.

9 Stawiski MA. Skin manifestations of leukemias and lymphomas. *Cutis* 1978; **21**: 814–8.

10 Ueda K, Kume A, Furukawa Y, Higashi N. Cutaneous infiltration in acute promyelocytic leukemia. *J Am Acad Dermatol* 1997; **36**: 104–6.

11 Kajisawa C, Matsui C, Morohashi M. A specific cutaneous lesion revealing myelodysplastic syndrome. *Eur J Dermatol* 1998; **8**: 517–8.

12 Traweek ST, Arber DA, Rappaport H, Brynes RK. Extramedullary myeloid cell tumors: an immunohistochemical and morphologic study of 28 cases. *Am J Surg Pathol* 1993; **17**: 1011–9.

13 Sisack MJ, Dunsmore K, Sidhu-Malik N. Granulocytic sarcoma in the absence of myeloid leukemia. *J Am Acad Dermatol* 1997; **37**: 308–11.

14 Dreizen S, McCredie KB, Keating MJ. Mucocutaneous granulocytic sarcomas of the head and neck. *J Oral Pathol* 1987; **16**: 57–60.

15 Husak R, Blume-Peytaki U, Orfanos CE. Aleukemic leukemia cutis in an adolescent boy. *N Engl J Med* 1999; **340**: 893–4.

16 Canioni D, Fraitag S, Thomas C *et al.* Skin lesions revealing neonatal acute leukemias with monocytic differentiation: a report of 3 cases. *J Cutan Pathol* 1996; **23**: 254–8.

17 Benez A, Metzger S, Metzler G, Fierlbeck G. Aleukemic leukemia cutis presenting as benign-appearing exanthema. *Acta Derm Venereol (Stockh)* 2001; **81**: 45–7.

18 Chang HY, Wong KM, Bosenberg M, McKee PH, Haynes HA. Myelogenous leukemia cutis resembling stasis dermatitis. *J Am Acad Dermatol* 2003; **49**: 128–9.

19 Metzler G, Cerroni L, Schmidt H *et al.* Leukemic cells within skin lesions of psoriasis in a patient with acute myelogenous leukemia. *J Cutan Pathol* 1997; **24**: 445–8.

20 Diaz-Cascajo C, Bloedern-Schlicht N. Cutaneous infiltrates of myelogenous leukemia in association with pre-existing skin diseases. *J Cutan Pathol* 1998; **25**: 185–6.

21 Urano Y, Miyaoka Y, Kosaka M *et al.* Sweet's syndrome associated with chronic myelogenous leukemia: demonstration of leukemic cells within a skin lesion. *J Am Acad Dermatol* 1999; **40:** 275–9.

22 Deguchi M, Tsunoda T, Yuda F, Tagami H. Sweet's syndrome in acute myelogenous leukemia showing dermal infiltration of leukemic cells. *Dermatology* 1997; **194:** 182–4.

23 Ohno S, Yokoo T, Ohta M *et al.* Aleukemic leukemia cutis. *J Am Acad Dermatol* 1990; **22:** 374–7.

24 Okun MM, Fitzgibbon J, Nahass GT, Forsman K. Aleukemic leukemia cutis, myeloid subtype. *Eur J Dermatol* 1995; **5:** 290–3.

25 Baksh FK, Nathan D, Richardson W, Kestenbaum T, Woodroof J. Leukemia cutis with prominent giant cell reaction. *Am J Dermatopathol* 1998; **20:** 48–52.

26 Tomasini C, Quaglino P, Novelli M, Fierro MT. 'Aleukemic' granulomatous leukemia cutis. *Am J Dermatopathol* 1998; **20:** 417–21.

27 Kaddu S, Beham-Schmid C, Zenahlik P, Kerl H, Cerroni L. CD56[+] blastic transformation of chronic myeloid leukemia involving the skin. *J Cutan Pathol* 1999; **26:** 497–503.

28 Chang H, Shih LY, Kuo TT. Primary aleukemic myeloid leukemia cutis treated successfully with combination chemotherapy: report of a case and review of the literature. *Ann Hematol* 2003; **82:** 435–9.

Chapter 19 Cutaneous lymphomas in immunosuppressed individuals (post-transplant lymphoproliferative disorders, HIV-associated cutaneous lymphomas)

Individuals who are immunosuppressed, either as a consequence of disease (e.g. human immunodeficiency virus [HIV] infection) or of specific treatment, are at higher risk of cutaneous and extracutaneous malignancies including lymphomas. Cutaneous lymphomas in immunocompromised patients have some peculiar aspects that deserve to be discussed in a separate chapter. The two main conditions discussed here are cutaneous post-transplant lymphoproliferative disorders and HIV-associated skin lymphomas. Other conditions such as methotrexate-associated lymphoproliferative disorders and lymphomas occurring in immunodeficient states other than HIV-related will not be discussed in detail. Cutaneous lymphomas in patients under methotrexate therapy have clinicopathological features similar to corresponding entities observed in patients who do not take the drug, the main difference being represented by a higher rate of association with Epstein–Barr virus (EBV) infection [1]. In over half of the cases the lesions regress upon withdrawal of methotrexate.

CUTANEOUS POST-TRANSPLANT LYMPHOPROLIFERATIVE DISORDERS

Lymphoproliferative disorders are one of the most common malignancies in recipients of solid organ and bone marrow transplantation, developing in approximately 2% (post-transplant lymphoproliferative disorders). They represent for the most part examples of EBV-associated lymphoproliferative disorders. Although cutaneous manifestations are rare, some patients may present with disease localized solely to the skin [2–8]. Most cases arise within the first year after organ or bone marrow transplantation, but the time interval

between transplantation and the onset of a post-transplant lymphoproliferative disorder may be much longer (several years).

Post-transplant lymphoproliferative disorders occur more often in recipients of heart–lung allografts, and less commonly in those who receive renal allografts. Other risk factors include primary infection with EBV following transplantation, infection with cytomegalovirus, T-cell-specific immunosuppression and younger age [9,10].

Post-transplant lymphoproliferative disorders are currently classified according to three major categories:
1 Early lesions (reactive plasmacytic hyperplasia, infectious mononucleosis-like).
2 Polymorphic post-transplant lymphoproliferative disorder.
3 Monomorphic post-transplant lymphoproliferative disorder [9,10].

Most monomorphic lesions exhibit a B-cell phenotype but in rare instances a T-cell phenotype has been observed.

Clinical features

Patients are adults or children who have received allogeneic solid organ or bone marrow transplantation and are under immunosuppressive treatment. Cutaneous lesions are variable, including erythematous plaques, nodules and tumours, sometimes ulcerated. They can be solitary, localized to a single anatomical region, or generalized. Concomitant involvement of other organs can be observed, and is usually associated with systemic symptoms, including elevated serum levels of lactic dehydrogenase. Precise staging investigations should always be performed, in order to evaluate the extent of involvement before planning the treatment.

Histopathology, immunophenotype and molecular genetics

Histopathological features vary according to the subtype of post-transplant lymphoproliferative disorder. Early lesions show polyclonal (rarely monoclonal) proliferations of mature plasma cells with rare immunoblasts. Polymorphic post-transplant lymphoproliferative disorder is characterized by the presence of a monoclonal infiltrate of B lymphocytes, comprising the whole spectrum of maturation and including plasma cells, immunoblasts and intermediate-sized lymphoid cells. In monomorphic post-transplant lymphoproliferative disorder, the histopathological picture is that of a malignant lymphoma (diffuse large B-cell lymphoma, Burkitt lymphoma, plasma cell myeloma or extramedullary plasmacytoma). Cases involving the skin present mostly with the features of diffuse large B-cell lymphoma. In rare cases a plasmablastic morphology can be observed, similar to cases arising in HIV-infected individuals [11].

In rare instances, the aspects may be those of a peripheral T-cell lymphoma not otherwise specified. Expression of α/β or γ/δ, as well as of CD4, CD8, CD30 and CD56, is variable in these cases. In a recent study, analysis of phenotypic and molecular features of a large group of cases confirmed the histogenetic diversity of different cases of monomorphic post-transplant lymphoproliferative disorders [12].

Treatment and prognosis

Reduction of immunosuppression, often associated with antiviral therapy, is the main strategy for treatment of post-transplant lymphoproliferative disorders [13–15]. Regression of the lesions may take place over a period of a few weeks up to a few months. Lesions that do not respond to these measures may be treated by more conventional modalities, including radiotherapy, interferon-α, anti-CD20 antibody (rituximab) and systemic chemotherapy.

Plasmacytic hyperplasia almost always responds completely to mild reduction of immunosuppression. The prognosis of polymorphic or monomorphic post-transplant lymphoproliferative disorders limited to the skin seems to be more favourable than that of extracutaneous post-transplant lymphoproliferative disorders.

CUTANEOUS LYMPHOMAS IN HIV-INFECTED INDIVIDUALS

The onset of cutaneous lymphomas caused by viral-induced

RÉSUMÉ

Cutaneous post-transplant lymphoproliferative disorder

Clinical — Children and adults. Onset of skin lesions usually within 1 year from organ transplantation. More frequent in recipients of heart–lung allografts. Three categories: plasmacytic hyperplasia, polymorphic or monomorphic post-transplant lymphoproliferative disorder.

Morphology — Mature plasma cells (plasmacytic hyperplasia); plasma cells, immunoblasts, intermediate cells (polymorphic type); clear-cut features of lymphoma (monomorphic type).

Immunology —
CD20, 79a +
LMP-1 +
EBER-1 +
CD3, 5 – (rare cases have a T-cell phenotype)

Genetics — Monoclonal rearrangement of the J_H gene (polymorphic and monomorphic types).

Treatment guidelines — Reduction of immunosuppression. Antiviral therapy. Cases that do not respond may be treated with rituximab, interferon-α, radiotherapy or systemic chemotherapy.

immunosuppression has been observed in individuals with acquired immunodeficiency syndrome (AIDS) [16,17]. It has been estimated that HIV-infected patients have a risk of developing a malignant lymphoma up to 200-fold higher than normal individuals. There are some overlapping features between the lymphomas arising in HIV+ patients and those observed after solid organ or bone marrow transplantation.

Cutaneous lesions may represent examples of 'common' skin lymphomas such as mycosis fungoides, CD30+ anaplastic large cell lymphoma or diffuse large B-cell lymphoma. In contrast to cutaneous lymphomas in non-infected individuals, however, mycosis fungoides represents a minority of the cases arising in HIV+ patients, whereas B-cell lymphomas are more common. The entity of plasmablastic lymphoma of the oral cavity has been reported mainly in HIV+ individuals, and seems to be associated with human herpesvirus 8 (HHV-8) infection [18,19]. Association with EBV has been documented in most cases of cutaneous B-cell lymphoma associated with HIV infection, and rarely also in cases of CD30+ anaplastic large cell lymphoma.

Clinical features

Patients are adults who are infected with HIV and have a very low CD4 count, but rarely children can be affected as well [16,20,21]. The onset of a cutaneous lymphoma may represent the first AIDS-defining illness in some of these patients. Cutaneous lesions are variable, depending on the type of cutaneous lymphoma, and are not different from those observed in non-HIV-infected individuals. Rarely, a post-transplant lymphoproliferative disorder-like polymorphic infiltrate may be observed [22]. Accurate staging investigations should be performed in order to evaluate the extent (if any) of extracutaneous involvement.

In patients with HIV infection, mycosis fungoides should be distinguished from benign CD8+ cutaneous infiltrates that may reveal similar clinicopathological features (see Chapter 20).

Histopathology, immunophenotype and molecular genetics

Histopathological, immunophenotypical and molecular genetic features are similar to those observed in the corresponding lymphoma entities arising in non-HIV-infected individuals. However, in cases of diffuse large B-cell lymphoma, plasmablastic differentiation (Fig. 19.1) and association with EBV (positivity for LMP-1 and/or EBER-1) are more commonly seen.

Although HHV-8 has a role in AIDS-associated primary effusion lymphoma, it seems that lymphomas arising in the skin in HIV patients are only rarely associated with HHV-8 infection, with the exception of oral plasmablastic lymphoma [16,19,23]. Infection with human T-lymphotropic virus 2 (HTLV-II) has been detected in one HIV patient with a cutaneous T-cell lymphoma [24].

Treatment and prognosis

Mycosis fungoides in HIV+ patients should be managed according to standard protocols (see Chapter 2) [16,25]. Other lymphomas may be treated with local radiotherapy. Antiviral treatment should be accurately verified.

As these lymphomas arise in patients who are profoundly immunocompromised, death often ensues, resulting from complications of AIDS rather than from direct lymphoma spread. In this context, the use of conservative strategies for treatment of the cutaneous lymphomas has been advocated [16].

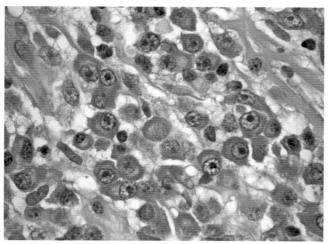

Fig. 19.1 Cutaneous diffuse large B-cell lymphoma in an HIV-infected individual. Note plasmablasts with eccentric nuclei, prominent nucleoli and abundant cytoplasm, admixed with plasma cells.

RÉSUMÉ

HIV-associated cutaneous lymphomas

Clinical	Adults with HIV infection and very low CD4 cell count (children rarely affected). Clinical features may be those of 'common' types of cutaneous lymphomas (e.g. mycosis fungoides, CD30+ anaplastic large cell lymphoma, diffuse large B-cell lymphoma).	
Morphology	Similar to the non-HIV-related counterparts; in diffuse large B-cell lymphomas plasmablastic morphology more common.	
Immunology	CD20, 79a	+ (B-cell types)
	CD3, 5	+ (T-cell types)
	CD30	+ (CD30+ anaplastic large cell lymphoma)
	LMP-1, EBER-1	+ (especially B-cell lymphomas)
	HHV-8	+ (oral plasmablastic lymphoma)
Genetics	Monoclonal rearrangement of the TCR or J_H genes.	
Treatment guidelines	Radiotherapy (solitary or localized lesions); mycosis fungoides should be managed according to standard treatment regimens; antiviral therapy should be verified.	

References

1 Harris NL, Swerdlow SH. Methotrexate-associated lymphoprolifer-ative disorders. In: Jaffe ES, Harris NL, Stein H, Vardiman JW, eds. *World Health Organization Classification of Tumours: Tumours of haematopoietic and lymphoid tissues.* Lyon: IARC press, 2001: 270–1.

2 Pacheco TR, Hinthner L, Fitzpatrick J. Extramedullary plasmacytoma in cardiac transplant recipients. *J Am Acad Dermatol* 2003; **49**: S255–8.

3 Seckin D, Demirhan B, Gülec TO, Arikan U, Haberal M. Post-transplantation primary cutaneous CD30 (Ki1)-positive large-cell lymphoma. *J Am Acad Dermatol* 2001; **45**: S197–9.

4 Ward HA, Russo GG, McBurney E, Millikan LE, Boh EE. Post-transplant primary cutaneous T-cell lymphoma. *J Am Acad Dermatol* 2001; **44**: 675–80.

5 Schumann KW, Oriba HA, Bergfeld WF, Hsi ED, Hollandsworth K. Cutaneous presentation of post-transplant lymphoproliferative dis-order. *J Am Acad Dermatol* 2000; **42**: 923–6.

6 Chai C, White WL, Shea CR, Prieto VG. Epstein–Barr virus-associated lymphoproliferative-disorders primarily involving the skin. *J Cutan Pathol* 1999; **26**: 242–7.

7 Gonthier DM, Hartman G, Holley JL. Post-transplant lymphopro-liferative disorder presenting as an isolated skin lesion. *Am J Kidney Dis* 1992; **19**: 600–3.

8 McGregor JM, Yu CCW, Lu QL et al. Post-transplant cutaneous lymphoma. *J Am Acad Dermatol* 1993; **29**: 549–54.

9 Harris NL, Swerdlow SH. Post-transplant lymphoproliferative dis-orders: summary of Society for Hematopathology Workshop. *Semin Diagn Pathol* 1997; **14**: 8–14.

10 Harris NL, Swerdlow SH, Frizzera G, Knowles DM. Post-transplant lymphoproliferative disorders. In: Jaffe ES, Harris NL, Stein H, Vardiman JW, eds. *World Health Organization Classification of Tumours: Tumours of haematopoietic and lymphoid tissues.* Lyon: IARC press, 2001: 264–9.

11 Nicol I, Boye T, Carsuzaa F et al. Post-transplant plasmablastic lym-phoma of the skin. *Br J Dermatol* 2003; **149**: 889–91.

12 Capello D, Cerri M, Muti G et al. Molecular histogenesis of post-transplantation lymphoproliferative disorders. *Blood* 2003; **102**: 3775–85.

13 Starzl TE, Nalesnik MA, Porter KA et al. Reversibility of lymphomas and lymphoproliferative lesions developing under cyclosporin-steroid therapy. *Lancet* 1984; **8377**: 583–7.

14 Green M. Management of Epstein–Barr virus-induced post-transplant lymphoproliferative disease in recipients of solid organ transplantation. *Am J Transplant* 2001; **1**: 103–8.

15 Blokx WAM, Andriessen MPM, van Hamersvelt HW, van Krieken JHJM. Initial spontaneous remission of post-transplantation Epstein–Barr virus-related B-cell lymphoproliferative disorder of the skin in a renal transplant recipient: case report and review of the literature on cutaneous B-cell post-transplantation lymphoproliferative dis-ease. *Am J Dermatopathol* 2002; **24**: 414–22.

16 Beylot-Barry M, Vergier B, Masquelier B et al. The spectrum of cuta-neous lymphomas in HIV infection: a study of 21 cases. *Am J Surg Pathol* 1999; **23**: 1208–16.

17 Kerschmann RL, Berger TG, Weiss LM et al. Cutaneous pre-sentations of lymphoma in human immunodeficiency virus disease: predominance of T-cell lineage. *Arch Dermatol* 1995; **131**: 1281–8.

18 Delecluse HJ, Anagnostopoulos I, Dallenbach F et al. Plasmablastic lymphomas of the oral cavity: a new entity associated with the human immunodeficiency virus infection. *Blood* 1997; **89**: 1413–20.

19 Cioc AM, Allen C, Kalmar JR et al. Oral plasmablastic lymphoma in AIDS patients are associated with human herpesvirus 8. *Am J Surg Pathol* 2004; **28**: 41–6.

20 Fardet L, Blanche S, Brousse N, Bodemer C, Fraitag S. Cutaneous EBV-related lymphoproliferative disorder in a 15-year-old boy with AIDS: an unusual clinical presentation. *J Pediatr Hematol Oncol* 2002; **24**: 666–9.

21 Gandemer V, Verkarre V, Quartier P, Brousse N, Blanche S. Lymphomes chez l'enfant infecte par le HIV-1. *Arch Pediatr* 2000; **7**: 738–44.

22 Nador RG, Chadburn A, Gundappa G et al. Human immuno-deficiency virus (HIV)-associated polymorphic lymphoproliferative disorders. *Am J Surg Pathol* 2003; **27**: 293–302.

23 Nakamura K, Katano H, Hoshino Y et al. Human herpesvirus type 8 and Epstein–Barr virus-associated cutaneous lymphoma taking anaplastic large cell morphology in a man with HIV infection. *Br J Dermatol* 1999; **141**: 141–5.

24 Poiesz B, Dube D, Dube S et al. HTLV-II-associated cutaneous T-cell lymphoma in a patient with HIV-1 infection. *N Engl J Med* 2000; **342**: 930–6.

25 Paech V, Lorenzen T, Stoehr A et al. Remission of cutaneous mycosis fungoides in a patient with advanced HIV-infection. *Eur J Med Res* 2002; **7**: 477–9.

Part 6 Pseudolymphomas of the skin

Chapter 20 Pseudolymphomas of the skin

Pseudolymphomas of the skin are benign lymphocytic proliferations that simulate cutaneous malignant lymphomas clinically and/or histopathologically [1–5]. The term pseudolymphoma is not specific but is merely descriptive as it encompasses reactive skin conditions with different aetiologies, pathogeneses, clinicopathological presentations and behaviours. Cutaneous pseudolymphomas are traditionally divided into T- and B-cell pseudolymphomas according to the histopathological and immunophenotypical features [6], although in many conditions this distinction is artificial. For example, pseudolymphomas induced by drugs may present with either a T- or a B-cell pattern and the same drug may induce different patterns in different patients. Thus, in what follows we classify cutaneous pseudolymphomas according to specific clinicopathological entities (Table 20.1).

In recent years, many reactive skin diseases have been added to the list of cutaneous pseudolymphomas, mainly because of the presence of histopathological features similar to those observed in malignant lymphomas of the skin. In contrast, several entities classified in the past as cutaneous pseudolymphomas have been reclassified as low-grade malignant lymphomas, based on clinicopathological and genetic features as well as on follow-up data. Nevertheless, most of the diseases reported as 'pseudolymphoma' in the past are benign reactive skin disorders and need to be clearly separated from cutaneous malignant lymphomas. In this context, the introduction of the concept of 'clonal dermatoses', that is, reactive skin conditions with monoclonal populations of T or B lymphocytes showing a possible evolution into clear-cut cutaneous malignant lymphoma, has brought confusion to an already confused field [7–9]. True 'evolution' from a clear-cut cutaneous pseudolymphoma into a malignant lymphoma of the skin is exceptional, if it occurs at all.

There are no exact data concerning the incidence, prevalence and geographical distribution of cutaneous pseudolymphomas. Cutaneous pseudolymphomas associated with infectious organisms (*Borrelia burgdorferi* lymphocytoma) commonly arise in regions with endemic *B. burgdorferi* infection. There has also been a rise in the number of cases of *Borrelia* lymphocytoma in countries where *Borrelia* species are absent, in patients returning from travels in endemic regions.

The clinical manifestations of cutaneous pseudolymphomas are protean. The lesions are often solitary although they may be regionally clustered or generalized in distribution. Cutaneous pseudolymphomas may also show the features of generalized erythroderma. The course of pseudolymphomas varies considerably. The lesions may persist for weeks, months or even years; they may resolve spontaneously and they may recur unpredictably.

Histological criteria for the diagnosis of cutaneous pseudolymphomas include two main features: (i) the architectural pattern of the infiltrates; and (ii) the cellular composition of those infiltrates, which frequently show a mixed character. These histological features then need to be compared carefully with the immunophenotypical data obtained on routinely fixed, paraffin-embedded sections [10–12]. The recent introduction of polymerase chain reaction (PCR) analysis of the rearrangement of the T-cell receptor (TCR) and immunoglobulin heavy-chain (J_H) genes allows the clonality of cutaneous T- and B-cell infiltrates to be established [13–16]. Although, as a rule, malignant lymphomas reveal a monoclonal population of lymphocytes whereas pseudolymphomas show a polyclonal infiltrate, it must be underlined that demonstration of monoclonality may be lacking in true malignant lymphomas and that a distinct proportion of cutaneous pseudolymphomas harbour a monoclonal T- or B-cell population. In this context, it must be clearly stated that differentiation of benign from malignant lymphoid infiltrates of the skin is possible only after a careful synthesis and integration of the clinical, histopathological, immunophenotypical and molecular features. In some cases, only careful follow-up will reveal the true diagnosis.

Table 20.1 Classification of cutaneous pseudolymphomas.

Clinicopathological entity	Simulated malignant lymphoma
Actinic reticuloid	Mycosis fungoides/Sézary syndrome
Lymphomatoid contact dermatitis	
Lymphomatoid drug reaction, T-cell type	
Solitary T-cell pseudolymphoma	
Lichenoid ('lymphomatoid') keratosis	
Lichenoid pigmented purpuric dermatitis (including lichen aureus)	
Lichen sclerosus et atrophicus	
CD8+ cutaneous infiltrates in HIV patients	
Pseudolymphomas in tattoos, T-cell type	
Pseudolymphomas at sites of vaccination, T-cell type	
Atypical lymphoid infiltrates (CD30+) associated with: orf, milker's nodule, herpes simplex/zoster, molluscum contagiosum	Lymphomatoid papulosis/anaplastic large cell lymphoma—CD30+
Arthropod reactions (including nodular scabies)	
Lupus panniculitis	Subcutaneous T-cell lymphoma
Lymphocytoma cutis	Follicle centre cell lymphoma
	Marginal zone B-cell lymphoma
	Large B-cell lymphoma
Lymphomatoid drug reaction, B-cell type	Follicle centre cell lymphoma
Pseudolymphoma after vaccination, B-cell type	Marginal zone B-cell lymphoma
Pseudolymphoma in tattoos, B-cell type	
Morphoea, inflammatory stage	Marginal zone B-cell lymphoma
Syphilis (secondary)	
'Acral pseudolymphomatous angiokeratoma' (small papular pseudolymphoma)	
Lymphocytic infiltration of the skin (Jessner–Kanof)	Chronic lymphocytic leukaemia, B-cell type
Inflammatory pseudotumour	Plasmacytoma
	Marginal zone B-cell lymphoma
Reactive angioendotheliomatosis	Intravascular large B-cell lymphoma

SPECIFIC CLINICOPATHOLOGICAL ENTITIES

Actinic reticuloid

The concept of chronic actinic dermatitis encompasses four chronic photodermatoses: persistent light reactivity, photosensitivity dermatitis, photosensitive eczema and actinic reticuloid [17–20]. Actinic reticuloid is a severe persistent photodermatitis that usually affects older men. The disease is characterized by extreme photosensitivity to a broad spectrum of UV radiation [21]. Clinically and histologically, it has many of the features of mycosis fungoides and Sézary syndrome. The patients present in the early stages with erythemas on the face and neck and on the back of the hands (Fig. 20.1). Ectropion may be present. As the eruption pro-

gresses, it becomes lichenified as a consequence of chronic scratching and scaly plaques may develop. In some areas, the lesions may consist of lichenoid papules. Recurrent erythroderma is common in these patients [22]. A 'leonine' face with deep furrowing of markedly thickened skin as well as diffuse alopecia can also be seen. Pruritus is generally severe and intractable and may lead to attempts at suicide. The disease is chronic and shows no tendency to spontaneous remission [23]. Although 'progression' into T-cell lymphoma has been reported, it seems more likely that these cases represented examples of mycosis fungoides from the onset, and that actinic reticuloid is not a potential precursor of cutaneous T-cell lymphoma [24,25].

Histological examination reveals dense, superficial or deep perivascular mixed-cell infiltrates of lymphocytes, histiocytes, plasma cells and eosinophils as well as some atypical mononuclear cells with hyperchromatic lobulated nuclei

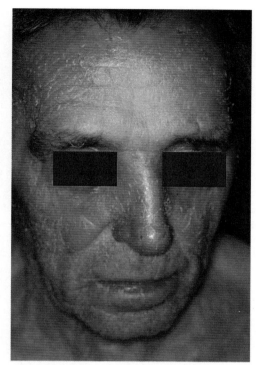

Fig. 20.1 Actinic reticuloid. Erythematous scaling lesions on the face.

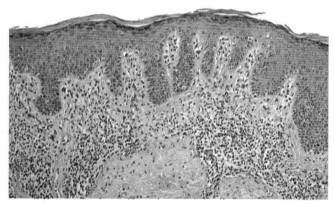

Fig. 20.2 Actinic reticuloid. Psoriasiform epidermal hyperplasia with band-like infiltrate of lymphocytes in the upper dermis. Note focal exocytosis of solitary lymphocytes.

(Fig. 20.2). In the upper part of the dermis, the infiltrate is band-like or patchy. The papillary dermis is usually thickened. Stellate and multinucleated fibroblasts are present. Exocytosis of lymphocytes within the hyperplastic epidermis can be found. When present, the features of lichen simplex chronicus superimposed upon an inflammatory process are helpful in distinguishing actinic reticuloid from mycosis

fungoides and Sézary syndrome. Immunohistology is characterized by the predominance of CD8+ T cells [26,27].

The clinical differentiation of actinic reticuloid from cutaneous T-cell lymphomas (mycosis fungoides and Sézary syndrome) can be difficult because circulating Sézary cells may be found in the peripheral blood of patients with actinic reticuloid [28]. A low helper : suppressor ratio in the peripheral blood has been found in patients with erythrodermic actinic reticuloid, as opposed to the high ratio commonly observed in patients with Sézary syndrome [29]. Unlike patients with mycosis fungoides and Sézary syndrome, on phototesting, patients with chronic actinic dermatitis are sensitive to UVB, UVA and, in most instances, to visible light. Fluorescent light may lead to an exacerbation of the disease. In patients with actinic reticuloid, the minimal erythema dose is lower than normal.

Treatment of chronic actinic dermatitis is difficult and numerous therapeutic approaches have been proposed [30]. Photoprotection is crucial. Any relevant associated contact or photocontact allergens have to be identified and avoided. Some patients have been reported to respond to corticosteroids, photochemotherapy with psoralen and UVA (PUVA), interferon-α or to a combination treatment with azathioprine, hydroxychloroquine and prednisone. Ciclosporin (sometimes combined with bath PUVA) or topical tacrolimus ointment (especially for facial lesions) also appears to be effective [31,32].

Lymphomatoid contact dermatitis

The term lymphomatoid contact dermatitis was coined by Gomez Orbaneja *et al.* [33] in 1976. These authors described four patients with persistent allergic contact dermatitis proved by patch tests. The clinical picture and histological features in their patients were highly suggestive of mycosis fungoides. Clinically, lymphomatoid contact dermatitis is characterized by pruritic erythematous plaques (Fig. 20.3). Generalized plaques or exfoliative erythroderma can be observed rarely. The lesions undergo phases of exacerbation and remission.

Histologically, lymphomatoid contact dermatitis resembles mycosis fungoides (Fig. 20.4) [34]. The differentiation is performed mainly on the basis of changes within the epidermis. In lymphomatoid contact dermatitis, there are usually only a few intraepidermal atypical lymphocytes that have no tendency to form 'Darier's nests' ('Pautrier's microabscesses'). Small intraepidermal collections of keratinocytes admixed with Langerhans cells and a few lymphocytes are common, and should not be misinterpreted as true 'Darier's nests' (Fig. 20.5). Staining for CD1a highlights Langerhans cells in these intraepidermal collections (Fig. 20.6). Analysis

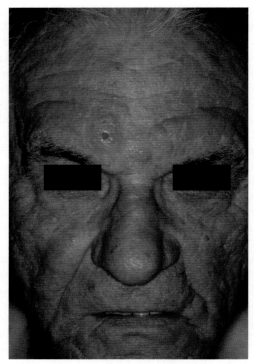

Fig. 20.3 Lymphomatoid contact dermatitis. Erythematous papules and small plaques on the forehead.

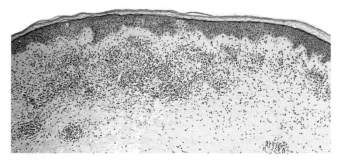

Fig. 20.4 Lymphomatoid contact dermatitis. Band-like infiltrate in the superficial dermis with focal spongiosis and intraepidermal collections of cells.

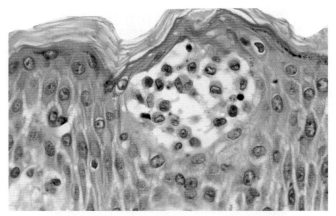

Fig. 20.5 Lymphomatoid contact dermatitis. Spongiotic vesicle with Langerhans cells, keratinocytes and a few lymphocytes simulating 'Darier's nests' ('Pautrier's microabscesses').

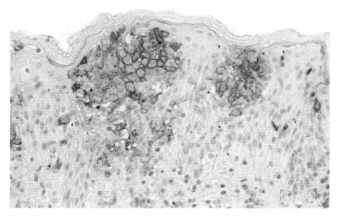

Fig. 20.6 Lymphomatoid contact dermatitis. Staining for CD1a reveals large numbers of Langerhans cells within the intraepidermal nests.

of TCR gene rearrangement commonly shows a polyclonal population of T lymphocytes in the skin lesions of lymphomatoid contact dermatitis. However, in the majority of patch test lesions in patients with 'conventional' contact dermatitis, monoclonality can be observed by Southern blotting, demonstrating that the finding of a clonal population of T lymphocytes in such patients does not have any diagnostic implications [35].

Patch tests to a variety of common antigens can give a positive reaction in lymphomatoid contact dermatitis and the diagnosis should be reserved for patients in whom the lymphomatoid skin lesions are caused by a positively reacting antigen. Although lymphomatoid contact dermatitis has been reported to evolve into true malignant lymphoma, it is more likely that such patients had malignant lymphoma from the outset. For the management of patients, a thorough search for antigens is necessary in order to interrupt the process. When contact with the responsible allergens is avoided, the lesions heal in a relatively short time.

Solitary T-cell pseudolymphoma

Solitary cutaneous lesions with clinicopathological features similar to those observed in mycosis fungoides have been observed in patients who are not obviously taking any drug (thus ruling out the diagnosis of lymphomatoid drug erup-

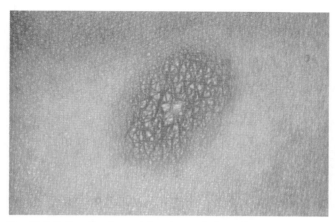

Fig. 20.7 Solitary T-cell pseudolymphoma. Solitary plaque on the breast.

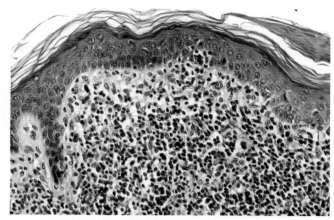

Fig. 20.9 Solitary T-cell pseudolymphoma. Note focal epidermotropism of lymphocytes (detail of Fig. 20.8).

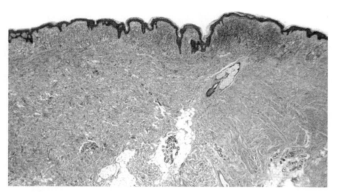

Fig. 20.8 Solitary T-cell pseudolymphoma. Dense band-like infiltrate in the upper dermis.

Lichenoid (lymphomatoid) keratosis

Lichenoid (lymphomatoid) keratosis is a benign epithelial neoplasm, related in some cases to seborrhoeic keratosis and lentigo actinica (Fig. 20.10) [39,40]. Patients are elderly adults with small scaly plaques located usually on the trunk. The histopathological features with dense band-like inflammatory lymphoid infiltrates and often epidermotropism of lymphocytes may be indistinguishable from those of mycosis fungoides (Fig. 20.11) [41]. Moreover, clonality of T lymphocytes can sometimes be found in these lesions. Accurate clinicopathological correlation is crucial to establish a correct diagnosis.

Differentiation of lichenoid (lymphomatoid) keratosis from solitary T-cell pseudolymphoma may be impossible in cases that do not show clear-cut features of an epithelial neoplasm, and the two conditions may be strictly related (see above).

tion; see p. 165). They represent distinct entities, which have been referred to as 'solitary T-cell pseudolymphoma' in the literature [36,37]. These lesions are frequently located on the breasts of adult women (Fig. 20.7). Histology reveals a band-like infiltrate in an expanded papillary dermis, sometimes with exocytosis of lymphocytes within the epidermis (Figs 20.8 & 20.9). In several patients, a monoclonal rearrangement of the TCR genes has been reported. Some of the cases reported in the past as 'unilesional' or 'solitary' mycosis fungoides may represent examples of solitary T-cell pseudolymphoma but at present it is not possible to establish with certainty whether they are wholly benign monoclonal lymphoid proliferations or represent a variant of cutaneous T-cell lymphoma with a very favourable course [38]. Surgical excision results in complete remission; recurrences are uncommon.

There may be some overlap between solitary T-cell pseudolymphoma and so-called lichenoid keratosis (see below).

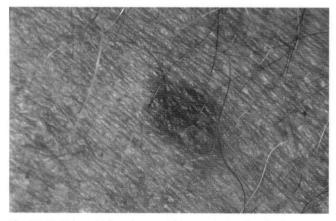

Fig. 20.10 Lichenoid (lymphomatoid) keratosis. Small scaly plaque on the breast.

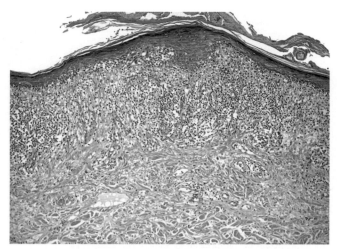

Fig. 20.11 Lichenoid (lymphomatoid) keratosis. Band-like infiltrate of lymphocytes with exocytosis in the lower layers of the epidermis.

Lichen aureus/lichenoid pigmented purpuric dermatitis

Lichen aureus is a benign skin condition characterized by asymmetrical persistent purpuric skin macules and thin plaques with a typical golden brown colour clinically (Fig. 20.12) and by a band-like lymphocytic infiltrate that may simulate mycosis fungoides histopathologically (Fig. 20.13) [42]. Patients are usually adults with asymmetrical, solitary or, more commonly, localized lesions. Molecular analyses may reveal T-lymphocyte clonality in some cases [42]. Accurate clinicopathological correlation is crucial to establish a correct diagnosis. Local steroid ointments or PUVA therapy can be used to treat lichen aureus.

A relationship between lichen aureus or lichenoid pigmented purpuric dermatitis and mycosis fungoides has been postulated (see Chapter 2) [42–45]. However, we would like to emphasize that lichen aureus is a wholly benign inflammatory disorder without any relationship to mycosis fungoides or any other cutaneous T-cell lymphoma. Cases of mycosis fungoides preceded by pigmented purpuric dermatitis probably represented examples of mycosis fungoides from the outset [46].

Lichen sclerosus

Sometimes, cases of lichen sclerosus on genital skin reveal histopathological features characterized by dense band-like lymphoid infiltrates and epidermotropism of lymphocytes that may be indistinguishable from those of mycosis fungoides (Figs 20.14 & 20.15) [47]. Moreover, T-lymphocyte clonality can be found in some of these cases [47,48]. The

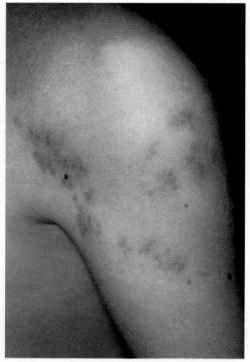

Fig. 20.12 Lichen aureus. Localized macules with characteristic brown–orange colour.

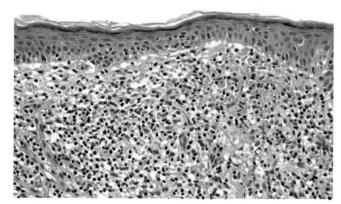

Fig. 20.13 Lichen aureus. Dense infiltrate of lymphocytes with prominent extravasation of erythrocytes and vacuolar changes of the basal keratinocytes.

finding of the typical hyalinization of the collagen is a useful clue for the diagnosis of lichen sclerosus but may be missing, especially in small biopsies. Accurate clinicopathological correlation is required to establish a correct diagnosis. In this context, a diagnosis of mycosis fungoides on genital skin should never be made without a precise correlation between

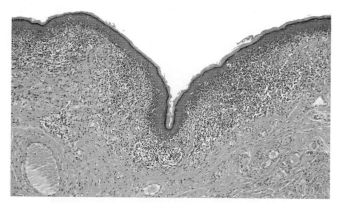

Fig. 20.14 Lichen sclerosus. Dense band-like infiltrate of lymphocytes with exocytosis within the lower layers of the epidermis.

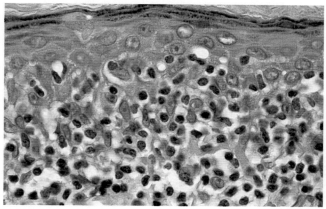

Fig. 20.15 Lichen sclerosus. Intraepidermal lymphocytes within the lower layers of the epidermis. Note some lymphocytes with perinuclear halo ('haloed lymphocytes') mimicking mycosis fungoides (detail of Fig. 20.14).

the histopathological and clinical features, even in cases that show monoclonality of the infiltrate.

CD8+ cutaneous infiltrates in HIV-infected patients

The onset of aggressive non-Hodgkin lymphomas, including skin lymphomas, has been described in patients with advanced HIV infection. In some patients, a cutaneous eruption clinically and histopathologically similar to mycosis fungoides but characterized by a predominance of CD8+ T lymphocytes has been observed [49,50]. The lymphocytes in these cases are polyclonal, indicating that this eruption is a cutaneous pseudolymphoma rather than a true T-cell lymphoma of the skin. CD8+ cutaneous infiltrates arise usually in HIV-infected patients with a profound CD4 lymphopenia and are con-

sidered as a bad prognostic sign for the underlying disease (the bad prognosis, however, may be linked to the very low CD4 count rather than to the skin lesions *per se*). PUVA, topical steroids and even chemotherapy have been used for the treatment of this uncommon condition [49]. Regression upon antiviral triple treatment has been observed [51]. A similar condition, but with monoclonal CD8+ T-lymphocytes, has been observed in common variable immunodeficiency.

CD30+ T-cell pseudolymphomas

In recent years, the presence of CD30+ large blasts has been observed in the skin in several reactive conditions including various viral infections (orf, milker's nodule, molluscum contagiosum, viral warts, herpes simplex, herpes zoster), arthropod reactions, scabies and drug eruptions (Figs 20.16–20.19) [52–56]. CD30+ cells have also been observed in lesions of hidradenitis and rhynophyma, as well as at the sites of cutaneous abscess and of injury caused by red sea coral. The finding may be related, at least in part, to improved methods

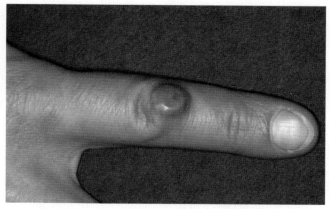

Fig. 20.16 Milker's nodule. Solitary nodule on the finger.

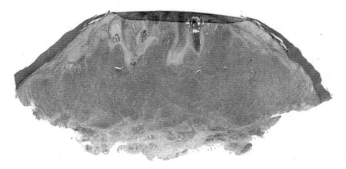

Fig. 20.17 Milker's nodule. Epidermal hyperplasia, large telangiectatic vessels and dense infiltrate of lymphocytes.

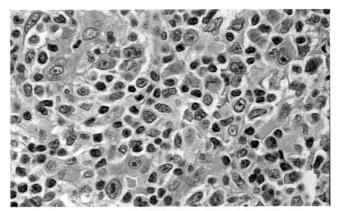

Fig. 20.18 Milker's nodule. Note presence of large blastic cells (detail of Fig. 20.17).

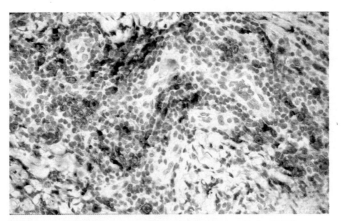

Fig. 20.19 Milker's nodule. Positivity of the larger cells for CD30 (same case as Figs 20.17 & 20.18).

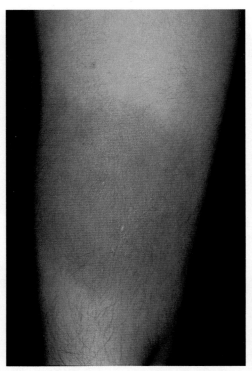

Fig. 20.20 Lupus panniculitis. Erythematous infiltrated plaque on the leg.

of antigen demasking and immunohistochemical staining of routinely fixed, paraffin-embedded sections of tissue (see Chapter 1).

Besides the presence of large atypical CD30+ cells, the histology in these lesions reveals the typical changes of the specific underlying disorder. Moreover, in these reactive conditions CD30+ lymphocytes are scattered throughout the infiltrate and are usually not arranged in clusters or sheets as observed in lymphomatoid papulosis or cutaneous anaplastic large cell lymphoma. However, in some cases differentiation may be very difficult or even impossible on histological and immunohistochemical grounds alone. Unlike the situation in lymphomatoid papulosis and cutaneous anaplastic large cell lymphoma, gene rearrangement studies in CD30+ pseudolymphomas reveal the presence of a polyclonal population of T lymphocytes.

The therapy of CD30+ pseudolymphomas depends on the specific diagnosis, and includes surgical excision, cryotherapy and antiviral treatment.

Lupus panniculitis

Patients with lupus erythematosus may rarely present with prominent involvement of the subcutaneous tissues, a condition that has been termed lupus panniculitis or lupus profundus. Lupus panniculitis reveals subcutaneous plaques and indurations, mostly located on the extremities, which can simulate clinically and histopathologically those observed in subcutaneous T-cell lymphoma (see Chapter 5) (Fig. 20.20) [57]. Antinuclear antibodies and other criteria for the diagnosis of systemic lupus erythematosus may be absent in some cases. Histology shows a predominantly lobular panniculitis, often with concomitant presence of broadened fibrotic septa. A useful feature for the differentiation of subcutaneous T-cell lymphoma from lupus panniculitis is the presence in the former of so-called 'rimming' of fat cells by pleomorphic atypical T lymphocytes that are positive for proliferation markers. It must be remembered that rimming of fat lobuli by lymphocytes is not a diagnostic feature *per se*, as it can be observed in several benign and malignant lymphoid infiltrates with involvement of the subcutaneous fat. In contrast to subcutaneous T-cell lymphoma, B cells, plasma cells and germinal centres are usually a prominent feature in lupus panniculitis (Figs 20.21 & 20.22). Moreover, the

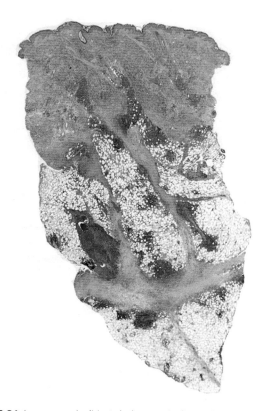

Fig. 20.21 Lupus panniculitis. Lobular panniculitis with dense lymphoid infiltrates and fibrotic septa.

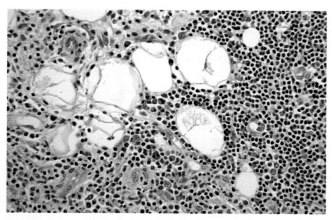

Fig. 20.22 Lupus panniculitis. Note mixed-cell infiltrate with lymphocytes, histiocytes, neutrophils and several plasma cells (detail of Fig. 20.21).

dermo-epidermal junction may show features of lupus erythematosus (interface dermatitis). Analysis of TCR gene rearrangement reveals polyclonal populations of T lymphocytes in lupus panniculitis, in contrast to subcutaneous T-cell lymphoma where monoclonality of T lymphocytes is found in most cases.

Treatment of lupus panniculitis is similar to that of other variants of lupus erythematosus. The lesions respond well to systemic steroids but recurrences are the rule.

Lymphomatoid drug reactions

A pseudolymphoma syndrome characterized by generalized lymphadenopathy, hepatosplenomegaly, leucocytosis, fever, malaise, arthralgia, severe oedema of the face and cutaneous lesions such as erythematous pruritic macules, papules and nodules has been described in patients treated with anticonvulsants, particularly hydantoin derivatives [58,59]. Many other drugs may induce lymphoid infiltrates in the skin that simulate malignant lymphoma clinically and/or histopathologically [37,60–62]. The external use of etheric plant oils may also cause lymphoproliferative reactions that mimic malignant lymphomas, clinically and histologically.

Lymphomatoid drug eruptions may present with a T- or a B-cell pattern, simulating either mycosis fungoides, Sézary syndrome, follicle centre cell lymphoma or marginal zone lymphoma [63–68]. A rare type of lymphomatoid drug eruption with many CD30+ cells may simulate the CD30+ cutaneous lymphoproliferative disorders [53]. It should be noted that the same drug may be responsible for cutaneous lesions with different histopathological features and phenotypes in different patients.

Clinically, patients present with generalized papules, plaques or nodules (Fig. 20.23) or even erythroderma. A digitate dermatitis-like pattern has also been observed [68]. Accentuation of skin changes in sun-exposed areas may occur.

Histologically, pseudolymphomatous drug eruptions are characterized by dense band-like nodular or diffuse infiltrates of lymphocytes, sometimes with atypical cells, revealing a T- or B-cell pattern (Figs 20.24–20.26). Eosinophils may or may not be present. In some cases, the histopathological changes may be those of lymphadenosis benigna cutis with formation of reactive germinal centres (Fig. 20.26). There is a polyclonal pattern of immunoglobulin light-chain expression. Molecular analysis of J_H and TCR genes usually shows a polyclonal pattern.

Lymphomatoid drug reactions invariably regress when the offending drug is withdrawn and recur if the same or a similar compound is reintroduced.

Rarely, the development of a true cutaneous lymphoma has been recorded in relation to the use of drugs that commonly induce lymphomatoid drug eruptions [69]. In these cases, the skin lesions do not regress upon discontinuation of the drug.

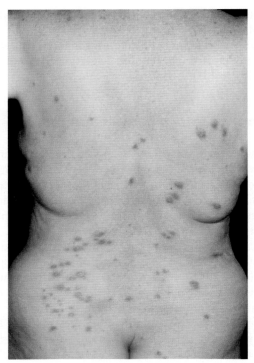

Fig. 20.23 Lymphomatoid drug eruption. Papules, plaques and nodules on the back.

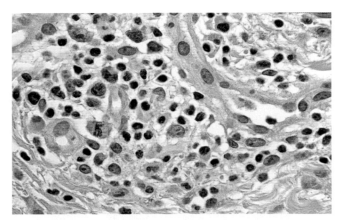

Fig. 20.25 Lymphomatoid drug eruption, T-cell type. Note several atypical lymphocytes and one mitotic figure (detail of Fig. 20.24).

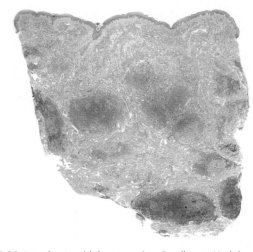

Fig. 20.26 Lymphomatoid drug eruption, B-cell type. Nodular infiltrates of lymphocytes with reactive germinal centres. (Courtesy of Dr Dieter Metze, Münster, Germany.)

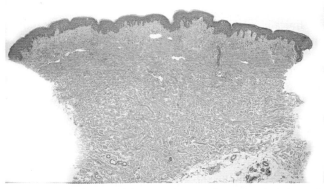

Fig. 20.24 Lymphomatoid drug eruption, T-cell type. Patchy lichenoid infiltrate of lymphocytes without epidermotropism within the superficial dermis.

Lymphocytoma cutis

Several synonyms have been used for lymphocytoma cutis including lymphadenosis benigna cutis, cutaneous lymphoplasia, cutaneous lymphoid hyperplasia and pseudolymphoma of Spiegler–Fendt. Various antigenic stimuli can induce these lesions: insect bites, drugs, vaccinations, acupuncture, wear-

ing of gold pierced earrings, medicinal leech therapy and tattoos [70–72]. One of the most common associations is found with the spirochaete *B. burgdorferi* [12,73].

Women are affected more commonly than men. There are numerous clinical presentations of lymphocytoma cutis. Frequently, a firm solitary lesion can be observed although lesions may be clustered in a region or, rarely, be scattered widely. There is usually a nodule or tumour although papules or plaques may also be observed. The colour varies from reddish brown to reddish purple. Scaling and ulceration are absent. Involvement of particular body sites (earlobe, nipple, scrotum) is almost pathognomonic of *B. burgdorferi*-associated lymphocytoma cutis (Figs 20.27 & 20.28) [73]. The *B. burgdorferi*-associated type of lymphocytoma cutis often occurs in children and is the most frequent pseudolym-

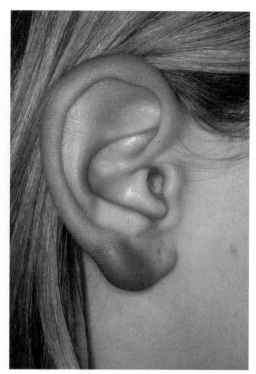

Fig. 20.27 Lymphocytoma cutis associated with infection by *Borrelia burgdorferi*. Erythematous nodule on the right earlobe.

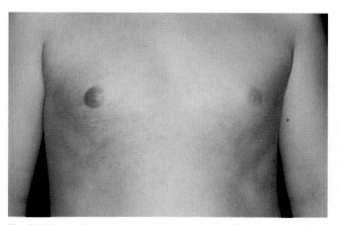

Fig. 20.28 Lymphocytoma cutis associated with infection by *Borrelia burgdorferi*. Erythematous nodule on the right nipple.

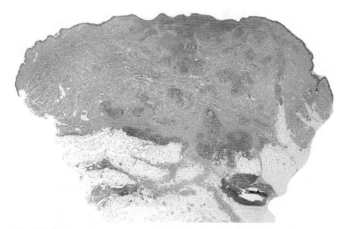

Fig. 20.29 Lymphocytoma cutis. Wedge-shaped infiltrate within the entire dermis. Note small regular germinal centres.

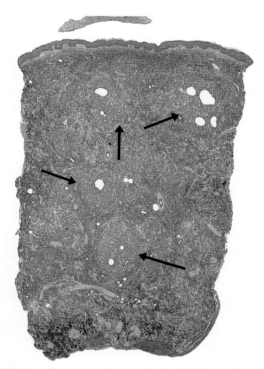

Fig. 20.30 Lymphocytoma cutis associated with infection by *Borrelia burgdorferi*. Dense diffuse lymphoid infiltrate with prominent follicular structures devoid of a mantle (arrows).

phoma in this age group in regions with endemic *B. burgdorferi* infection.

Histological examination shows dense, nodular, mixed-cell infiltrates, often with the formation of lymphoid follicles (Fig. 20.29). Although the infiltrates may be 'top-heavy', in *B. burgdorferi*-associated lymphocytoma cutis there are frequently dense diffuse lymphoid infiltrates involving the entire dermis and superficial subcutaneous fat (Fig. 20.30). In addition, in these lesions the reactive germinal centres are commonly devoid of mantle zones and may show confluence simulating the picture of a large B-cell lymphoma (Fig. 20.31) [73,74]. Plasma cells and eosinophils are found in almost all cases as well as a distinct population of T lymphocytes, features that represent useful clues for the differential diagnosis.

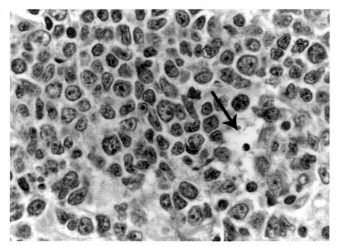

Fig. 20.31 Lymphocytoma cutis associated with infection by *Borrelia burgdorferi*. Large blastic cells (centroblasts, large centrocytes) admixed with 'tingible body' macrophages characterized by large empty spaces with nests of apoptotic cells (arrow).

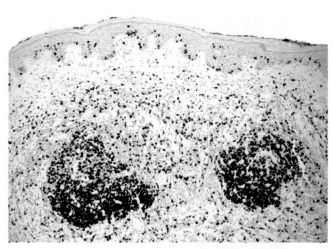

Fig. 20.33 Lymphocytoma cutis associated with infection by *Borrelia burgdorferi*. Germinal centres with normal (high) proliferation rate. Note absence of mantle and polarization of the staining reflecting the presence of normal dark and light areas within the germinal centres.

Immunohistology reveals a normal phenotype of germinal centre cells (CD10$^+$, Bcl-6$^+$, Bcl-2$^-$), normal (high) proliferation, and polytypical expression of immunoglobulin light-chains (Figs 20.32 & 20.33). Molecular analysis of the J_H gene rearrangement shows a polyclonal pattern in most (but not all) cases [12].

Lymphocytoma cutis may resolve spontaneously in several months or years. Small nodules can be removed by surgical excision, and local injection of corticosteroids or interferon-α may result in regression. Cryosurgery has also been applied with success [75]. Patients with lesions of lymphocytoma cutis and evidence of *B. burgdorferi* (detection of serum antibodies by enzyme-linked immunosorbent assay [ELISA] or immunoblotting or of *Borrelia* DNA by PCR) can be treated with doxycycline or erythromycin. In refractory lesions, a very effective treatment method is radiotherapy.

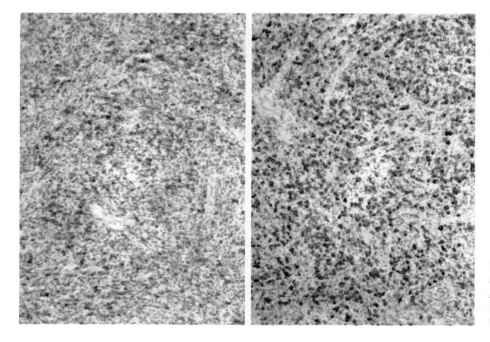

Fig. 20.32 Lymphocytoma cutis associated with infection by *Borrelia burgdorferi*. Polyclonal expression of immunoglobulin light chains kappa and lambda.

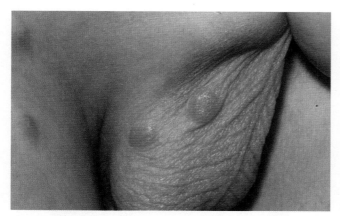

Fig. 20.34 Typical lesions of nodular scabies on the genital area.

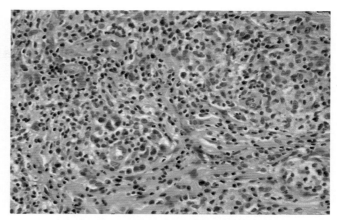

Fig. 20.36 Nodular scabies. Note some atypical lymphocytes (detail of Fig. 20.35).

Persistent nodular arthropod bite reactions

The most typical example of this group of lymphomatoid infiltrates is nodular scabies but many other arthropods can induce skin lesions that may simulate malignant lymphoma histopathologically. Clinically, in nodular scabies, elevated round or oval bright reddish papules and nodules occur most frequently on the genitalia, elbows and in the axillae (Fig. 20.34). The lesions are found in approximately 7% of patients with scabies. The nodules are very pruritic and may persist for many months.

The mite and its parts are seldom identified in the long-standing papules or nodules of scabies. The clinical differential diagnosis includes prurigo nodularis and malignant lymphoma; some lesions of secondary syphilis may be diagnosed incorrectly as a pseudolymphoma of this type.

Histologically, dense superficial and deep perivascular predominantly lymphohistiocytic infiltrates with plasma cells and varying numbers of eosinophils are seen (Figs 20.35 & 20.36) [76]. Eosinophils are also scattered among collagen bundles. Prominent vessels with thickened walls lined by plump endothelial cells are nearly always found. The epidermis may be slightly spongiotic, hyperplastic and hyperkeratotic. Large atypical lymphocytes can be observed. The histological features of nodular scabies may mimic those of mycosis fungoides, lymphomatoid papulosis or Hodgkin lymphoma. Occasionally, a B-cell pattern analogous to lymphocytoma cutis can be recognized in persistent nodular arthropod bite reactions.

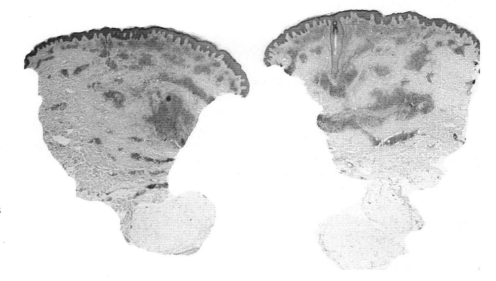

Fig. 20.35 The nodular lesions of scabies infiltrate deeply into the dermis and are composed of a mixture of lymphocytes, macrophages, plasma cells and eosinophils.

Immunohistological investigations reveal that T lymphocytes predominate in nodular scabies. Although previous reports claimed that the use of antibodies for CD30 differentiated the skin lesions of persistent arthropod bites from those of lymphomatoid papulosis because the first are negative, in contrast to the latter that are positive [77], in truth in some cases of scabies the CD30 antigen can be seen in the large lymphoid cells.

Antiscabietic therapy is usually ineffective in cases caused by *Sarcoptes scabiei*. Large nodules may be excised surgically. Intralesional injection of corticosteroids may be helpful. Spontaneous resolution in time is the rule.

Pseudolymphomas at sites of vaccination

Rarely, a florid inflammatory reaction develops at sites of vaccinations. Clinically, lesions may show either superficial papules or nodules, or subcutaneous tumours [70]. The histopathological pattern may be lichenoid, simulating that seen in mycosis fungoides, or nodular with the formation of germinal centres, simulating a follicle centre cell lymphoma (Fig. 20.37). It is believed that pseudolymphomas after vaccination represent a form of local reactive hyperplasia or a persisting delayed hypersensitivity reaction to a vaccine constituent. Lesions may arise after injection of different vaccines including those used for allergen hyposensitization [78]. We have observed the onset of bilateral lesions of lymphocytoma cutis at the skin sites of different injections of early summer meningoencephalitis (früh Sommer Meningoencephalitis—FSME) vaccinations performed after an interval of over 1 year.

Lesions tend to persist unchanged for months or years. Intralesional steroids may be ineffective.

Pseudolymphomas in tattoos

Besides granulomatous infiltrates, inflammatory reactions to tattoos may sometimes reveal lymphoid follicular structures or a mycosis fungoides-like pattern (Figs 20.38 & 20.39) [72,79–81]. Red tattoo pigment (cinnabar) is most frequently (but not always) responsible for the lymphomatoid infiltrate. The presence of pigment suggests the correct diagnosis. A well-documented case of cutaneous lymphoma arising in a tattoo has been reported, so careful follow-up of these lesions is necessary [82]. The management of pseudolymphomas in tattoos can be very difficult because of the large areas of skin involved in some patients. Intralesional steroid injections, laser vaporization or surgical excision of small lesions may be used for treatment.

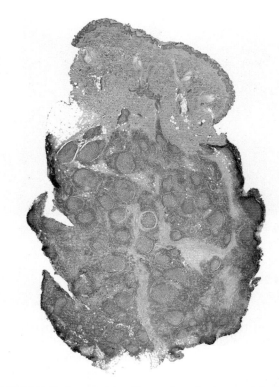

Fig. 20.37 Follicular pseudolymphoma after subcutaneous injection of vaccine. Dense nodular infiltrate of lymphocytes with follicular pattern.

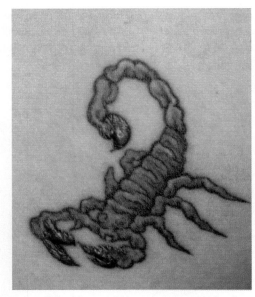

Fig. 20.38 Pseudolymphoma within a tattoo. Onset of a plaque in the red pigmented area of the tattoo.

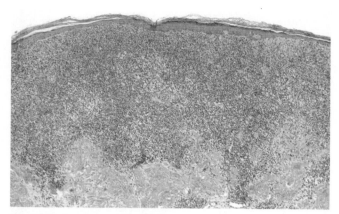

Fig. 20.39 Pseudolymphoma within a tattoo. Dense infiltrate of lymphocytes simulating a cutaneous lymphoma.

Acral pseudolymphomatous angiokeratoma (small papular pseudolymphoma)

Acral pseudolymphomatous angiokeratoma (termed originally 'acral pseudolymphomatous angiokeratoma in children'; APACHE) is characterized by unilateral clustered red violaceous papules and small nodules usually located on the hands and feet of children [83–87]. The aetiology is unknown. Histopathological investigations reveal a dense nodular lymphoid infiltrate with occasional plasma cells and eosinophils (Fig. 20.40). A proliferation of capillaries can be observed. The term angiokeratoma is misleading; based on the distinctive clinicopathological features the more correct (but nonspecific) designation 'small papular pseudolymphoma' has been suggested for this benign lymphoproliferative disease

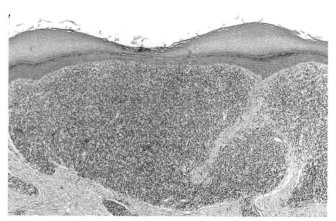

Fig. 20.40 Acral pseudolymphomatous angiokeratoma (small papular pseudolymphoma). Nodular lymphoid infiltrate in the superficial and mid-dermis of acral skin.

[84]. Lesions can be treated by cryotherapy, surgical excision or laser vaporization.

Localized scleroderma/morphoea

In the inflammatory stage of connective tissue diseases, especially in localized scleroderma, dense lymphoid infiltrates may be observed, simulating cutaneous lymphomas histopathologically [88,89]. Plasma cells are almost invariably present and reveal a polyclonal pattern of immunoglobulin light-chain expression. Correlation with the clinical picture confirms the diagnosis. Treatment does not differ from the conventional therapy of the underlying disease.

Secondary syphilis

Rarely, cutaneous lesions in secondary syphilis may show dense lymphoplasmacellular infiltrates simulating histopathologically the picture of a marginal zone B-cell lymphoma (Figs 20.41 & 20.42) [90,91]. These plasma cells always reveal a polyclonal pattern of immunoglobulin light-chain

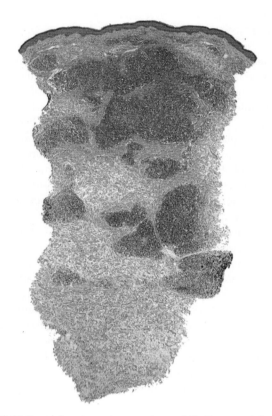

Fig. 20.41 Pseudolymphoma in secondary syphilis. Dense nodular lymphoid infiltrates throughout the entire dermis.

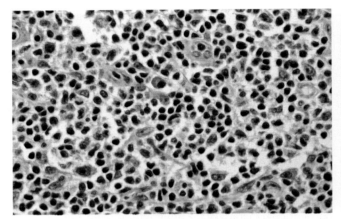

Fig. 20.42 Pseudolymphoma in secondary syphilis. Lymphocytes and histiocytes admixed with several plasma cells (detail of Fig. 20.41).

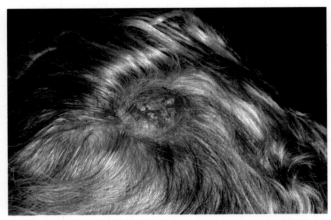

Fig. 20.43 Inflammatory pseudotumour of the skin (inflammatory myofibroblastic tumour). Large reddish tumour on the scalp with crusts.

expression. Correlation with the clinical picture and positivity of serological tests for syphilis confirm the diagnosis. Antibiotic treatment leads to a rapid resolution of the lesions.

Cutaneous inflammatory pseudotumours

Cutaneous inflammatory pseudotumour is a term encompassing at least two main entities: plasma cell granuloma and inflammatory myofibroblastic tumour. In particular, plasma cell granuloma can simulate the histopathological picture of cutaneous plasmacytoma or marginal zone lymphoma with prominent plasma cell differentiation [92]. Cutaneous plasma cell granuloma and inflammatory myofibroblastic tumour should probably not be lumped within the same diagnostic group [93,94]. Some cases of plasma cell granuloma may represent postinfective reactions (Epstein–Barr virus, *Borrelia*, mycobacteria, human herpesvirus-8).

Clinically, patients with plasma cell granuloma present with firm cutaneous or subcutaneous nodules of long duration. Lesions of inflammatory myofibroblastic tumour are generally more superficial and may show focal ulceration (Fig. 20.43). On histopathological examination, circumscribed nodules with thick hyalinized collagen bundles and a dense inflammatory infiltrate with lymphocytes, sheets of plasma cells and occasionally germinal centres can be observed in cutaneous plasma cell granuloma (Fig. 20.44). In cutaneous inflammatory myofibroblastic tumour, fascicles of large spindle cells are admixed with large clusters of plasma cells (Fig. 20.45). Immunohistology reveals polyclonal expression of immunoglobulin light-chains. Molecular analyses do not reveal monoclonality of the infiltrate.

Surgical excision of the lesions results in cure.

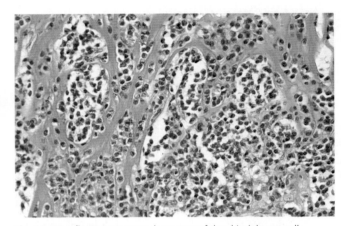

Fig. 20.44 Inflammatory pseudotumour of the skin (plasma cell granuloma). Fibrotic areas with numerous plasma cells.

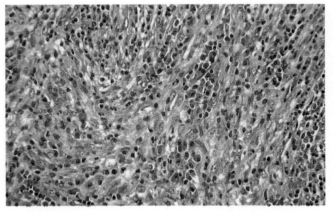

Fig. 20.45 Inflammatory pseudotumour of the skin (inflammatory myofibroblastic tumour). Numerous large spindle cells admixed with plasma cells, small lymphocytes and neutrophils.

Lymphocytic infiltration of the skin

Lymphocytic infiltration of the skin (Jessner–Kanof) can be confused histopathologically with lesions of B-cell chronic lymphocytic leukaemia (B-CLL). The coexpression of CD20, CD5 and CD43 on the B cells of B-CLL as well as the detection of a monoclonal rearrangement of the J_H gene, in contrast to the predominance of polyclonal T lymphocytes in lymphocytic infiltration of the skin, help to distinguish these diseases. It has been recently proposed that lymphocytic infiltration of the skin and lupus erythematosus tumidus represent one and the same disease [95].

Reactive angioendotheliomatosis

In rare cases, an intravascular proliferation of endothelial cells and/or histiocytes may mimic the histopathological picture of intravascular large cell lymphoma (intravascular angioendotheliomatosis, intravascular histiocytosis) (see Chapters 8 and 15) (Fig. 20.46) [96,97]. Lesions may arise on the backgound of disparate conditions including chronic cutaneous infections, autoimmune disorders or other systemic diseases [98]. Immunohistological and molecular analyses allow a clear-cut distinction from angiotropic lymphomas. Management of the lesions is dependent on the associated disorder but sometimes skin lesions do not show improvement upon treatment [98].

Other cutaneous pseudolymphomas

Besides the cutaneous pseudolymphomas discussed in the

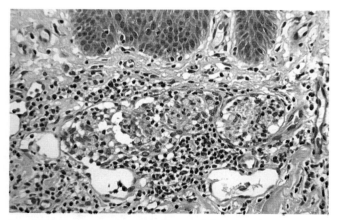

Fig. 20.46 Reactive angioendotheliomatosis (intravascular histiocytosis). Dilated blood vessels in the superficial dermis, some filled with large histiocytes, simulating the picture of intravascular large cell (angiotropic) lymphoma.

previous paragraphs, the occurrence of other skin conditions simulating clinically and/or histopathologically cutaneous lymphomas has been reported sporadically. Cases of inflammatory lesions of vitiligo and of eruption of lymphocyte recovery with histopathological features mimicking those of mycosis fungoides have been observed [99,100]. A condition termed 'annular lichenoid dermatitis of youth' has been reported recently as a simulator of mycosis fungoides, but it may in truth represent a variant of this disease in children [101]. Besides the entities listed in the paragraph on CD30+ cutaneous pseudolymphomas (see p. 163), we have rarely observed the presence of dense lymphoid infiltrates with scattered CD30+ cells in skin lesions of mycotic infections. True B-cell pseudolymphomas have been observed at the site of previous herpes zoster eruptions [102]. However, it must be stressed that only a few cases of clear-cut pseudolymphoma have been documented in association with herpes zoster and that most cases reported as such in the past represented in truth specific infiltrates of B-CLL (see Chapter 14). Atypical lymphoid proliferations can be observed also in patients with chronic discoid lupus erythematosus, but other features typical of lupus dermatitis allow one to make the correct diagnosis. Besides lymphocytoma cutis, infection by *Borrelia burgdorferi* may cause pseudolymphomatous infiltrates (mimicking marginal zone B-cell lymphoma) in patients with acrodermatitis chronica atroficans, but plasma cells are polyclonal in this condition. Marginal zone B-cell lymphoma and/or cutaneous plasmacytoma may be differential diagnostic concerns also in cases of so-called cutaneous plasmacytosis, a condition reported almost exclusively in Japan and associated with polyclonal plasma cell infiltrates in the skin [103].

It should also be recalled that molecular analyses demonstrated on many occasions that a monoclonal population of lymphocytes can be detected in several benign skin conditions besides cutaneous lymphomas—lichen planus for example [104]. It is crucial to keep in mind this possibility when evaluating molecular analyses of TCR and J_H gene rearrangement in skin infiltrates.

Finally a few words should be devoted to pityriasis lichenoides et varioliformis acuta (PLEVA) (Mucha-Habermann disease) as in recent years the nosology of this disease has often been debated [105–107]. Many reports demonstrated that in some cases the T-lymphocytes of PLEVA are monoclonally rearranged [104,105]. Evolution of PLEVA into cytotoxic mycosis fungoides has been documented and some authors suggested that the disease may represent yet another variant of the cutaneous T-cell lymphomas [108]. On the other hand, in some reports of 'atypical' PLEVA the exact diagnosis and classification of the cases was questionable (see p. 51). However, it seems possible that at least one variant of PLEVA, the so-called febrile ulceronecrotic type, may be related to the cutaneous cytotoxic lymphomas [109,110]. In fact patients may die of this disease (although not from lymphoma-specific causes) and the clinicopathological features resemble those of other cytotoxic lymphomas (although the infiltrates are never as dense or as deep, nor is cytomorphology as atypical). A definitive conclusion cannot be reached at present. In this context patients with classical PLEVA should not be over-diagnosed nor treated as having a cutaneous T-cell lymphoma as the disease is most likely of an inflammatory (or infectious) nature and behaves in a benign fashion. In contrast, patients with the febrile ulcero-necrotic variant of PLEVA should be monitored carefully and may require more aggressive treatment, such as methotrexate.

References

1 Clark WH, Mihm MC, Reed RJ, Ainsworth AM. The lymphocytic infiltrates of the skin. *Hum Pathol* 1974; **5**: 25–43.

2 Connors RC, Ackerman AB. Histologic pseudomalignancies of the skin. *Arch Dermatol* 1976; **112**: 1767–80.

3 LeBoit PE. Cutaneous lymphomas and their histopathologic imitators. *Semin Dermatol* 1986; **5**: 322–33.

4 Kerl H, Ackerman AB. Inflammatory diseases that simulate lymphomas: cutaneous pseudolymphomas. In: Fitzpatrick TB, Eisen AZ, Wolff K *et al.*, eds. *Dermatology in General Medicine*, 4th edn. New York: McGraw-Hill, 1993: 1315–27.

5 Caro WA, Helwig EB. Cutaneous lymphoid hyperplasia. *Cancer* 1969; **24**: 487–502.

6 Smolle J, Torne R, Soyer HP, Kerl H. Immunohistochemical classification of cutaneous pseudolymphomas: delineation of distinct patterns. *J Cutan Pathol* 1990; **17**: 149–59.

7 Siddiqui J, Hardman DL, Misra M, Wood GS. Clonal dermatitis: a potential precursor of cutaneous T-cell lymphomas with varied clinical manifestations. *J Invest Dermatol* 1997; **108**: 584.

8 Wood GS, Ngan BY, Tung R *et al.* Clonal rearrangements of immunoglobulin genes and progression to B-cell lymphoma in cutaneous lymphoid hyperplasia. *Am J Pathol* 1989; **135**: 13–9.

9 Nihal M, Mikkola D, Horvath N *et al.* Cutaneous lymphoid hyperplasia: a lymphoproliferative continuum with lymphomatous potential. *Hum Pathol* 2003; **34**: 617–22.

10 Cerroni L, Kerl H. Diagnostic immunohistology: cutaneous lymphomas and pseudolymphomas. *Semin Cutan Med Surg* 1999; **18**: 64–70.

11 Cerroni L, Goteri G. Differential diagnosis between cutaneous lymphoma and pseudolymphoma. *Anal Quant Cytol Histol* 2003; **25**: 191–8.

12 Leinweber B, Colli C, Chott A, Kerl H, Cerroni L. Differential diagnosis of cutaneous infiltrates of B lymphocytes with follicular growth pattern. *Am J Dermatopathol* 2004; **26**: 4–13.

13 Wood GS. T-cell receptor and immunoglobulin gene rearrangements in diagnosing skin disease. *Arch Dermatol* 2001; **137**: 1503–6.

14 Bakels V, van Oostveen JW, van der Putte SCJ, Meijer CJLM, Willemze R. Immunophenotyping and gene rearrangement analysis provide additional criteria to differentiate between cutaneous T-cell lymphomas and pseudo-T-cell lymphomas. *Am J Pathol* 1997; **150**: 1941–9.

15 Medeiros LJ, Picker LJ, Abel EA *et al.* Cutaneous lymphoid hyperplasia: immunologic characteristics and assessment of criteria recently proposed as diagnostic of malignant lymphoma. *J Am Acad Dermatol* 1989; **21**: 929–42.

16 Rijlaarsdam JU, Bakels V, van Oostveen JW *et al.* Demonstration of clonal immunoglobulin gene rearrangements in cutaneous B-cell lymphomas and pseudo-B-cell lymphomas: differential diagnostic and pathogenetic aspects. *J Invest Dermatol* 1992; **99**: 749–54.

17 Ive FA, Magnus IA, Warin RP, Wilson Jones E. 'Actinic reticuloid': a chronic dermatosis associated with severe photosensitivity and the histological resemblance to lymphoma. *Br J Dermatol* 1969; **81**: 469–85.

18 Norris PG, Hawk JLM. Chronic actinic dermatitis: a unifying concept. *Arch Dermatol* 1990; **126**: 376–8.

19 Lim HW, Morison WL, Kamide R *et al.* Chronic actinic dermatitis: an analysis of 51 patients evaluated in the United States and Japan. *Arch Dermatol* 1994; **130**: 1284–9.

20 Toonstra J. Actinic reticuloid. *Semin Diagn Pathol* 1991; **8**: 109–16.

21 Giannelli F, Botcherby PK, Marimo B, Magnus IA. Cellular hypersensitivity to UV-1: a clue to the aetiology of actinic reticuloid? *Lancet* 1983; **321**: 88–91.

22 Toonstra J, Wildschut A, Boer J *et al.* Actinic reticuloid. *J Am Acad Dermatol* 1989; **21**: 205–14.

23 Dawe RS, Crombie IK, Ferguson J. The natural history of chronic actinic dermatitis. *Arch Dermatol* 2000; **136**: 1215–20.

24 Bilsland D, Crombie IK, Ferguson J. The photosensitivity dermatitis and actinic reticuloid syndrome: no association with lymphoreticular malignancy. *Br J Dermatol* 1994; **131**: 209–14.

25 Jensen NE, Sneddon IB. Actinic reticuloid with lymphoma. *Br J Dermatol* 1970; **82**: 287–91.

26 Heller P, Wieczorek R, Waldo E *et al.* Chronic actinic dermatitis: an immunohistochemical study of its T-cell antigenic profile, with comparison to cutaneous T-cell lymphoma. *Am J Dermatopathol* 1994; **16**: 510–6.

27 Toonstra J, van der Putte SCJ, van Wichen DF *et al.* Actinic reticuloid: immunohistochemical analysis of the cutaneous infiltrate in 13 patients. *Br J Dermatol* 1989; **120**: 779–86.

28 Neild VS, Hawk JLM, Eady RAJ, Cream JJ. Actinic reticuloid with Sézary cells. *Clin Exp Dermatol* 1982; **7**: 143–8.

29 Chu AC, Robinson D, Hawk JLM *et al.* Immunologic differentiation of the Sézary syndrome due to cutaneous T-cell lymphoma and chronic actinic dermatitis. *J Invest Dermatol* 1986; **86**: 134–7.

30 Ferguson J. The management of the photosensitivity dermatitis and actinic reticuloid (PD/AR) syndrome. *J Dermatol Treat* 1990; **1**: 143–5.

31 Granlund H, Reitamo S. Cyclosporin A in the treatment of chronic actinic dermatitis. *Eur J Dermatol* 1992; **2**: 237–41.

32 Uetsu N, Okamoto H, Fujii K, Doi R, Horio T. Treatment of chronic actinic dermatitis with tacrolimus ointment. *J Am Acad Dermatol* 2002; **47**: 881–4.

33 Gomez Orbaneja J, Iglesias Diez L, Sanchez Lozano JL, Conde Salazar L. Lymphomatoid contact dermatitis. *Contact Dermatitis* 1976; **2**: 139–43.

34 Ackerman AB, Breza TS, Capland L. Spongiotic simulants of mycosis fungoides. *Arch Dermatol* 1974; **109**: 216–20.

35 Wolff-Sneedorff A, Thomsen K, Secher L, Lange Vejlsgaard G. Gene rearrangement in positive patch tests. *Exp Dermatol* 1995; **4**: 322–6.

36 van der Putte SCJ, Toonstra J, Felten PC, van Vloten WA. Solitary non-epidermotropic T cell pseudolymphoma of the skin. *J Am Acad Dermatol* 1986; **14**: 444–53.

37 Rijlaarsdam JU, Willemze R. Cutaneous pseudo-T-cell lymphomas. *Semin Diagn Pathol* 1991; **8**: 102–8.

38 Cerroni L, Fink-Puches R, El-Shabrawi-Caelen L *et al.* Solitary skin lesions with histopathologic features of early mycosis fungoides. *Am J Dermatopathol* 1999; **21**: 518–24.

39 Al-Hoqail I, Crawford RI. Benign lichenoid keratoses with histologic features of mycosis fungoides: clinicopathologic description of a clinically significant histologic pattern. *J Cutan Pathol* 2002; **29**: 291–4.

40 Glaun RS, Dutta B, Helm KF. A proposed new classification system for lichenoid keratosis. *J Am Acad Dermatol* 1996; **35**: 772–4.

41 Kossard S. Unilesional mycosis fungoides or lymphomatoid keratosis? *Arch Dermatol* 1997; **133**: 1312–3.

42 Boyd AS, Vnencak-Jones CL. T-cell clonality in lichenoid purpura: a clinical and molecular evaluation of seven patients. *Histopathology* 2003; **43**: 302–3.

43 Barnhill RL, Braverman IM. Progression of pigmented purpura-like eruptions to mycosis fungoides: report of three cases. *J Am Acad Dermatol* 1988; **19**: 25–31.

44 Crowson AN, Magro CM, Zahorchak R. Atypical pigmentary purpura: a clinical, histopathologic, and genotypic study. *Hum Pathol* 1999; **30**: 1004–12.

45 Toro JR, Sander CA, LeBoit PE. Persistent pigmented purpuric dermatitis and mycosis fungoides: simulant, precursor, or both? A study by light microscopy and molecular methods. *Am J Dermatopathol* 1997; **19**: 108–18.

46 Viseux V, Schoenlaub P, Cnudde F *et al.* Pigmented purpuric dermatitis preceding the diagnosis of mycosis fungoides by 24 years. *Dermatology* 2003; **207**: 331–2.

47 Citarella L, Massone C, Kerl H, Cerroni L. Lichen sclerosus with histopathologic features simulating early mycosis fungoides. *Am J Dermatopathol* 2003; **25**: 463–5.

48 Lukowsky A, Muche JM, Sterry W, Audring H. Detection of expanded T cell clones in skin biopsy samples of patients with lichen sclerosus et atrophicus by T cell receptor-γ polymerase chain reaction assays. *J Invest Dermatol* 2000; **115**: 254–9.

49 Guitart J, Variakojis D, Kuzel T, Rosen S. Cutaneous CD8⁺ T cell infiltrates in advanced HIV infection. *J Am Acad Dermatol* 1999; **41**: 722–7.

50 Zhang P, Chiriboga L, Jacobson M *et al.* Mycosis fungoides-like T-cell cutaneous lymphoid infiltrates in patients with HIV infection. *Am J Dermatopathol* 1995; **17**: 29–35.

51 Schartz NEC, De la Blanchardiere A, Alaoui S *et al.* Regression of CD8⁺ pseudolymphoma after HIV antiviral triple therapy. *J Am Acad Dermatol* 2003; **49**: 139–41.

52 Gallardo F, Barranco C, Toll A, Pujol RM. CD30 antigen expression in cutaneous inflammatory infiltrates of scabies: a dynamic immunophenotypic pattern that should be distinguished from lymphomatoid papulosis. *J Cutan Pathol* 2002; **29**: 368–73.

53 Nathan DL, Belsito DV. Carbamazepine-induced pseudolymphoma with CD-30 positive cells. *J Am Acad Dermatol* 1998; **38**: 806–9.

54 Rose C, Starostik P, Bröcker EB. Infection with parapoxvirus induces CD30-positive cutaneous infiltrates in humans. *J Cutan Pathol* 1999; **26**: 520–2.

55 Kim KJ, Lee MW, Choi JH *et al.* CD30-positive T-cell-rich pseudolymphoma induced by gold acupuncture. *Br J Dermatol* 2002; **146**: 882–4.

56 Moreno-Ramirez D, Garcia-Escudero A, Rios-Martin JJ, Herrera-Saval A, Camacho F. Cutaneous pseudolymphoma in association with molluscum contagiosum in an elderly patient. *J Cut Pathol* 2003; **30**: 473–5.

57 Magro CM, Crowson AN, Kovatich AJ, Burns F. Lupus profundus, indeterminate lymphocytic lobular panniculitis and subcutaneous T-cell lymphoma: a spectrum of subcuticular T-cell lymphoid dyscrasia. *J Cutan Pathol* 2001; **28**: 235–47.

58 Choi TS, Doh KS, Kim SH *et al.* Clinicopathological and genotypic aspects of anticonvulsant-induced pseudolymphoma syndrome. *Br J Dermatol* 2003; **148**: 730–6.

59 Schreiber MM, McGregor JG. Pseudolymphoma syndrome: a sensitivity to anticonvulsant drugs. *Arch Dermatol* 1968; **97**: 297–300.

60 Magro CM, Crowson AN, Kovatich AJ, Burns F. Drug-induced reversible lymphoid dyscrasia: a clonal lymphomatoid dermatitis of memory and activated T cells. *Hum Pathol* 2003; **34**: 119–29.

61 Ploysangam T, Breneman DL, Mutasim DF. Cutaneous pseudolymphomas. *J Am Acad Dermatol* 1998; **38**: 877–905.

62 Crowson AN, Magro CM. Antidepressant therapy: a possible cause of atypical cutaneous lymphoid hyperplasia. *Arch Dermatol* 1995; **131**: 925–9.

63 Aguilar JL, Barcelo CM, Martin-Urda MT *et al.* Generalized cutaneous B-cell pseudolymphoma induced by neuroleptics. *Arch Dermatol* 1992; **128**: 121–3.

64 Kardaun SH, Scheffer E, Vermeer BJ. Drug-induced pseudolymphomatous skin reactions. *Br J Dermatol* 1988; **118**: 545–52.

65 Magro CM, Crowson AN. Drugs with antihistaminic properties as a cause of atypical cutaneous lymphoid hyperplasia. *J Am Acad Dermatol* 1995; **32**: 419–28.

66 Rosenthal CJ, Noguera CA, Coppola A, Kapelner SN. Pseudolymphoma with mycosis fungoides manifestations, hyperresponsiveness to diphenylhydantoin, and lymphocyte dysregulation. *Cancer* 1982; **49**: 2305–14.

67 Rijlaarsdam JU, Scheffer E, Meijer CJLM, Kruyswijk MRJ, Willemze R. Mycosis fungoides-like lesions associated with phenytoin and carbamazepine therapy. *J Am Acad Dermatol* 1991; **24**: 216–20.

68 Mutasim DF. Lymphomatoid drug eruption mimicking digitate dermatosis: cross reactivity between two drugs that suppress angiotensin II function. *Am J Dermatopathol* 2003; **25**: 331–4.

69 Sangueza OP, Cohen DE, Calciano A, Lee M, Stiller MJ. Mycosis fungoides induced by phenytoin. *Eur J Dermatol* 1993; **3**: 474–7.

70 Stavrianeas NG, Katoulis AC, Kanelleas A, Hatziolou E, Georgala S. Papulonodular lichenoid and pseudolymphomatous reaction at the injection site of hepatitis B virus vaccination. *Dermatology* 2002; **205**: 166–8.

71 Smolle J, Cerroni L, Kerl H. Multiple pseudolymphomas caused by Hirudo medicinalis therapy. *J Am Acad Dermatol* 2000; **43**: 867–9.

72 Rijlaarsdam JU, Bruynzeel DP, Vos W, Meijer CJLM, Willemze R. Immunohistochemical studies of lymphadenosis benigna cutis occurring in a tattoo. *Am J Dermatopathol* 1988; **10**: 518–23.

73 Colli C, Leinweber B, Müllegger R et al. Borrelia burgdorferi-associated lymphocytoma cutis: clinicopathologic, immunophenotypic, and molecular study of 106 cases. J Cutan Pathol 2004; 31: 232–40.

74 Grange F, Wechsler J, Guillaume JC et al. Borrelia burgdorferi-associated lymphocytoma cutis simulating a primary cutaneous large B-cell lymphoma. J Am Acad Dermatol 2002; 47: 530–4.

75 Kuflik AS, Schwartz RA. Lymphocytoma cutis: a series of five patients successfully treated with cryosurgery. J Am Acad Dermatol 1992; 26: 449–52.

76 Fernandez N, Torres A, Ackerman AB. Pathologic findings in human scabies. Arch Dermatol 1977; 113: 320–4.

77 Smoller BR, Longacre TA, Warnke RA. Ki-1 (CD30) expression in differentiation of lymphomatoid papulosis from arthropod bite reactions. Mod Pathol 1992; 5: 492–6.

78 Goerdt S, Spieker T, Wölffer LU et al. Multiple cutaneous B-cell pseudolymphomas after allergen injections. J Am Acad Dermatol 1996; 34: 1072–4.

79 Kahofer P, El-Shabrawi-Caelen L, Horn M, Kern T, Smolle J. Pseudolymphoma occurring in a tattoo. Eur J Dermatol 2003; 13: 209–12.

80 Amann U, Luger T, Metze D. Lichenoid-pseudolymphomatöse Tätowierungsreaktion. Hautarzt 1997; 48: 410–3.

81 Di Landro A, Marchesi L, Valsecchi R, Motta T, Locati F. Pseudolymphomatous reaction to a red pigment in tattoo. Eur J Dermatol 1997; 7: 235–7.

82 Sangueza OP, Yadav S, White CR Jr, Braziel RM. Evolution of B-cell lymphoma from pseudolymphoma: a multidisciplinary approach using histology, immunohistochemistry, and Southern blot analysis. Am J Dermatopathol 1992; 14: 408–13.

83 Hara M, Matsunaga J, Tagami H. Acral pseudolymphomatous angiokeratoma of children (APACHE): a case report and immunohistologic study. Br J Dermatol 1991; 124: 387–8.

84 Kaddu S, Cerroni L, Pilatti A, Soyer HP, Kerl H. Acral pseudolymphomatous angiokeratoma. Am J Dermatopathol 1994; 16: 130–3.

85 Marukami T, Ohtsuki M, Nakagawa H. Acral pseudolymphomatous angiokeratoma of children: a pseudolymphoma rather than an angiokeratoma. Br J Dermatol 2001; 145: 512–4.

86 Ramsay B, Dahl MCG, Malcom AJ, Wilson Jones E. Acral pseudolymphomatous angiokeratoma of children. Arch Dermatol 1990; 126: 1524–5.

87 Lee MW, Choi JH, Sung KJ, Moon KC, Koh JK. Acral pseudolymphomatous angiokeratoma of children (APACHE). Ped Dermatol 2003; 20: 457–8.

88 Magro CM, Crowson AN, Harrist TJ. Atypical lymphoid infiltrates arising in cutaneous lesions of connective tissue disease. Am J Dermatopathol 1997; 19: 446–55.

89 Brazzelli V, Vassallo C, Ardigo M, Rosso R, Borroni G. Unusual histologic presentation of morphea. Am J Dermatopathol 2000; 22: 359.

90 Hodak E, David M, Rothem A, Bialowance M, Sandbank M. Nodular secondary syphilis mimicking cutaneous lymphoreticular process. J Am Acad Dermatol 1987; 17: 914–7.

91 McComb ME, Telang GH, Vonderheid EC. Secondary syphilis presenting as pseudolymphoma of the skin. J Am Acad Dermatol 2003; 49: S174–6.

92 Hurt MA, Santa Cruz DJ. Cutaneous inflammatory pseudotumor: lesions resembling 'inflammatory pseudotumors' or 'plasma cell granulomas' of extracutaneous sites. Am J Surg Pathol 1990; 14: 764–73.

93 El Shabrawi-Caelen L, Kerl K, Cerroni L, Soyer HP, Kerl H. Cutaneous inflammatory pseudotumor—A spectrum of various diseases? J Cut Pathol in press.

94 Kerl H, Cerroni L. The morphologic spectrum of cutaneous inflammatory pseudotumors. Am J Dermatopathol 2001; 23: 545–6.

95 Weber F, Schmuth M, Fritsch P, Sepp N. Lymphocytic infiltration of the skin is a photosensitive variant of lupus erythematosus: evidence by phototesting. Br J Dermatol 2001; 144: 292–6.

96 Rieger E, Soyer HP, LeBoit PE et al. Reactive angioendotheliomatosis or intravascular histiocytosis?: an immunohistochemical and ultrastructural study in two cases of intravascular histiocytic cell proliferation. Br J Dermatol 1999; 140: 497–504.

97 Lazova R, Slater C, Scott G. Reactive angioendotheliomatosis: case report and review of the literature. Am J Dermatopathol 1996; 18: 63–9.

98 McMenamin ME, Fletcher CD. Reactive angioendotheliomatosis: a study of 15 cases demonstrating a wide clinicopathologic spectrum. Am J Surg Pathol 2002; 26: 685–97.

99 Petit T, Cribier B, Bagot M, Wechsler J. Inflammatory vitiligo-like macules that simulate hypopigmented mycosis fungoides. Eur J Dermatol 2003; 13: 410–2.

100 Gibney MD, Penneys NS, Nelson-Adesokan P. Cutaneous eruption of lymphocyte recovery mimicking mycosis fungoides in a patient with acute myelocytic leukemia. J Cut Pathol 1995; 22: 472–5.

101 Annessi G, Paradisi M, Angelo C et al. Annular lichenoid dermatitis of youth. J Am Acad Dermatol 2003; 49: 1029–36.

102 Wolff HH, Wendt V, Winzer M. Cutaneous pseudolymphoma at the site of prior herpes zoster eruption. Arch Dermatol Res 1987; 279: S52S–4.

103 Uhara H, Saida T, Ikegawa S et al. Primary cutaneous plasmacytosis: report of three cases and review of the literature. Dermatology 1994; 189: 251–5.

104 Schiller PI, Flaig MJ, Puchta U, Kind P, Sander CA. Detection of clonal T-cells in lichen planus. Arch Dermatol Res 2000; 292: 568–9.

105 Dereure O, Levi E, Kadin ME. T-cell clonality in pityriasis lichenoides et varioliformis acuta: A heteroduplex analysis of 20 cases. Arch Dermatol 2000; 136: 1483–6.

106 Kadin ME. T-cell clonality in pityriasis lichenoides. Evidence for a premalignant or reactive immune disorder? Arch Dermatol 2002; 138: 1089–90.

107 Magro C, Crowson AN, Kovatich A, Burns F. Pityriasis lichenoides: a clonal T-cell lymphoproliferative disorder. Hum Pathol 2002; 33: 788–95.

108 Tomasini D, Zampatti C, Palmedo G, Bonfacini V, Sangalli G, Kutzner H. Cytotoxic mycosis fungoides evolving from pityriasis lichenoides chronica in a seventeen-year-old girl. Dermatology 2002; 205: 176–9.

109 Fink-Puches R, Soyer HP, Kerl H. Febrile ulceronecrotic pityriasis lichenoides et varioliformis acuta. J Am Acad Dermatol 1994; 30: 261–3.

110 Rivera R, Ortiz P, Rodriguez-Peralto JL, Vanaclocha F, Iglesias L. Febrile ulceronecrotic pityriasis lichenoides et varioliformis acuta with atypical cells. Int J Dermatol 2003; 42: 26–8.

Index

Note: page numbers in **bold** refer to tables, those in *italics* refer to figures